the brain revolution

the brain revolution

THE FRONTIERS OF MIND RESEARCH

Marilyn Ferguson

TAPLINGER PUBLISHING COMPANY | NEW YORK

First Edition

Published in the United States in 1973 by
TAPLINGER PUBLISHING CO., INC.
New York, New York

Published simultaneously in the Dominion of Canada by
Burns & MacEachern, Ltd., Ontario

Library of Congress Catalog Card Number: 72-2178

ISBN 0-8008-0961-0

Designed by Mollie M. Torras

for my husband,
my mother,
and in memory of my father

acknowledgments

There are, in the world of science, men and women of uncommon curiosity and creativity. Their breakthroughs are celebrated in the pages of this book. I hereby express my gratitude to these exceptional people—for interviews, for correspondence, for time, and counsel.

There are friends who are uncommonly stimulating, whose interest and excitement would sustain the weariest writer in his dullest hour. I thank them. And I have been extremely lucky in having a husband and a mother who helped maintain a semblance of civilization around me during the research and writing of this book. I am indebted to my brother Rick, who first suggested that I explore the phenomena of meditation. I want to thank my father-in-law, Noel Ferguson, of the University of Houston, and my brother-in-law, Gary G. Ferguson, of Northeast Louisiana University, for their criticism and suggestions.

And I am grateful for the encouragement and enthusiasm of the late Richard Taplinger, a brilliant publisher and a warm human being.

MARILYN FERGUSON

Los Angeles
May 1973

Publisher's Note:

For greater readability, numbered references have been omitted from the text. An extensive bibliography at the back of the book includes the sources of information, chapter notes, and suggested reading for those who may wish to pursue a topic further.

Mind has mountains;
cliffs of fall
Frightful, sheer, no-man-fathomed.
—GERARD MANLEY HOPKINS

The potentialities of development in human souls are unfathomable.
—WILLIAM JAMES

contents

introduction

For perhaps two hundred years rational science painstakingly cleansed the civilized world of magic and superstition. For a time it seemed well on its way to reducing a mechanistic universe to an understandable equation. Then came Einstein, with his "holy curiosity," and physicists began talking about curved space, antimatter, relative time, and the nonreal world. More recently the discoveries in other branches of science are contributing to a composite picture of man more startling, more miraculous, than science fiction.

The most astonishing reality of all appears to be the potential of the human brain. Science and the humanities have converged in the most unexpected way. In order to describe the wonders they have come upon, brain researchers have begun quoting Buddha and William Blake. And poets and mystics, long fearful of the dehumanizing aspects of science, now cite laboratory reports to verify what they had long held as intuitive knowledge.

Although the great change under way has been called the consciousness movement, the term consciousness has been much abused, and movement is inadequate to describe the impact of a scientific revolution.

This book will emphasize the findings of the laboratory and their implications. As Abraham Maslow observed, although our visionary artists and mystics may be correct in their insights they can never make the whole of mankind sure. "Science" he wrote, "is the only way we have of shoving truth down the reluctant throat."

The findings of brain research and allied disciplines are revolutionizing scientific theory and society. They are setting off chain reactions in medicine, psychiatry, and education. Theories of the nature of intelligence are being turned upside down. There is an enormous groundswell of scientific interest in practices considered quackery a brief decade ago, in altered states of consciousness, unorthodox healing, and parapsychology. And so many improbable theories have proved to be genuine insights that one noted scientist said of a colleague's purported conclusion, "It isn't crazy enough to be true."

Our specialists too often have not reported their stunning discoveries to the lay public. Often the news that trickles through has been oversimplified or distorted and its real impact lost.

When the findings from various specialties are pieced together, there emerges a picture of human capabilities and complexities as unlike the popular concept of man as the sun is unlike a 100-watt bulb. The purpose of this book is to furnish a coherent account of this emerging concept. The material has been drawn from interviews, seminars, conferences, lectures, technical literature, and correspondence, the fruits of research by thousands of scientists in many countries.

Some popular accounts have given the scientific explosion a "Brave New World" coloration. They predict head transplants, genetic tampering to produce a superbrain, lovemaking by electronic stimulation of the brain.

This is romantic nonsense—and not crazy enough to be true. We already have the superbrain. We have had it all along. That's what the brain revolution is all about.

I.

the whirlpool

Man's . . . body and proud brain are mosaics of the same elemental particles that compose the dark, drifting clouds of interstellar space. —LINCOLN BARNETT

1

THE PHENOMENA

We had stumbled on one of those natural paradoxes which are the surest signs of hidden truth. —W. GREY WALTER, THE LIVING BRAIN

The adult human brain, resembling an oversized pinkish-gray walnut, weighs less than three pounds. It has been called "the most complex piece of matter in the universe." A computer sophisticated enough to handle the functions of a single brain's ten billion cells would more than cover the face of the earth. More mysterious than Mars, harder to plumb than the Mindanao deeps, the brain has been only tentatively charted.

Like the early explorers of the New World, our most brilliant brain researchers have barely made out the peaks and coastal regions. Though they can only speculate about what lies in the heartland they have found a region greater and stranger than their wildest imaginings. "There will be no end to this enterprise, at least for centuries," said Sir John Eccles, the Australian neurophysiologist who won the Nobel prize in 1963.

As the research expands, the phenomena multiply geometrically, forcing constant revision of existing theories. The investigators must somehow deal with the new data, a task that grows more formidable with every discovery. One researcher compared the progress to the clearing of a great forest. The wider the clearing, the greater the contact with the unknown. Nowhere in science is this more evident than in the exploration of the human brain.

Human volunteers in biofeedback laboratories are learning consciously to control their brain waves, perspiration, blood pressure, digestive juices, and heart rate. The rat has learned even more exotic tricks, such as the ability to blush in one ear only. Other rats, rewarded by stimulation of the brain's pleasure centers, learned to slow their heartbeat so effectively that several died of cardiac arrest.

In other laboratories, medical researchers have learned that it is sometimes better to enhance the body's pain signals rather than dull them, because the brain will automatically repress some pain when it reaches a certain level. And in cases of intractable pain, implanted transistors scramble the signals and fool the brain, which then interprets the nerve messages as a tingle.

Twenty minutes of meditation, the ancient Eastern technique of passive concentration, alters oxygen consumption, blood flow, and can dramatically reduce the level of blood lactate, a substance associated with anxiety symptoms. Reaction time is shortened and auditory perception measurably sharpened immediately after a period of meditation.

Surgery patients under general anesthesia apparently hear what is said in the operating room. Under postsurgical hypnosis they can frequently reconstruct the operating team's conversation. Other studies have shown that consciousness persists even in deep sleep. In one experiment, some volunteers were consistently able to awaken within ten minutes of a target time with no environmental clues.

Injected with substances isolated from the urine of schizophrenics, laboratory volunteers have begun to hallucinate. Sociopaths—those whose crimes against society are pathological in origin—fail to show a distinctive brainwave pattern associated with expectancy and found in the electroencephalograms (EEGs) of all normal persons.

The human brain is sensitive to weak magnetic fields. It reacts to stimuli too faint to be registered in consciousness. It can literally hear light waves and experience visual effects from sound waves. Mental activities can influence a nimbus of energy made visible by a high-frequency electrical field. The glittering surround, called bioplasma by Russian researchers, is also known as the Kirlian effect.

In Czech and later in New York parapsychological laboratories, scientists demonstrated that human beings react physically to mental activities of those to whom they have strong emotional or biological ties. In one experiment, a young man sat quietly for a time, then was silently shown a mathematical problem. As he mentally computed the answer, equipment in another room measured a sudden increase in the blood volume of his mother's capillaries.

Early-learning researchers have experimental evidence that human infants are born with a preference for pattern and prefer complex patterns to plain colors. Neurologists have hypothesized a scanning device in the human brain, a mechanism that searches for pattern the way radar scans.

Left to his own devices, the typical child the world around walks at approximately thirteen months. But the women in one East African tribe traditionally pay close attention to their infants' needs and eagerness to explore. They help them to sit or stand. A typical baby may walk at seven months and use sentences months earlier than European or American children. Nor is this a genetic fluke. Babies of the same tribe, if reared by Europeans or Europeanized natives, show no such precocious development.

Citing a colleague's statement that the DNA * in the cells of a single human being would stretch across the solar system if laid end to end, one scientist said, "The potential inherent in such an endowment beggars the imagination."

But life on the molecular level is so alien to our daily concepts that the brain boggles at its own unseen transactions. Erwin Schrödinger, Nobel prizewinning physicist, warned in 1951 that there is no true model of reality. "We can think it, but however we think it, it is wrong; not perhaps quite as meaningless as a 'triangular circle,' but much more so than a 'winged lion.'" As our mental eye penetrates into smaller and smaller distances and shorter and shorter times, Schrödinger said, we find nature behaving very strangely.

Schrödinger feared that it might be fifty years before the educated layman grasped the implications of modern science: that reality is a convenient fiction. He said, "There is always a cer-

---

* Deoxyribonucleic acid, the molecules containing the genetic code.

tain time-lag between the views held by learned men and the views held by the general public about the views of those learned men."

Of the popular but naïve reductionism, Arthur Koestler said, "You can always detect it by the phrase 'nothing but.' Man is nothing but a complex biochemical system or nothing but a computer. The whole idea is a hangover from 19th Century physics, which the physicist has long since abandoned."

Although most of us are complacent in our assumption that science is gaining on the unknown, scientists are acknowledging that man's own brain is complex beyond any hope of complete understanding. But the research described in the following chapters suggests that the good news is more than we dared hope for.

2

FIRST CLUES:
THE WHIRLPOOL

. . . it all comes down to this fabulous electronic dance.

—ALAN WATTS

"Oh, I'm sorry—I've done for you!" Loren Eiseley spoke spontaneously to the blood that gushed from his mouth onto the sidewalk after he had suffered a bad fall.

"I was quite sane," Eiseley said, "only it was an oddly detached sanity, for I was addressing the blood cells, phagocytes, platelets . . . dying like beached fish on the hot pavement. . . . I had caused to the universe I inhabited as many deaths as the explosion of a supernova in the cosmos."

Picturing the body's dynamics at the cellular level gives one a firmer grasp of how the brain can maintain its almost omnipotent control over the physiological processes and at the same time be affected by trauma, malnutrition, light, and geomagnetic fields. A physicist has suggested that we think of ourselves as standing in a sea of radiation: sonic, gravitational, electromagnetic. And each of us is a microcosm of that sea, a shifting, exploding, decaying universe.

If the body were truly fixed, it would be incomprehensible that mind could influence matter, and vice versa. But it becomes increasingly clear that no line can be drawn between psyche and soma, mind and body. A continuum, a flux of staggering complexity, emerges. As John Pfeiffer expressed it, "Your body does not contain a single one of the molecules that were you seven years ago."

Pfeiffer and other scholars have likened the body to a whirl-pool. The spinning vortex of the whirlpool maintains its out-ward form, but its components change unceasingly. In man, three million red blood cells vanish and are replaced every second. According to the researchers Howard Rasmussen and Maurice Pechet, even the bones are rebuilt, "as if each bone were an elaborate Gothic structure in which a resident engi-neer, in response to changes in stresses, continually directs the replacement of supporting arches with new ones providing a slightly different center of trust."

Whether stimulated by a drop in the January temperature or a rise in the level of uric acid, man's complex responses are processed in the brain. The brain is a sentry, always vigilant. Many brain cells are more active in sleep than during waking consciousness.

The brain's mysterious directorates move molecules. By its thousands of hormones, enzymes, and transmitters, the brain at-tempts to maintain homeostasis: a state of physiological bal-ance. It monitors the respiration rate and cardiac rate. The brain alone decides when a female should ovulate, when a man should step up his testosterone production. It stimulates physi-cal growth or inhibits it.

But starved of its only fuel, sugar, the brain produces bizarre behavior indistinguishable from psychosis. Should some subtle metabolic disorder occur in brain chemistry, the individual might lapse into coma. If certain brain cells have been re-moved, the laboratory cat will remain awake until it drops dead from exhaustion.

Man, that whirlpool of electrons, is also astonishingly vulner-able to light, to magnetic fields, free electricity, and extraterres-trial forces. His brain responds to a sea of radiation, and by its responses controls his every function. He is a field of energies moving inside a larger fluctuating system of energies.

One example of this vulnerability: In 1968, hospitals around the country began treating jaundiced newborn infants with al-most continuous light. The bright light helped clear the nude babies' bodies of bilirubin, a substance that causes brain dam-age if the concentration becomes high enough. Because the traditional treatment has involved the replacement of the babies' blood, nearly every U.S. hospital adopted light therapy.

But in 1971 the nation's pediatricians were warned that the light-treated babies were showing every sign of retarded growth. The steady light, eighteen hours daily for a week or so, apparently upset delicate biological rhythms dependent on alternating light and darkness. Joan Hodgman, chief of the newborn services at the Los Angeles County-University of Southern California Medical Center, said that the babies had smaller head size and gained weight poorly. Gerard Odell of Johns Hopkins reminded pediatricians that "visible light energy is part of the same spectrum as x-rays and cosmic rays."

One clue to the light-related phenomena is the pineal gland, the legendary third eye. In mammals the pineal receives its information through the visual system. It inhibits the activity of sexual hormones, for instance, much as a dam controls a river. If a young child's pineal gland is invaded by a tumor, the result may be sexual precocity. (Congenitally blind girls first menstruate an average of two years earlier than sighted girls, probably because their pineal glands, deprived of light, fail to suppress development.)

The brain itself is *also* capable of light perception. This was first suggested in controversial reports during the 1930s, and was recently proved at the University of Texas at Austin. Certain behavior in birds is dependent on fluctuations of light and darkness. Michael Menaker blinded sparrows to see if this behavior would then disappear. It didn't. Even through the feathers and layers of skin atop their heads, their brains perceived light *the equivalent of bright moonlight.*

Artificial light cycles can so accelerate a bird's biological rhythms that it will fly north when it should fly south. Continuous light halts ovulation in rats and can keep rabbits in constant heat. Because it appears that light may also influence ovulation in human beings, researchers are checking into the possibility that light therapy could be used as a contraceptive —or to enhance fertility.

The relationship between human chemistry and light is also evident in individuals who suffer from severe cataracts. According to a German study, such persons have an array of metabolic disorders. When their eyesight is restored, their rhythms return to normal. Even in individuals with normal vision, the daily rhythm of adrenal hormones is upset by laboratory conditions of steady light or darkness.*

Theorists about man's rhythms fall into two camps. One school holds that an inner clock establishes the rhythms. The other, pointing to the circadian (approximately daily) nature of many cycles and the effects of the moon and sunspots, attributes our rhythms to fluctuations of earth's magnetic field and planetary force fields. Rapidly growing evidence suggests that both theories are partially right.

The idea of an internal biological clock is hardly new. Around the turn of the century, two researchers working independently came up with the premise that human physical strength and emotionality ebb and flow on 23- and 28-day cycles, and that the timing of those cycles is launched at birth. Wilhelm Fleiss, a physician and close friend of Freud, and Hermann Swoboda of the University of Vienna believed that in the traumatic moment of birth there are so many sudden changes that an entirely new series of rhythms is set in motion:

> . . . massive stimulation of all the sensory organs and of the nervous system, and sudden and drastic changes in all the vital functions. At no subsequent time in life will the individual experience such profound and rapid readjustment. The body is squeezed and pushed and pulled, perhaps slapped. . . . Air abruptly enters the lungs, drying and chilling the delicate membranes. The body has weight; bright lights, harsh sounds. . . . All the functions performed by the placenta must be taken over by the infant's own organs.†

Sophisticated biologists have dismissed the 23-day and 28-day cycles as naïve and perhaps oversimplified, but they acknowledge a kernel of truth in the biorhythm theory. Using Fleiss's biorhythm mathematics, researchers at Humboldt University in Berlin reported that one-fourth of the accidents involving workers on agricultural machinery took place on a triple critical day, a configuration of biorhythmic cycles that occurs, on the average, once a year.

* Discussed more fully by Gay Gaer Luce in *Body Time,* her comprehensive book about biological rhythms.

† *Is This Your Day?* by George Thommen.

Innate rhythms may exist, but life is also profoundly influenced by surrounding energy fields. Even when kept in closed rooms, such creatures as rats, oysters, and fiddler crabs are attuned to changes in lunar and geomagnetic fields. Birds and insects are sensitive to earth's weak magnetic field. According to Russian scientists, artificially increasing the magnetic field enhances telepathy in human beings, and sunspots and thunderstorms interfere with telepathy. There is evidence that surgical and postsurgical bleeding is worse during the full moon. Sunspot activity affects man's blood serum, a phenomenon that led Miki Takata, a Japanese researcher, to describe the human being as "a living sundial."

A French researcher has compiled a monumental study that suggests an almost outrageous possibility. Michel Gauquelin believes that individuals may inherit from their parents a sensitivity to certain configurations in the heavens. No believer in astrology per se, he speculates that the genetic code for each person might contain a releaser, a mechanism initiating labor and birth, which is likelier to be triggered by one configuration of planetary force fields than another. He reported a correspondence between the "birth sky" of parents and children so striking that the odds were 500,000 to one against its occurrence by chance. That is, on the birthdays of parent and child, the juxtaposition of planetary force fields was very much alike. *Today's Health,* published by the American Medical Association, said, "If Gauquelin's preposterous statistics have never been explained, neither have they been explained away."

Franz Mesmer insisted in 1766 that celestial bodies affect life on earth. Mesmer spoke of a hypothetical subtle fluid that sounds surprisingly like the plasma state of matter postulated by modern physicists; and he believed that in the human body there are "poles, diverse and opposed, which can be communicated, changed, destroyed, and reinforced."

Mesmer's theories were crude but perhaps visionary. The curious electrical and electronic properties of man are now attracting keen scientific interest. Many researchers are concerned about the possible adverse effects of power pollution—the free electricity that is a by-product of urban generators. Others are exploring the healing possibilities in artificial energy fields.

The extreme sensitivity of human beings to electromagnetic

and magnetic energy has been shown by a number of studies. Burton Milburn, then at the University of California at Los Angeles, pulsed weak magnetic fields at the heads of volunteers. After a while some of the volunteers could detect consistently these minute changes, only four times stronger than earth's own weak magnetic field. Those who succeeded said that they noticed a faint tingling in the area of the nose and upper lip as the magnetic pulsations began. In another study, human subjects learned to fall asleep on sensing a change in the magnetic field.

Scientists can cancel the effects of earth's own field to create what they call a null field. Such an environment has strange effects on human beings. For example, ordinarily one sees moving pictures as separate—that is, flickering—until they reach the rate of twenty per second. The flicker fusion rate in a null magnetic field is *ten* per second. In other words, there is a loss of precision in our visual perception when we are denied earth's weak magnetic field. In mice, the null field causes premature deaths, aging, inactivity, cannibalism of the newborn.

Research by the Army's Advanced Material Concepts Agency in Alexandria, Virginia, suggested that the ancient art of dowsing probably exploits human sensitivity to low electromagnetic fields. Such sensitivity may enable the dowser to locate water, buried metal, or buried electrical lines. In one study, 80 percent of the subjects reportedly could dowse using an L-shaped rod, compared to 20 percent who could use a forked twig successfully.

In 1972 the Defense Department finally lifted the secrecy classification on a study conducted by Duke University for the government during the Korean conflict. Troops were successfully trained to dowse for land mines. Similar dowsing has been employed in Vietnam, by civilian geologists searching for water or metal, and by employees of public utilities companies, who sometimes find dowsing faster and more accurate than relying on metal detectors.

Sometimes called radiesthesia, the strange ability of human beings to detect electromagnetic energy has captured the interest of physicists and electronics engineers all over the world. As James Beal of NASA's Space Flight Center put it, "We are all tuned in. . . ." Beal pointed out that because each cell is a tiny, complex electrical system, external energy may have a more profound effect than we have supposed. Russian researchers report that the hypothalamus is the brain structure most sensitive to electromagnetic fields. They also say that damage to the hypothalamus increases this sensitivity.

Part of the limbic system or so-called emotional brain, the hypothalamus is involved in such critical areas as sexuality, appetite, pain, and pleasure. Malfunctions of its chemistry have been blamed for mental disorders. The purported sensitivity of this structure to energy fields might be involved in another eye-opening finding. After studying the pattern of 28,000 admissions to psychiatric hospitals, a team at the Upstate Medical Center, State University of New York, Syracuse, found a striking correlation between acute psychosis and changes in the intensity of the geomagnetic field. The odds against chance occurrence were 10,000 to one!

Magnetic storms also seem to affect the suicide rate. Behavior disturbances in schizophrenics seem to vary with changes in the cosmic ray levels, which, in turn, result from solar flares. And Arnold Lieber of the University of Miami reported that a survey covering Dade County statistics for fifteen years showed a "scientifically sound" relationship between phases of the moon and the murder rate.

Lieber said, "I feel that eventually we're going to show that any organism, human or animal, is an integral part of the universe and responds to changes like variations in the solar cycle and the lunar cycle." He pointed out that the human body and the surface of the earth have a comparable composition: 80 percent water, 20 percent mineral. Other scientists have pointed out that our bodies may have their own tidal systems.

Is man transistorized? A solar cell? After studying the accumulated research and the results of his own experiments, Robert O. Becker has postulated a theory about the brain that could explain a host of phenomena now baffling science. If Becker and several other investigators are right, our nervous system is not dependent solely on the weak, slow electrical impulses from cell to cell. It has the characteristics of a semi-conductor—that is, it behaves in many ways like a transistor or solar cell. The glial cells of the nervous system may actually act as liquid crystals in resonance with surrounding energy fields. If this is true, the nervous system is capable of magnifying electrical effects over a million times in amplitude.

Based on work in his own laboratory, Becker, research orthopedic surgeon at the State University of New York, sees this solid-state electronic current as a critical factor in determining the sensitivity of nerve cells—the threshold at which they respond by firing. (The brain's ten billion nerve cells function by passing along tiny electrical impulses. Each cell is a minute generator, creating the electrical energy necessary to pass an impulse on to the next cell.)

He believes that the brain contains a midline structure with a stronger direct-current (DC) field than the rest of the nervous system. He also thinks that the intensity and perhaps the polarity of this current directly determine the level of consciousness.

By placing a magnetic field oriented at right angles to the brainstem, Becker caused unconsciousness in animals; their brainwave patterns went from waking to comatose. And the process can be reversed. By applying direct current to the frontal region of the brain, Becker could arouse chemically anesthetized animals. It was as if he had found an off-on switch for consciousness.

Data from our unmanned satellites suggest that the planet itself may operate as a direct-current generator. James Van Allen, discoverer of the radiation belts, has said that the effect may be as high as 50,000 volts.

A number of scientists have suggested that it is not coincidental that the brain's predominant rhythm—its rate of electrical firing—is about eight to twelve pulses per second, similar to the rate of earth's magnetic pulsations, which range from eight to sixteen cycles per second, peaking at ten. They believe that low-frequency radiation from the planet may have biologically entrained the human brain. Since life on earth evolved in an electromagnetic field, these energies may be our natural genetic medium.

Becker has suggested that the brain's own steady-state bioelectric energy field might constitute an ancient communications system. This field, he said, has already been correlated with growth, tissue repair, tumors, sleep, and human behavior. Perhaps it is a central intelligence network that senses injury to the cells and sends out orders for repair. If other scientists replicate Becker's findings, we may learn more about the brain's role in healing.

In an experiment that stunned the scientific community, Becker demonstrated the relationship between regeneration and electrical energy. Many lower creatures, such as the salamander, can regenerate an amputated limb. Becker thought that mammals could do the same if there were energy enough at the point of amputation. He cut off the forelimbs of rats up to the shoulder. Then he applied a delicately controlled current to the stumps. *The rats regrew their limbs beyond the knee.*

In other experiments, energy introduced into the stomach via electrodes has helped heal ulcers. Power packs have stimulated the rapid regeneration of bones that had stubbornly refused to mend. (Becker himself discourages such experimentation on human beings because of the possible risk of cancer.)

The relationship of energy fields to disease is bewildering. It appears that artificial fields can enhance health or they can cause serious damage. Madeleine and J. M. Barnothy of the University of Illinois injected twenty-two mice with a highly malignant cancer, then treated half the mice with high-intensity magnetic fields. Five of the treated mice rejected the already well-developed tumor. Four were eventually completely healed. When the experiment was repeated, none of the mice survived, but the treated mice lived longer than the untreated. Although their tumors had continued to grow after treatment began, there was no evidence of metastasis, the spreading to other sites that is the scourge of cancer therapy.

The Barnothys believe that the magnetic field increased the animals' immune responses. In other experiments they found that magnetic fields influenced the ovarian cycle, the development of tissue, and aging. Varying the strength of the field could change the effects from beneficial to injurious.

Kirlian photography, sometimes called aura photography, is a lensless process developed by Soviet researchers. An object is placed on film in a high-frequency electrical field. Living organisms such as plants and people produce a remarkable effect, a glittering, multicolored field of light, the "aura" that has captured the public imagination. Soviet physicists believe that this field effect is caused by "a cold emission of electrons" and is the secondary effect of an unknown primary energy. This energy has been likened to the ancient concept of *qi* or prana, an organizing life-force.

Since the Kirlian effect was first internationally publicized, several colleges and universities in the West have devised equipment to obtain similar "pictures," but the Russian state of the art, with thirty years' head start, is vastly more sophisticated.

Human subjects wear elastic dielectric garments in some Soviet laboratories, so that their energy fields can be observed in action rather than on the plates. The researchers report that the bioplasma, their name for the glittering radiation, gives evidence of disease long before it would be seen in conventional diagnosis. This work supports the controversial but venerable theory that an organizing radiation field plays a part in the growth and health of living things.

The striking correlation of Kirlian flare points to traditional acupuncture points has inspired many clinical applications in the Soviet Union and Czechoslovakia. The tobiscope, a device that measures electrical changes on the surface of the skin, lights up as it is passed over the acupuncture points. The experiments have used electronic and even laser stimulation at such points. A mild laser beam directed at a point over the lips reportedly stops an epileptic seizure.

The most provocative report from the Kirlian scientists is their ranking of the strength of stimuli applied to the points. Chemicals, such as adrenaline, are the weakest stimuli, followed by physical pressure, needles, electrical impulses, and laser beams. The most powerful stimulus of all, as observed by changes in the bioplasma, is human volition. If the subject quietly directs his thought toward a specific part of the body, the bioplasma shows corresponding changes.

Laboratories in Japan, the United States, and France have been experimenting with the Kirlian effect. Thelma Moss and Kendall Johnson at the University of California at Los Angeles and Douglas Dean at the Newark College of Engineering have obtained a number of photographs demonstrating a sharp correspondence between shifts in the state of mind and the appearance of the energy field. The UCLA researchers call their process radiation field photography.

Another provocative finding: Human beings in artificially ionized environments show many of the effects seen in altered states of consciousness: greater strength, shorter reaction time, rapid healing, reduction of pain, and a tranquilizing or mood-brightening effect.

This negative ionization may speed up the oxidation of one of the brain chemicals, serotonin, acting in the same way as reserpine, a tranquilizing drug. The EEG, or electroencephalogram, also shows changes when negative ions are introduced into the air. The visual purple, a substance critical in vision, is rapidly restored. There is also an antiaging effect. Negative ionization halved the errors in time scores in test groups of old rats.

The human brain seems to radiate energy of its own. According to one study, the brain's cerebral cortex actually emits near-infrared radiation. Electrical stimulation of the brain alters this radiation. The limbic brain, an older structure, radiates light about ten times brighter than starlight.

Man's alpha-pattern brainwave seems to create a magnetic field of its own. David Cohen, then at the University of Illinois, discovered the small, fluctuating magnetic field produced by alpha-rhythm activity (one of the patterns of electrical activity measured by the EEG). Cohen later devised equipment to produce a magnetoencephalogram (MEG), a measurement that may help round out our crude picture of what the brain is doing.

Johannes Kepler, sixteenth-century astronomer, wrote: "Everything that is, or that happens in the sky, is felt in some hidden fashion by earth and nature." It has been said that the entire universe is affected by the displacement of a single particle. By keeping in mind our dynamic nature, we can more readily grasp and accept the almost incredible discoveries about the brain.

3

BIOFEEDBACK:
MASTERMINDING THE BODY

It's as if your body has always been on automatic pilot, and suddenly you find you can take over the controls.

—LABORATORY VOLUNTEER

In the late 1960s a handful of scientists in laboratories in several countries demonstrated beyond doubt that men and animals can learn conscious control over their most remote inner processes. A graph, a tone, or a light furnish the feedback to guide them.

The implications are so startling, so urgent, that biofeedback therapy has become a reality almost before the original experiments have been replicated. Biofeedback institutes have already opened on the East and West coasts of the United States. Hospitals and clinics around the world have set up electronic apparatus for experimental training. The list of ills successfully treated reads like the spiel of a snake-oil peddler: cardiac arrhythmias and angina pectoris, migraine and tension headaches, impotence, and even epileptic seizures.

As the biofeedback pioneer Neal Miller of Rockefeller University wryly observed, there is a question whether people can learn control as well as rats can. "I believe that in this respect they are as smart as rats," Miller said. "But as a recent critical review points out, this has not yet been completely proved."

A monkey has learned to fire a single nerve cell to obtain a reward. At Queen's University in Kingston, Ontario, John Basmajian trained human subjects to discharge a single motor-nerve cell, selected from the brain's ten billion cells. Miller's rats learned to form urine at greater or lesser rates, to redden one ear and blanch the other, to increase or decrease the blood in their intestinal lining.

Remarkable—but there has, after all, existed a great body of popular literature giving the lie to the dogma that, as Miller put it, the "stupid" autonomic nervous system was incapable of sophisticated, voluntary control. For more than two hundred years British colonials had soberly recorded the feats of Indian yogis who appeared to have almost miraculous control. Harry Houdini, the American magician, had mastered his stomach viscera so adroitly that he could vomit up a key to free himself from his underwater chains. Many actors and actresses have learned to weep on command.

Miller points out that there was never a strong foundation of evidence for the premise that the brain cannot voluntarily control the inner processes. Early experiments had been inconclusive. Pavlov's salivating dogs, granted, had proved a type of visceral learning, but this was termed "classical conditioning." As such it was considered an altogether different type of learning.

For more than a decade Miller could not interest his students, nor even paid assistants, in his theory. "I almost always ended up by letting them work on something they didn't think was so preposterous," Miller said. His first "encouraging but inconclusive early results" were described at the 18th International Congress of Psychology in Moscow in 1966.

In 1967 Miller and Alfredo Carmona rewarded one group of dogs for spontaneous salivation, another for decreasing their salivation. Another associate, Jay Trowill, had begun experimenting with rats paralyzed by curare, the deadly dart poison of South American natives. The rats were maintained on artificial respiration, since the curare paralyzes the respiratory activity, and were rewarded for speeding up or slowing down their hearts. The curare guaranteed that they could not "cheat" by using the musculature in the heart region. Scientists had long insisted that yogis who stopped their hearts were merely performing a powerful muscular maneuver. The animals were rewarded by electric stimulation of their brains' pleasure centers. Later, to prove that brain stimulation was not the only effective reward, the researchers trained a group of rats to control their heart rate by rewarding them with shock avoidance.

Over the next two years Miller and Leo DiCara undertook a variety of feedback training experiments at Yale. Having learned from Russian scientists that a dog can detect the exact placement of tiny water-filled balloons in its rectum, they placed such balloons inside rats. They measured and rewarded the control of intestinal contractions.

In other experiments, rats rewarded for urine formation apparently learned to change the rate of blood flow through the kidneys, which changed the rate of filtration. Other rats learned to control the amount of blood in their stomach walls. Then Miller and DiCara proved conclusively that the control was more than a simple change in heart rate or blood pressure. They trained rats to increase the blood flow to one ear and not the other. Later animals were trained specifically to control blood pressure independent of heart rate and vice versa.

Other scientists had been exploring the possibilities of human training. As early as 1958, M. I. Lisina, a Russian psychologist, had reported her attempts to teach dilation and constriction of blood vessels to human subjects. Significantly, she said that she was not successful until she let the subjects watch the recording of their vascular changes.

Earlier yet, in 1910, Johannes Schultz of Switzerland had developed a technique he called autogenic training. Somewhat reminiscent of both yoga and self-hypnosis, autogenic training involved learning to control blood flow. Even blood sugar and white cell count are affected by the exercises, according to later studies. Autogenic training became a major factor in European medicine and psychotherapy. By the 1960s more than six hundred publications about autogenic training were in print, less than a dozen of them in English.

In 1965, Elmer and Alyce Green at the Menninger Foundation began teaching Kansas housewives, college students, and children to vary their hand temperatures by using autogenic techniques. A feedback device accelerated the learning process. If the subjects could see when they were succeeding and when they were missing, they learned control in days or hours, a fraction of the time it had taken Johannes Schultz's typical patients. Feedback seemed the vital factor.

By the early sixties, a few scattered experimenters had announced success in human control of heart rates. In 1962, Peter

Lang at the University of Pittsburgh devised an apparatus he described as "similar to the driving-skill booths at penny arcades." The subjects drove their hearts between two vertical lines on the screen. They had to maintain their heart rate within an astonishingly narrow range—as low as ninety milliseconds—to stay within the line. Lang and Michael Hnatiow, his co-worker, found that their human subjects needed no reward other than the amusement of the game.

Meanwhile, Joe Kamiya had begun experimenting with brainwave feedback at the University of Chicago, bootlegging the project while officially working under a grant to study sleep. His student volunteers soon learned to discriminate between alpha and nonalpha brainwave activity, and Kamiya discovered that his subjects could maintain the alpha state or turn it off if they had adequate feedback, usually a tone.

Those who learn control by feedback can seldom explain their techniques. The sensations involved are so subtle and ineffable that they can only be felt and dimly identified. Miller pointed out that nerves not only run from the brain to the visceral organs but vice versa. Yet, except in extreme cases, such as a stomachache, we are not aware of sensations from these organs. He likened the situation to that of a basketball player trying to make a basket while blindfolded. The feedback devices, such as light, tone, or reward, remove the blindfold. "If patients can learn to detect internal changes, they can practice visceral control just as a basketball player practices his shots."

A child gets environmental feedback if he calls a cow a dog, Miller said. But because there has been no way to check on what's happening inside him, he has not been trained to identify his visceral processes. We are all novices when it comes to accurate visceral perception. "But with the help of modern instrumentation, perhaps we can be trained to become experts."

Drawing attention to the Oriental tradition of power over the body's internal functions, Miller speculated that the reason curarized rats learn more quickly than noncurarized may be more than coincidentally similar to yoga. "It's interesting that yogis practice absolutely regular breathing and muscular relaxation, and monotonously concentrate their attention on a single point to eliminate external distractions. Our paralyzed rats are given absolutely regular breathing by the artificial-respiration machine. Their muscles are relaxed because curare paralyzes them. And they are trained in a sound-deadened box."

Noncurarized rats learn much more slowly, as does noncurarized man. Miller suggested that some centering technique, such as hypnosis, might simulate the curarized state.

The parallel with eastern disciplines is drawn with increasing frequency in biofeedback literature. It may be significant, too, that Johannes Schultz included a series of "meditative exercises" in his autonomic training program. Perhaps the most curious twist occurred at the 1970 World Conference on Scientific Yoga held in New Delhi. One of the speakers, Swami Rama, flew to India from the Menninger Foundation, where his remarkable control of autonomic processes had been the subject of research. The yogi took two of Menninger's biofeedback machines to India for their possible usefulness in training young yogis in the rudiments of control.

In Baltimore, Bernard Engel, a physiological psychologist, and Eugene Bleecker, a cardiovascular specialist, have successfully trained heart patients to control such abnormalities as atrial fibrillation and premature ventricular contraction. The patient watches a box at the foot of his hospital bed. As the heart rate is monitored, the box flashes yellow ("maintain speed"), red ("slow the heart rate"), or green ("speed it up"). Many of the patients have learned to manage their heart rates at home. Similar results have been obtained by researchers at Rockefeller University, New York Hospital-Cornell Medical Center, and in private clinics.

Subjects at Lafayette Clinic in Detroit, Harvard Medical School, and Rockefeller University have learned to bring their blood pressure down steadily and substantially and to keep it down. Psychologically oriented critics who feared symptom substitution have no grounds for concern thus far. Individuals who learn to undo or improve one disease don't seem to substitute another. Chances are an individual with a neurotic need for his disease would not have worked to achieve visceral control in the first place.

Stress-related illness is not necessarily neurotic. One analogy might be a parking lot. In an emergency situation (stress), one car is parked astraddle two spaces. After that the other cars entering the lot park off-center in both directions because of that one emergency. If at some point the malparked car is driven away, the pathology of the parking lot remains. The proprietor, however, might clear away all the cars, restoring order. The parking lot would not necessarily be scarred by its history.

If any chronic ailment would seem intractable to unlearning, it should be the tension headache—especially if one assumes, as many psychologists do, that the headache offers escape or excuse. Nonetheless, Thomas Budzynski, Johann Stoyva, and Charles Adler at the University of Colorado have taught many volunteers to eliminate or reduce chronic tension headaches by learning to relax the frontalus muscle. With an electromyelogram (EMG) feedback, the subject can monitor his muscle tension. Seven out of twenty volunteers at Menninger's achieved zero muscle tension and a simultaneous euphoric, floating sensation. Without feedback it is all but impossible to reduce tension to zero.

Volunteers who learn muscular control frequently report a curious side effect. Minor stresses in their daily lives no longer upset them. This phenomenon may be due to a by-product, relaxation training. One soon learns that anxiety aborts the subtle changes he must make to maintain the light or tone feedback.

Budzynski and Stoyva cite the theory of the Swiss researcher W. R. Hess that the body's reactions are paired. In the stress response, high muscle activity and high sympathetic activity are linked. In relaxation, low striate muscle activity and parasympathetic nervous system activity are associated. For example, in learning to bring the needle across the dial, the muscular biofeedback trainee automatically controls to some extent the deep-brain structures involved in slowing respiration and heart rate.

Wolfgang Luthe speculates that the therapeutic key in autogenic training is that the subject learns to modify the relationship between his so-called higher and lower nervous systems. This allows natural forces in the body to regain their capacity for self-regulation. It is a swing back in the direction of health —the opposite of the negative adaptation that follows prolonged stress. Luthe emphasizes that the change is never one-sided. Mind and body change as one, in whichever direction they move.

Elmer Green of Menninger's has postulated what he calls the

"psychophysiological principle." It is already much-quoted in biofeedback circles:

> Every change in the physiological state is accompanied by an appropriate change in the mental-emotional state, conscious or unconscious . . . and conversely, every change in the mental-emotional state, conscious or unconscious, is accompanied by an appropriate change in the physiological state.

Green compared this closed-loop system to the thermostat on a furnace. Even as an outside force—one's hand—manipulates the furnace, so the body can be manipulated by volition. Will is the meta-force, or outside force, in biofeedback training.

Green, Joseph Sargent, and E. Dale Walters of Menninger's report considerable success in teaching migraine sufferers a simple technique to forestall the excruciating headaches. In the grand tradition of science, the trick was a chance discovery. In an early study, the experimenters noticed that a volunteer made a sudden recovery from a migraine attack at the same time she successfully willed a temperature increase in her hands—ten degrees in two minutes. Since migraines involve an initial distention of blood vessels in the head, there seemed a strong possibility that drawing blood into the hands might prevent the headache. Of the first hundred subjects trained, ninety learned to control the headaches without drugs.

Oddly enough, although subjects in their preliminary study have been surprisingly successful in warding off migraines, the hand-warming technique has little or no effect on sinus or tension headaches. Tension headaches apparently require the more specific relaxation of the frontalus muscle, another indication that biofeedback techniques can be highly specific.

Unexpected uses have been found for clinical biofeedback. Through breatholyzer scores, alcoholics are learning to sense the level of alcohol in their blood. If they guess incorrectly, they are given an uncomfortable electric shock. Reportedly, a drinker who masters the art can maintain a socially acceptable high without getting drunk.

Neal Miller has suggested that chronic illness may be the result of negative biofeedback learning. His example is a child so distraught at the idea of going to school unprepared for a test that he may turn pale. His mother, alarmed at his pallor, insists that he stay home. If the scene is repeated often enough, the child may unconsciously learn a cardiovascular symptom that plagues him for life. A different parent, unimpressed by a wan face, might sympathize instead with gastric distress. The rewarded child would eventually learn that symptom. Lasting emotional as well as physical damage might ensue. Rats trained to speed their hearts were so emotional that they performed poorly in maze tests.

These phenomena are not really new, of course, but until now scientists had lacked rigorous laboratory techniques for pinpointing the awesome role of the brain in health and disease.

4

STRESS AND HEALING

*A new and sensible variant of faith healing may be on its way . . .
a whole new area of medical research is opened by the control of
the autonomic system.* —NIGEL CALDER, THE MIND OF MAN

The most minutely examined interaction between brain and
body is the so-called stress syndrome, the fight-or-flight response. This reaction is a dangerous anachronism from the days
when our ancestors were confronted by savage animals or other
clear-cut threats to survival. As the cerebral cortex registers a
threat, its alarm triggers a flurry of preparations in more ancient brain sites. Adrenaline pours forth, gastric juices seethe,
muscles tense, the heart races.

Our forebears had to scramble away from predators or club
an enemy into unconsciousness. But contemporary man can neither flee from his problems nor physically battle his adver-
saries. He is repeatedly primed for a burst of activity that
would be impractical.

Hans Selye, the Canadian researcher who pioneered stress-
syndrome research, maintains that "no living organism can
exist continuously in a state of alarm." The body's intricate
feedback mechanisms eventually are exhausted. Prolonged
stress results in what Selye calls the general adaptation syndrome. The defensive reactions wear down, and man's precious
homeostasis, his physiological balance, is upset.

Prolonged stress has been blamed for most of the ills of
modern man: cardiovascular disease, ulcers, asthma, migraine,
ulcerative colitis, hypertension. The chain of biochemical factors
responsible for mental disease can be set off by stress and the
general adaptation syndrome.

At Columbia University, scientists demonstrated the effects

of stress as neatly as if they had pressed a button. Two hours after feeding dogs and cats a high-cholesterol diet, they electrically stimulated two brain regions commonly responsive to stress. During the stimulation, which lasted no longer than four minutes, clear plasma turned milky from an increase in lipids (fatty substances).

The role of psychological stress in disease is evident in a recent study of air traffic controllers. Of 111 controllers, 66 had gastrointestinal illness. Of those, 36 had peptic ulcers. Their poor health was blamed on a single factor: their fear of causing a midair collision.

The origin of disease is like the optical illusion of a staircase that can be viewed from topside or underside. Neither view is more valid than the other. In man, the mind can alarm the body until the sugar-metabolizing mechanism fails or malfunctions. The undernourished brain then slumps into depression, becomes rattled, or occasionally soars into madness. Conversely, the pancreas might be insulted by a pregnancy or an automobile accident. In this case the psychological effects are secondary.

In popular usage the term psychosomatic has come to mean "all in the head," but so-called psychosomatic illnesses can be devastating, even fatal. What the brain experiences is real in the only meaningful sense of the word. At Harvard Medical School, Gary Schwartz showed that human subjects could generate cardiac responses and other autonomic changes by self-induced thoughts.

Psychosomatic health is a field of intense contemporary interest. Many researchers are now asking what makes an individual well. As René Dubos put it, "If we depend exclusively on defense measures, we shall increasingly behave like hunted creatures, running from one therapeutic or protective device to another, each more complex and costly than the one before."

Among the unorthodox but effective approaches to health is Structural Integration, more commonly known as rolfing. Ida Rolf's approach is to separate the muscle groups that have become bound together over the years by the body's temporary stresses: injury, anxiety, tension. Psychologist Sam Keen described his experience with rolfing:

My chest wouldn't yield. Each time a hand approached it I went into panic and felt pain. The disarming of the emotional-physical defenses in this area involved both memory and manipulation. In the seventh hour of processing, pressure on a muscle in my shoulder released a memory of childhood conflict with a person I loved deeply—a memory that had become incysted in my chest. I wept. The release of the memory, and the grief it occasioned, eased the panic and tension that had made me unable to bear manipulative work on my chest. At the end of that hour I was able, for the first time, to fill my lungs in one smooth movement.

With my release from this, I experience a new openness, ease and expansiveness. . . . I find myself warming to opinions, persons and events that not long ago would have raised my hackles. Something new is happening and my head will have to get used to it.

Once again, the tandem: a profound change in the body and a simultaneous psychological release. It seems irrelevant whether the body is dealt the first cleansing blow or whether, as in the altered states of consciousness, the brain receives the impact.

Ida Rolf, who developed her technique in the 1920s, maintains that the process results in a reawakening. Basically the theory says that the individual's posture becomes misaligned over the years. If he breaks an ankle as a child, for example, his body temporarily adopts a new arrangement to accommodate the laws of gravity and favor the injured joint. The solution may become permanent. Or he adopts a defensive posture in early life because of anxiety or insecurity. This too becomes a part of him. The muscle groups, which should remain autonomous, become tightly bound to each other in short, inelastic connective tissue, the fascia. Rolfing, an admittedly painful process, is the systematic manipulation of the connective tissue to free the muscles.

A UCLA study measured fourteen individuals before and after they underwent the ten basic rolfing sessions. Telemetry packs measured signals from the subjects' shoulders, neck, back, and hips. After rolfing they walked, sat, and threw with a lower expenditure of energy, and it was inferred that the nervous system control was moved from the brain's cortex to the spine. That implies a reversal of some of the motor patterns involved in aging, when many activities shift from spinal to cortical control. The subjects' brainwave patterns also changed. According to the researchers, their measurements suggest that rolfing "creates a more spontaneous, open, rhythmic reaction to the environment and to one's own . . . sensations."

Rolfing, the Alexander technique, dance therapy, bioenergetics, hara, and other somatic approaches had been anticipated by Wilhelm Reich's orgone therapy; and before Reich, many Indian, Chinese, and Japanese methods presumed a simultaneous healing of body and soul.

There is mounting evidence that even cancer is linked to emotional stress. Claus Bahnson, director of behavioral sciences at Eastern Pennsylvania Psychiatric Institute in Philadelphia, reported that cancer patients seem to share certain characteristics not found to such a striking degree in individuals ill with heart disease and other diseases.

The cancer-prone tend to bottle up emotions to a striking degree, he said. And this seems to tie in with findings about the body's stress hormones. Those who do not express emotions openly tend to build up these hormones. That buildup, in turn, has a suppressive effect on the body's immunity system.

Evidence from two sources points to a portion of the hypothalamus as the brain region involved in immunity. Elena Kornevac of the USSR reported that stimulating that region increased animals' ability to make antibodies. And two American researchers, Joseph Meites of Michigan State University and James Clemens of the National Institutes of Health, found that they could reduce the incidence of breast cancer in rats by burning out a tiny section of the hypothalamus. They speculated that a hormone factor in the hypothalamus may be essential to tumor growth.

Scientists have said that everyone probably has cancer once or twice in his lifetime. It only becomes a clinical disease when the immune system fails to destroy the tumor early in its development. Suppose cancer patients could learn to consciously activate their immune systems? If the central nervous system contains the bioelectric wherewithal to mastermind healing, can this ability be consciously manipulated?

Over the centuries there have been many claims of tumor regression by hypnosis or by so-called faith healing. Mesmer and other early hypnotists insisted that they had cured malignancies.

Carl Simonton, now head of the immunology laboratory at Travis Air Force Base in California, as well as a member of the board of directors and executive committee of the American Cancer Society, once studied the personal characteristics of the "miraculous" 2 to 5 percent of all cancer patients, those who experience spontaneous remission. He interviewed them and their doctors and relatives. He also interviewed the doctors and families of cancer patients who had succumbed. As the case histories accumulated he found a distinct pattern. The spontaneous-remission patients were optimistic, positive individuals.

Years later, when Simonton was experimenting with various types of biofeedback training, he was reminded of his cancer study. Suppose cancer patients could learn consciously to activate their immune systems?

Simonton and his co-workers treated fifty consecutive patients with traditional therapy such as drugs and radiation in combination with suggestion and visualization. The patients were told in simple language how the body's immune mechanism works. They were asked to imagine the white cells carrying off dead cancer cells. This visualization procedure was to be practiced three times daily. Meanwhile, the staff rated the patients' cooperativeness on a five-point scale.

The fifty patients' response to treatment—that is, the measurable regression of tumors—was markedly better than would have been expected from traditional treatment alone. Of the twelve whose tumor regression was judged excellent, eight had been given less than a fifty-fifty chance of successful treatment. Not only did the inner visualization seem to have an effect, but the best results were seen in the patients who had been rated most highly motivated.

A New Jersey physician, Howard Smith, has reported that hypnotic suggestion was apparently instrumental in regressing tumors in his patients. Naturally, researchers are always concerned lest publicity raise false hopes, but Smith and Simonton have spoken out in the hope that their colleagues might be encouraged to conduct their own research.

Clarence Cone, head of the Molecular Biophysics Laboratory

at NASA's Langley Research Center, made headlines in 1970 when he produced evidence that cell division is precisely controlled by the electrical voltage across the surface membrane. By inhibiting the activity of DNA, the high negative voltages in normal cells block division. Cancer cells have an abnormally low negative voltage. It appears that malignant cells proliferate because they are permanently depolarized. Cone has already found that even brain cells, which ordinarily do not regenerate, can be made to divide in the laboratory if they are kept in a depolarized state for long enough.

Whether these surface changes are caused by an irritant or by the cancer virus, according to Cone's theory, the lowered energy level of the cells now feeds back to sustain the metabolic pathways that produced it in the first place.

Using a highly refined version of Kirlian photography, Soviet scientists say that they can detect cancer by observing changes in what they call the bioplasma long before the disease would be discovered by routine diagnostic methods.

In a Molière play, a patient was recovering by following an unorthodox method of treatment. His doctor scolded, "Sir, it would be better to die according to the rules than to live in contradiction to the Faculty of Medicine."

In 1970 a distinguished group of American physicians and scientists founded the Academy of Parapsychology and Medicine, hoping to draw their colleagues into the investigation of unorthodox medicine and the mind's role in healing. Headquartered in Los Altos, California, the academy has sponsored seminars, workshops, and symposia on such subjects as acupuncture, biofeedback training, and psychic healing. Every event has attracted overflow crowds. An acupuncture symposium at Stanford, immediately preceding the annual convention of the American Medical Association, drew so many physicians that it had to be rescheduled for a larger auditorium.

Perhaps the work of the Academy of Parapsychology and Medicine will fulfill Thomas Hanna's hope that men of unexpectedly broad knowledge will devise treatment for the whole man, even if they must resort to unorthodox tools.

5

5

INNER CONTROL OF PAIN

The fiercest agonies have shortest reign.

—WILLIAM CULLEN BRYANT, MUTATION

A tool-and-die maker hurt his hand one afternoon. After examining the injured fingers, the company doctor sent him home. By early evening the man was moaning, and his wife suggested somewhat facetiously that he might try an old Zen technique she had just read about. He muttered that this was no time to be funny. Aspirin didn't touch the excruciating pain, and by eight o'clock he was all but screaming in agony. Desperate, he said, "Tell me about that Zen business again. . . . I'll try anything!"

She explained that young monks are told that if they have an urge to scratch their flesh they should instead say, "Itching, itching," and if they feel pain they are to experience the pain fully, immerse themselves in it, and chant, "Paining, paining."

The anguished man gave himself to the technique with a vengeance. He said later, "I talked to the damned fingers as if they were spoiled kids. I admired the quality of the pain. I gave it my full attention. And then, just like that, it vanished. It was like flipping a switch." *

Peter Mezan, a writer doing an article on the psychiatrist

---

* The reader can subjectively test the paining-paining technique. When pain reaches consciousness, close your eyes and consciously attempt to enhance and intensify it. Experience it completely, and imagine drawing it up toward the brain. Sustain the intensification for half a minute. When you stop, the pain may well be gone.

R. D. Laing, spent considerable time with him. One night he found himself in a meditation circle at Laing's home. He wrote:

> There is a terrifically painful corn that simply will not let me past, it is making such a racket. For the next ten minutes or so I give myself over to that corn, all the attention I can muster. . . . At first, the harder I concentrate, the more intense the pain seems to become, until I am virtually alone and excruciated with it; then, after a while it ceases to be a pain exactly . . . and then, suddenly, it seems, it ceases altogether.

A similar incident is related in *The Quiet Mind,* the journal of John E. Coleman, an ex-CIA agent. In an Eastern monastery he experienced physical pain: "It was like fire, burning and scorching. Suddenly, like a bolt of lightning, something snapped, and when the search [for relief] stopped, there was relief."

The phenomenon of pain that suddenly stops after having become almost unbearable might be explained by the recent "gate-control theory of pain." Admittedly speculative, the theory devised by Ronald Melzack and Patrick Wall accounts for paradoxes that have perplexed researchers. The simplest previous approach had been the so-called specificity theory that assumed simple pathways from receptor to brain: Match burns skin, skin receptors flash message to brain much as telephone wires carry signals, brain registers pain.

But the specificity theory could not explain such bizarre puzzles as phantom-limb pain. It is estimated that 30 percent of all amputees report pain in their nonexistent limbs, and 10 percent experience suffering for many years. Their reports are so similar that one can hardly account for this phenomenon as mere hallucination.

Nearly all amputees report feeling the limb after surgery. They describe its sensations and movements as being precisely like those of a normal limb. They may even clench a missing fist, Melzack reports, or try to scratch a missing finger:

> As time passes, however, the limb begins to change shape. The leg or arm becomes shorter and may even fade away altogether, so that the phantom foot or hand seems to be hanging in mid-air. . . . If the patient wears an artificial limb, however, the

phantom usually remains vivid and may correlate perfectly with the movement and shape of the artificial limb.

Most extraordinary of all, severing pathways between the stump and the brain relieves the pain little if at all. *It frequently worsens it.* And other areas of the anatomy, referred to as trigger zones, may be drawn into a fray, so that bumping the amputee's right elbow sets off pain in his phantom left leg. In causalgia, a similar mysterious pathology, a site that has once been injured becomes increasingly sensitive until even a feather's touch or a gentle breeze can send the sufferer into agonized screams.

There is another confounding question: What of psychological anesthesia? For example, the badly wounded soldier who is so exhilarated to be alive after battle that he experiences no pain from his injury, but yelps when given a morphine injection? And even if battle anesthesia could be explained away as a version of self-hypnosis—not that that explains anything— Melzack and Wall call attention to Pavlov's conditioned dogs. If the dogs were shocked, burned, or cut, then immediately given food, they soon stopped responding to the stimuli as pain.

Some pain theorists had held that pattern is the key, and that the pathological pain states are due to the destruction of a system that normally prevents the summation of firing nerve cells; that is, a random discharge of the cells would not add up to a sensation of pain as would their simultaneous firing. Melzack and Wall believe that the pattern theory stops short of a satisfactory explanation. Their gate-control theory deals with the marvelous complexity of a perception—pain—that we think of as relatively simple.

The nerves in a limb contain fibers that set off activity in pools of nerve cells in the spinal cord. The larger fibers conduct impulses quickly. The small fibers conduct more slowly. After a limb is amputated, about half the cut nerve fibers in the stump die. Unfortunately, those that regenerate are usually the small, slowly conducting fibers. These small fibers react to stimulation, such as bumping the stump, by producing synchronous volleys rather than a dispersed pattern typical of nerve cells whose fiber sizes are varied. It is something like rhythmic drumming rather than a full, complex orchestration.

Earlier Melzack and his colleagues had measured the electrical activity of the sensory system in the brain of a cat being gently massaged. Rubbing for ten to fifteen seconds produced very transient changes. But in anesthetized cats, the same brief rubbing resulted in brain changes lasting as long as half an hour. From this they concluded that even moderate anesthesia can interfere with a natural mechanism that usually shuts off brain activity as soon as the stimulus is removed. They assumed that the persistent activity is due to an arrangement of nerve fibers described as a "reverbatory circuit" by another pain theorist, W. K. Livingston.

Because the inhibition of pain depends on the level of input, the short, slow, surviving fibers at the amputee's stump might not be powerful enough to close the gate: to trigger inhibition at the various spinal levels and up into the brain. Therefore the volleys of activity would go on and on, unchallenged. It would be only a matter of time until the stump nerve cells (neurons), like a guerrilla band, would recruit other populations of neurons in adjacent areas of the nervous system.

Once activity patterns are established in the brain, severing the pathways in the spinal cord will not help. The brain creates its own images of the body parts. A phantom-limb pain pattern might be compared to the so-called epileptic mirror focus. Damaged cells in one hemisphere of the brain somehow trigger a mirror-image epileptic pattern in the opposite hemisphere. Even when the original damaged area is surgically removed, the mirror focus may continue to cause seizures for many months.

Some of the cells in the brain's thalamus and cortex receive information about very large sensory fields, according to Melzack, sometimes half or more of the body surface. He speculates that stimuli from distant skin areas could set off sustained activity in the brain. That activity would then translate as phantom limb pain. This could explain how trigger zones can develop far from the stump.

If the gate-control theory of pain is valid, one should be able to bring about inhibition by intensifying phantom-limb pain. Melzack injected salt solution into the base of the spine of amputees, producing "a sharp, localized pain that radiates into the phantom limb. It lasts only about ten minutes, yet it may produce dramatic relief for hours, weeks, sometimes indefinitely."

On the other hand, decreasing the sensory input may help, too, by letting the reverberatory circuits finally run down. The amputee should avoid using the stump for a time to accomplish this.

The theory holds that gate-closing can occur at various points in the central nervous system; also that psychological factors such as experience, attention, and emotion influence pain . . . by acting on the gate-control system. And that the brain can reset the level at which the gates will inhibit pain. Interestingly, pain relief often comes when the sufferer quits struggling, when he resigns himself. It is as if resistance itself helps perpetuate the pain, perhaps by inhibiting the activity of the longer nerve fibers. Surrender may enable them to join the fray, thereby closing the gate in the higher nervous system.

The gate-control model explains several pain mechanisms, but the nature of pain itself remains a mystery. Just as an explosion would be soundless without a brain to interpret the sound waves, pain exists not as an entity but as the brain's translation of electrochemical activity in the nervous system.

Interfering with the brain's analysis of signals is the modus operandi of a number of pain-killing advances, among them electronic anesthesia, acupuncture anesthesia, LSD for terminal cancer pain, alpha brainwave conditioning, surgical excision of the brain's hippocampus, the implantation of electrodes that scramble the pain signals or shock the brain mechanisms; and techniques like the Lamaze method that train the cortex to interpret the signals as something other than pain.

Although clinical experiments with LSD fell off sharply after reports of chromosome damage, the powerful psychedelic is still being used in psychotherapy and for the management of terminal cancer. It is administered to cancer patients partly for its psychological effects and partly because it seems to increase pain tolerance. Studies of the effects of LSD on terminal cancer patients were conducted by Eric Kast at Cook County Hospital in Chicago and by Walter Pahnke at Sinai Hospital in Baltimore. Kast said:

> The preterminal patient suffers "pain," to be sure, like metastatic bone pain, but he is also depressed, nauseated, uncomfortable, distended, wet, and afraid. He feels the need for flexion; and he

must escape from his whole body. . . . LSD is capable of reconciling the patient with a mutilated body image. . . . The reconciliation was accompanied by such relief and joy that it was decided to enlarge the scope of the investigation.

A patient in the Baltimore study had inoperable cancer of the pancreas and was described as "more like a whimpering animal than a human being." Narcotics no longer relieved her pain. Her agony so upset her family that the husband asked Pahnke directly one day if mercy killing might not be the most humane solution. Several days after a euphoric experience under LSD, the patient asked if her illness was terminal and calmly accepted the answer. She returned to her home, and during the months before she died her pain was manageable with narcotics.

Unlike narcotic drugs, LSD has no dulling effect. Pahnke compared the escape of narcotics with the enhanced awareness that sometimes follows a psychedelic experience. LSD may enable patients to spend their last days alert rather than heavily sedated.

Fernand Lamaze, a French physician, evolved a technique sometimes confused with Grantly Dick Read's so-called painless childbirth. Psychoprophylaxis, Lamaze's system, manipulates brain events more than did the Read method, which was largely concerned with the elimination of fear. Lamaze maintained that the signals arriving at the brain from a contracting uterus will almost inevitably be interpreted as pain unless the patient's brain has undergone "apprenticeship," which consists primarily of learning to convert the uterine contractions to the status of signals.

Pierre Vellay, a physician and Lamaze proponent, explained that if woman's role is passive, "the field of her cerebral activity is left entirely free to carry out incoherent actions that could only bring about pain." The woman in labor must absorb herself in some strong and coherent activity, which in the Lamaze method is hyperventilation and deliberate muscular contraction.

Pain may be subject to cancellation. That is the theory of researchers at Oxford and the University of Sheffield who are studying, of all things, the nature of being tickled. They speculate that the reason one cannot tickle oneself is that one knows where he will be tickled, and the brain cancels the effect. Theoretically, a similar mechanism could be effective in pain control.

At Harvard, Vernon Mark, a neurologist, and Frank Ervin, a neurosurgeon, explored the possibilities of electronic control of pain. They implanted electrodes in the brains of cancer patients. The electrodes were attached to a portable device the patients could carry in their pockets. By pressing a button they sent electrical current directly into the brain. For most patients the current controlled pain for several hours, and they no longer needed morphine derivatives.

Doctors at Duke University Medical Center have implanted platinum electrodes and a radio receiver beneath the skin on the spinal cord. Most of the patients implanted were suffering from spinal injuries, multiple disc operations or other severe back pain, and sometimes cancer. When they experienced the first wave of pain, they placed an antenna over the implanted receiver. A radio signal from a battery-powered transmitter activated the receiver, and the radio signals interfered with the pain messages. Instead of pain, the patient felt tingling.

Robert Heath at Tulane University has alleviated terminal cancer pain by implanting as many as 125 electrodes in the brain. Heath inserted some of the electrodes in the brain's so-called pleasure center, the septal region.

Actually, there are many pleasure centers in the brain. And there is no single pain center. As Ronald Melzack said, "The concept is pure fiction unless virtually the whole brain is considered to be the 'pain center,' because the thalamus, the limbic system, the hypothalamus, the brainstem reticular formation, the parietal cortex, and the frontal cortex are all implicated." Some surgeons have experimented with removing the brain's hippocampus, since it seems to be important in the interpretation of pain. However, this is rather drastic, even in the case of the terminally ill, because that structure is also vital to memory.

At the moment the most promising advance of all is acupuncture anesthesia. How it works, no one can say with any certainty. The method is a variation on traditional acupuncture, which involves the insertion of needles into the skin at various depths and at various points identified by Chinese medical tradition. These points supposedly lie along energy meridians traversing the body. Acupuncture has been used in China for at least 2300 years, in Japan for 300 years, and in Europe for half a century.

But it was not until the 1960s that Chinese doctors began using acupuncture as an anesthetic. For reasons unknown, the insertion of a needle at a certain point produces profound anesthesia in distant regions, an effect lasting for many hours. The sensation is described as "numbness, distention, heaviness, and hotness."

Acupuncture may change the quality of pain stimuli reaching the brain. Scientists at Peking Medical College have reported that it lowers the cerebral induction voltage. The pathways involved defy conventional anatomical theory because they do not always coincide with the nerve network. A needle placed at a certain point in the ear changes the electrical resistance over the abdomen.

At first Westerners tended to dismiss the reports on acupuncture anesthesia as either sham or hypnosis. This latter possibility amused the Chinese, who pointed to the frequent use of acupuncture anesthesia in veterinary medicine. The American medical establishment, usually known for its conservatism, officially recognized the important possibilities in acupuncture with surprising haste, perhaps because a number of distinguished physicians were among the first enthusiastic observers in 1971 and 1972. Paul Dudley White, the eminent cardiac specialist, was so impressed with the possibilities for pain relief that he turned from the treatment of heart disease to the study of chronic pain and its alleviation. White House physician Walter Tkach described the Chinese technique as "very superior to our method of anesthesia." Samuel Rosen, a well-known Boston otologist, paraphrased Lincoln Steffens' famous remark about Russia. "Gentlemen," he said, "I have seen the past, and it works."

The advantages of acupuncture anesthesia are many. It can be administered to patients in chronic pain without the risk of addiction associated with chemical relief. Chemical anesthesia for surgical patients carries many side effects, among them the depression of heart rate and breathing, possible interference with the body's immune response (meaning a lower resistance to infection). Aftereffects typically include nausea, vomiting, grogginess, weakness. A small percentage of patients die as a result of anesthesia. With acupuncture, the patient is alert throughout the operation. He is usually ambulatory at once, and often returns to his room unassisted.

When the technique was first introduced, the needles were manipulated by hand. As many as eight attendants were needed in some operations, which meant quite a crowd around the operating table. Later the needle-twirling was automated. And, as the technique was refined, the number of needles necessary was steadily reduced, until now many major operations are performed with a single needle for anesthesia.

And there is evidence that some individuals have trained themselves to produce anesthesia whenever they choose to. Surprisingly often, the electroencephalogram shows a predominant alpha rhythm during the self-induced anesthesia. The people capable of this voluntary pain control usually explain that they have detached themselves from the afflicted body area.

In a laboratory at the Menninger Foundation, Jack Schwartz, an Oregon naturopath, plunged a large needle through his biceps. The EEG recorded a steady alpha rhythm. Schwartz laid a burning cigarette on his flesh. Still the alpha activity was not disrupted. At New York University, a Peruvian, Ramon Torres, maintained alpha brainwaves while ramming a sharpened bicycle spoke through his cheeks. In India, two yogis showed predominant alpha activity while holding their left hands in frigid (4 degrees C.) water for nearly an hour.

What it means is anyone's guess. One possibility is that the steady alpha reflects an unusual relationship between old and new regions of the brain, and that the usual mechanisms for pain interpretation are otherwise engaged. Or it may mean that the brain has closed down incoming signals from elsewhere in the body. For whatever reason, pain and high-amplitude (electrically large) alpha waves seem to be mutually exclusive.

The brain's own methods of turning off pain might have been explored and developed long ago had it not been for the introduction of chloroform as an anesthetic in 1847. Hypnosis had flourished, and doctors all over Europe were exploring its potential. But chloroform seemed the answer to a surgeon's prayers. There was no lengthy induction, as in hypnosis; no chance that the patient would not be susceptible. By the time the risks of chemical pain-killers and general anesthesia were recognized, hypnosis had become an entertainment. It was not until the past two decades that it regained official medical recognition.

Ironically, the recent research hints that simple suggestion is sufficient to induce anesthesia. Subjects were asked to imagine that the ice water in which they were to thrust their hands felt quite pleasant. They were as successful as the subjects who had been hypnotized, and they endured the water well beyond the normal tolerance period. Control subjects could not bear the pain.

Georgi Lozanov, head of the Suggestology Institute in Sofia, Bulgaria, introduced "waking suggestion" as anesthesia in major surgery. The surgical patients, guided by Lozanov, learned to anesthetize themselves.

Whatever the mechanics, it becomes increasingly clear that the brain can experience pain—or choose not to.

II.

breakthrough:
the altered states of consciousness

Of all the hard facts of science, I know of none more solid and fundamental than the fact that if you inhibit thought (and persevere) you come at length to a region of consciousness below or behind thought . . . and a realization of an altogether vaster self than that to which we are accustomed. And since the ordinary consciousness, with which we are concerned in ordinary life, is before all things founded on the little local self, and is in fact self-consciousness in the little, local sense, it follows that to pass out of that is to die to the ordinary self and the ordinary world.

It is to die in the ordinary sense, but in another sense, it is to wake up and find that the 'I,' one's real, most intimate self, pervades the universe and all other beings. . . .

So great, so splendid is this experience, that it may be said that all minor questions and doubts fall away in face of it; and certain it is that in thousands and thousands of cases the fact of its having come even once to a man has completely revolutionized his subsequent life and outlook on the world.

—EDWARD CARPENTER (1844–1929)

6

ALTERED STATES AND
THE LIMBIC BRAIN

The further limits of our being plunge into an altogether other dimension of existence from the sensible and merely "understandable" world.
— WILLIAM JAMES

Describing the altered states of consciousness is like trying to swim in quicksand. Even ordinary consciousness is not understood. Its origin, how mind came to be aware of itself, recedes into an infinity of mirrors.

Overnight, it seems, a mild but steady interest in psychology and in the occult has been transmuted into a burning interest in what has been called "the new consciousness," "higher states of consciousness," and "the supraconscious."

What are the altered states? What brings them on, and of what use are they?

Altered states of consciousness can be triggered by hypnosis, meditation, psychedelic drugs, deep prayer, sensory deprivation, and the onset of acute psychosis. Sleep deprivation or fasting can induce them. Epileptics and migraine sufferers often experience an altered awareness in the aura that precedes attacks. Hypnotic monotony, as in solo high-altitude jet flight, may bring on an altered state. Electronic stimulation of the brain (ESB), alpha or theta brainwave training, clairvoyant or telepathic insights, muscle-relaxation training, isolation (as in Antarctica), and photic stimulation (light flicker at certain speeds) may bring on a sharp change in consciousness.

Recent research has not only spelled out features of the altered states but also points to the brain structures involved in nonordinary consciousness. Artificially stimulated, the limbic brain seems to produce many of the phenomena associated with altered states. These classical characteristics of the qualitative change that marks an altered state are perhaps best demonstrated by examples.

In the following accounts notice the family resemblances: loss of ego boundaries and sudden identification with all of life (a melting into the universe); lights; altered color perception; thrills; electrical sensations; sense of expanding like a bubble or bounding upward; banishment of fear, particularly fear of death; roaring sound; wind; feeling of being separated from physical self; bliss; sharp awareness of patterns; a sense of liberation; a blending of the senses (synesthesia), as when colors are heard and sights produce auditory sensations; an oceanic feeling; a belief that one has awakened; that the experience is the only reality and that ordinary consciousness is but its poor shadow; and a sense of transcending time and space.

Descriptions of spontaneous mystical experience:

> All delight and power, all things living, all time fused in a brief second. I heard nothing; it was as if I were surrounded by golden light. . . .
>
> . . . .
>
> It seemed to me that in some way I was extending into my surroundings and becoming one with them.
>
> . . . .
>
> Time and space did not exist. After passing through the 'darkness,' I emerged alone into radiant white light. . . .

Altered states of consciousness (known among researchers as ASCs) induced by psychedelic drugs:

> I was for four hours in a state of total homogeneous light, bliss, and then I recall starting to come down, and this huge red wave rolled in across the room.
>
> . . . .
>
> I saw sparkling lights flashing across the darkness. [The container] began to glow, a dull purple which turned to a deep cherry red, and the heat of it overwhelmed me.
>
> . . . .
>
> I looked into the glass of water. In its swirling depths was a vortex which went down into the center of the world and the heart of time . . . an unexpected sound would bring back [visual illusions]. Colors seemed unusually bright. . . .
>
> . . . .

There is an awareness of eternal energy, often in the form of intense white light. . . . One sees quite clearly that all existence is a single energy, and that this energy is one's own being. Of course, there is death [but] basically there is nothing to worry about, because you yourself are the eternal energy of the universe.

. . . .

I felt a surge of power, much like a strong electrical current, flowing through my right arm and hand. There remained a sensation of numbness in the arm and hand for some fifteen minutes afterward.

The next accounts describe the exhilaration that sometimes precedes acute psychosis:

Colors become impressive to him, they lose their boundaries and seem to flow. In these states his sense of communion and community is enhanced.

. . . .

Colors seem to hold great and uncanny significance . . . everything takes on significance and patterns. I feel surges of warmth. I feel my tactile senses are enhanced as well as my visual ones, to a point of great power.

. . . .

There was no such thing as an inanimate object. Animate and inanimate seemed to merge, one into the other; I could speak to all things. . . . Opposites are reconciled, and the peace that passes understanding remains supreme. In it there is no death. . . .

Tennyson and several other literary figures of his day practiced a technique uncannily like the classic mantra yoga, which involves the silent repetition of a word to achieve an altered state. Tennyson repeated his name silently to himself. He once wrote of this induced state:

. . . individuality seemed to dissolve and fade away into boundless being; and this is not a confused state but the clearest of the clear, the surest of the sure, the weirdest of the weirdest, utterly beyond words—where death was an almost laughable impossibility.

Tennyson told friends that he experienced a roaring in his ears, flashes of light, and a general feeling of enlargement, followed by tears.

Kundalini yoga, a comprehensive Tibetan system involving

diet, meditation, and rigorous physical discipline, produces powerful effects. Mayne E. Coe, an American scientist, meticulously practiced the kundalini techniques in an attempt to understand the nature of the legendary energy. Reporting on Coe's experiments, Vincent Gaddis said, "One evening, without warning, while he was sitting relaxed in his chair, a powerful current passed downward through his entire body. He could feel it in his muscles. . . ."

In *Kundalini: Evolutionary Energy in Man,* Gopi Krishna described his long-awaited awakening of the kundalini.

> Suddenly, with a roar like that of a waterfall, I felt a stream of liquid light entering my brain through the spinal cord. The illumination grew brighter and brighter, the roaring louder. I experienced a rocking sensation and then felt myself slipping out of my body, entirely enveloped in a halo of light. . . . I felt the point of consciousness that was myself growing wider, surrounded by waves of light.

Gopi Krishna's experience occurred seventeen years after he first began meditating, although he had regularly experienced milder phenomena. Yet several inexperienced volunteers achieved an alteration of consciousness in an experiment designed by Arthur J. Deikman. Deikman's subjects spent fifteen minutes daily focusing their attention on a blue vase. They reported that the color became bluer, more intense, luminous, and that the vase sometimes changed shape. One said, "I felt this whole complete other plane where I was nothing. . . . I wasn't aware of my body. It could have not been there and I wouldn't be surprised."

The same subject reported after another session:

> The vase started radiating. I was aware of what seemed like particles . . . seemed to be coming from the highlights and right to me. I was fascinated with that. I felt it was radiating heat. I felt warmth from it and then realized that . . . everything was dark all around. . . . I felt that there was light coming down from above, too.

Another subject recalled that a landscape he looked at after the vase meditation was "transfigured" and that the fields had "a kind of luminescence."

The aura that precedes epileptic convulsions can be so euphoric that children and adolescents have been known to induce a seizure deliberately. Margiad Evans, a British writer who gave a personal account of epilepsy in *A Ray of Darkness,* alluded to a number of phenomena typical of the altered states of consciousness:

> I had experiences like 'yogiism.' . . . Once I saw an aura of a dog . . . I had visions of unity. Time has come to mean nothing to me. I slip out of its meshes as a sardine through a herring net. . . . I had the feeling that I was split into two or more entities. . . .
>
> Lights like comets dangled before me, slow at first and then gaining a fury of speed and change, whirling color into color, angle into angle. They were all pure ultra unearthly colors, mental colors, not deep visual ones. There was no glow in them but only activity and revolution.

W. Grey Walter, the noted neurologist, developed a method for testing the susceptibility of subjects to epilepsy. His test used the subject's own brainwave rhythms to establish the rate of a flickering light. Photic stimulation commonly sets off epileptic seizures, and flicker synchronized to the subject's own brain rhythms evokes epileptic-type discharges in more than 50 percent of normal young adults.

Walter and his colleagues decided to try their new machine on themselves.

> We all noticed a peculiar effect. . . . This effect was a vivid illusion of moving patterns. . . . Usually it is a sort of pulsating check or mosaic, often in bright colors. At certain frequencies —around ten per second *—some subjects see whirling spirals, whirlpools, explosions, Catherine wheels.
>
> . . . Some have seen profuse patterns of many colors, sometimes stable, sometimes moving. . . . Some describe feelings of swaying, of jumping, even of spinning and dizziness. Some people feel a tingling and prickling of the skin. . . .

Some subjects experienced organized hallucinations, complete scenes. Disturbances in the sense of time were reported. In one memorable account, "Yesterday was at one side, instead of behind, and tomorrow was off the port bow."

* The alpha rhythm.

Episodic dyscontrol is a syndrome related to the epilepsies in which the sufferer is compulsively violent from time to time. He may experience strange sensations at one side of his head or *déjà vu,* and he often reports seeing flashing lights.

In sensory deprivation experiments, subjects are isolated from sound, from patterned light (they may see diffused light), and sometimes from tactile sensations. They may be mittened or even immersed in tepid water. Remarkable perceptual changes take place. Some subjects see flashes of light. Others see geometric patterns, for example, squares, circles, and latticework. More complex hallucinations include animated scenes. One subject became immortal in sensory-deprivation circles by his report of "a procession of squirrels with sacks over their shoulders marching purposefully." Another began to see flashing spots that changed first into "banners of dreamlike colors which were moving back and forth" and later became "kind of dreamlike images."

John Lilly, the neurobiologist, was a subject in a sensory-deprivation experiment in water. Immersed and isolated, he felt as if he were the center of the universe. Later he spoke of "parking my body and traveling," and said, "When you're in the tank, you are certain of the reality of what you are experiencing."

Michel Siffre, a French speleologist, isolated himself in an underground cave for months. "Very soon I lost all notion of colors, particularly confusing green with blue," he wrote in his diary. Later: "I saw a multitude of flashing lights when I shut my eyes or peered intently into the darkness."

Occasionally a dream spills over into consciousness to produce a waking altered state. One dreamer described her experience to Marghanita Laski, the author of *Ecstasy,* a monumental study of mystical states.

It was as if a star was suddenly broken and poured out showers of light . . . brittle, cascading up and down. As if a rock, crystal, star, some substances broke, shattered, and all these streams, lines, poured up from it.

Everything [upon awakening] for a little while seems wonderful, lighter, brighter. On going downstairs (house somewhat shabby), even the carpet seems a better blue.

In his research on "vivid, poignant, shaking" peak experiences, the late psychologist, Abraham Maslow, found that virtually everyone has had an exalted, expanded period of consciousness but that many people forget such episodes or attach no significance to the transient alteration. The common triggers for such experiences are music, unexpected beauty, electrifying emotion, an extraordinary piece of luck, exhilaration after a difficult accomplishment. Trancelike daydreaming and road hypnosis are altered states, as is orgasm.

Only a scant handful of articles have touched upon the possible physiology involved in altered states. For one thing, until quite recently investigators have usually treated the ASCs as if they existed independent of the brain. "The self-transcending emotions are still the stepchild of psychology," Arthur Koestler wrote, "in spite of their evident reality."

Because pathology is usually a more tempting avenue of research than health, the brain's transcendent powers were long ignored by science. But now brain research is centering on the limbic region, the terra incognita most likely involved in the phenomena of the altered states of consciousness.

Thousands of scientific papers, most of them recent, deal with various parts of the limbic brain. However, these structures are no more understood by virtue of the observations than solar energy is understood by a child's awareness that it gives forth light and warmth. The limbic region is sometimes called the emotional brain, the nose brain, the smell brain, and the rhinencephalon. Early investigators had wrongly assumed that its primary function was to interpret olfactory sensations.

Analogies are crude at best in describing the brain. The cerebral hemispheres are usually likened to the two halves of a walnut. (It helps to picture the walnut as flattened underneath.) In profile, the disembodied brain would appear to blossom from the brainstem, a thick, trunklike structure ascending from the spinal cord.

The brainstem differentiates into a center for arousal and alerting, the reticular formation. The reticular formation then merges into the limbic system. Because these two systems encompass many of the same structures as if they were joint facilities, it is impossible to draw sharp lines between them.

The largest structure of the limbic system is the U-shaped hippocampus, which spans the underside of the cerebral cortex and is essential to learning. It processes data from short-term to long-term memory. The amygdala rests at the ends of the hippocampus. Stimulation in this small structure can produce anything from blind rage to euphoria.

Some authorities include all or part of the hypothalamus and a portion of the thalamus in the limbic system because of bundles of interconnecting nerves. The passionate hypothalamus is capable of generating hunger, thirst, sex drives, and exquisite pleasure. The thalamus just above it is a primitive analyzer of sensation. Because of its proximity, the brain's temporal lobe is sometimes referred to as part of the limbic system.

Brain researchers speak of "the fascinating activities of the limbic system," "the mysteries of the limbic system." Most believe that evolution of the emotional brain enabled mammals to progress beyond the programmed behavior of reptiles. Paradoxically, in man the limbic brain became more complex even as the neocortex—the new brain—was evolving. It was as if the original ground-level house was being redecorated at the same time new construction progressed on the second floor. Just as earlier the mammalian limbic brain had been added above the reptilian brain, nature stacked the neocortex over the limbic structures.

In man neither the old nor the new can function independently. Man's more complex, integrated processes have given him dominion of the planet, but he is more vulnerable to brain damage than the lower mammals. Removal of the entire neocortex would leave a cat or dog relatively unchanged, but a human being undergoing such surgery would never speak, walk, or feed himself again. Similarly, removing the hippocampus has little effect on an animal's ability to retain new information. A human being without his hippocampus may be unable to tell you where he lives or how old he is.

The limbic system accounts for most of the bewildering phenomena of the altered states. Euphoria, for example: Positive sensations ranging from mild pleasure to intense joy can be produced by electronic stimulation almost anywhere in the limbic system. As little as thirty seconds' stimulation results in mood changes that may persist for hours, even days. Self-stimulating animals have demonstrated that the profound pleasure has virtually no satiation point. A cat or monkey will press a bar 10,000 times an hour, for hours on end, to get such stimulation.

Focal brain seizures in the limbic brain can produce homicidal outbursts, but surgeons contemplating removal of the damaged cells are uneasy. The amygdala is often implicated in violent animal behavior, yet some parts of it produce gentleness. In human beings, stimulation creates a pleasant detachment similar to the effects of marijuana. Epileptic discharges in the upper half of the limbic brain sometimes produce ecstasy. Removal of some cells could eliminate an inhibiting factor, giving the others what one surgeon called "unbridled release."

James Olds found that hungry rats were deterred from obtaining food if they had to cross a grid giving off 60 microamperes of electricity. To obtain brain stimulation, on the other hand, rats have crossed grids charged with 450 microamperes.

"We couldn't go higher than that," Olds said. "Because of their electrodes, the shock would knock them out." When they regained consciousness, the rats would resume their path toward the brain reward. In other studies rats stimulated themselves until finally they were thrown about the box by violent motor seizures. As soon as they recovered, they would scurry back to the bar.

"At times we have been able to give stimuli so high above the seizure threshold," Olds said, "that they no longer produced seizures. These were apparently the most rewarding stimuli used to date." Olds described a colleague's project in which rats were given only one hour daily in which to eat or to stimulate their brains. One rat starved to death, and thereafter the experimenters withdrew the rats from the study once they dropped to 70 percent of body weight.

Stimulation of the limbic region often moves human subjects to say that they are "split apart" or witnessing themselves. A 28-year-old man, victim of a head injury, experienced spells of recurring violence, impulsiveness, gibberish. Stimulated in the hippocampus and amygdala, he remarked, "I feel quite amused. I don't know how to explain this—it's as though I can see myself."

He was one of several patients who underwent limbic stimulation. Boston researchers found that stimulation produced an array of effects: "complicated mood and intellectual alterations, depersonalization, a sense of unreality, trancelike state, displacement, bizarre distortion of bodily position, extrapersonal space."

The distortion of bodily space is often reported in altered states and is a very real danger to military jet pilots. Flying alone, they commonly experience what is known as the break-off phenomenon. The pilot may suddenly have the impression that he is floating or that the plane is turning. If he tries to correct for the imagined turn, he may send the plane into a dangerous spin. In one study in which the pilots were promised anonymity, the majority reported frequent instances of break-off, and several admitted that it was their reason for flying.

Floating is commonly reported by participants in muscle-relaxation and alpha biofeedback training. It is a typical meditation phenomenon. Mystics frequently speak of enlarging, of loss of body sensations, bubbling up, or becoming airborne. Sensory-deprivation subjects may lie quietly in their isolation chambers, then suddenly feel as if they have risen several inches and are buoyant.

Stimulation in the limbic brain sometimes produces heart and respiration changes or limb movements. Altered breathing, particularly a sudden cessation of breath, is also a common phenomenon in nonordinary consciousness. A typical description is in Raynor Johnson's study of mysticism, *Watchers on the Hills:* "Then a wave—an odd word to use, but I don't know how to explain it—started at my feet and moved rapidly upward with peculiar pulling sensations at different parts of my body. As the wave reached my lungs, I struggled for breath, but to no avail." Cessation of breathing is so routine in some meditation techniques that there is standard advice for handling it: consciously reestablish breathing, then resume meditating.

Light phenomena can be produced by electrical stimulation of the brain, though not necessarily in the limbic region. The Swiss researcher, W. R. Hess, noted his patients' responses:

> The visual experience changes, in such a way that she now sees white marks . . . at the same time a red point could appear. The contents of consciousness . . . corresponded in some cases to moving, starlike shapes. Other patients saw dancing or flickering

lights in white or yellow. In rare cases there were also red points on the stimulated side.

The brain-stimulation observations correspond to the reports of light in altered states. White light is the most common, yellow or golden is occasionally mentioned, and only rarely are there instances of pink or red light.

Brain stimulation can engender remarkable alertness, comparable to the reports of being "awake for the first time" in an altered state. When the reticular formation is stimulated, withdrawn psychotic patients may suddenly brighten and begin chatting intelligently. The abrupt change from withdrawal to animation is reminiscent of the talking dolls with taped voices and a pull string. The patient's speech often becomes clearer.

Déjà vu is the eerie, overpowering sensation that a current event has somehow happened before and in precisely the same way. This puzzling phenomenon has been reported in nearly all categories of altered states. Here again, brain stimulation achieves a similar effect. Only half a second's stimulation in the hippocampus and amygdala produce *déjà vu* (or familiarity, as it is called by some researchers). Jose Delgado of Yale noticed that patients stimulated in a certain region would listen to the subsequent exchange between themselves and the doctor with an air of amusement and bewilderment. "But this has all happened before. I knew what you were going to say before you said it." * This sense of familiarity is a hallmark of mystical

* Patients with temporal lobe epilepsy who experience *déjà vu* are more likely to have their lesions on the right. Perhaps coincidentally, the right hemisphere in the brain is nonverbal and more intuitive, artistic, emotional, and is likelier to produce alpha waves.

J. E. Orme of Middlewood Hospital in Sheffield, England, discussed the relationship of *déjà vu* to time theory in his scholarly *Time, Experience and Behavior.* He cited the work of R. Efron, who found that the brain hemispheres don't necessarily process a message simultaneously. In a right-handed subject, a stimulus delivered to the left half of the body isn't available to the left hemisphere for two to six milliseconds.

Efron speculates that, since the speechless right hemisphere first receives the signal from the left side of the body, it is unable to verbalize the sensation. The delay is the time it takes for the information to be passed to the talkative left hemisphere. If a lesion further delays the transfer, perhaps everything seems to be happening twice, like instant replay. This explanation falls short of accounting for the subjective feeling that one is recalling the distant past. Also, the *déjà vu* phenome-

experience. An increased incidence of *déjà vu* in daily consciousness is also reported by meditators.

Stimulation of the brain's temporal lobe, immediately adjacent to the limbic system, produces another effect typical of the altered states: past incidents, often of a trivial nature, are relived, almost as if a videotape were being run. Wilder Penfield, a famous neurosurgeon, discovered the phenomenon while exploring the brains of epileptics to zero in on the sites of their seizures. He found that electronic probing of specific points in the temporal lobe set off a rerun of past events.

The scenes seem to play back chronologically and in the same length of time as the originals. Moving the electrode triggers an entirely different chain of memories. A patient might, for example, recall standing outside a farmhouse on a summer morning. He would hear music from the radio, smell the odor of manure, feel a breeze. If the surgeon shifts the electrode slightly, the patient may suddenly find himself at his tenth birthday party.

The limbic brain is apparently the liaison between the ancient reptilian brain that controls the so-called autonomic responses and the modern brain, the neocortex. Its ability to modify the autonomic nervous system, for ill and for good, appears to be the key to disease and health. Limbic structures can alter metabolism, oxygen consumption, thirst, and appetite. They can slow or speed the heart, lower or elevate blood pressure. They can alter sex hormones, induce spontaneous ovulation, block ovulation, and produce erection in a male.

They can facilitate healing and increase resistance; facilitate or block learning and memory; launch the fight-or-flight defenses or counteract them; intensify sensory awareness or block it; facilitate motor activity or inhibit it; induce high excitement or sleep.

No doubt the neocortex has been sending random messages via the limbic brain all along. Fear or worry in the neocortex apparently activates the hot line to the limbic brain, which then stirs up the autonomic functions. Result: ulcers, heart disease, hypertension, chronic fatigue.

Neurotransmitters are concentrated in the limbic brain, par-

---

non is sometimes accompanied by a wave of ineffable poignance; the "memory" seems to be in an emotional context.

ticularly in the hippocampus. They are the substances that permit the nerve cells to fire (discharge electrically), sending their messages along the brain pathways. Norepinephrine (NE) is significantly affected by limbic stimulation. It is not only a transmitter but apparently controls growth hormone, shown by experiments to promote healing, lower cholesterol, increase resistance to infection, and speed up metabolism.

Of all the cells in the body, certain cells in the hippocampus have been found to be the most sensitive to another transmitter, acetylcholine (ACh). Small quantities of ACh excite these cells to the level of sustained epileptic discharge. The dizzying repertoire of the limbic system is demonstrated here. NE tends to constrict blood vessels, ACh to dilate them.

The limbic brain controls the infamous stress syndrome. When alarm is registered, the message is channeled to the hypothalamus, which signals the pituitary to secrete ACTH (adrenocorticotropic hormone). As the ACTH level rises, agitating the heart rate, blood pressure, and digestive juices, the adrenal glands begin to produce their hormones, which counteract ACTH. The limbic brain regulates these substances.

Stimulation originating within the brain is of a much more subtle nature than that produced by the electrical probes of the laboratory. By comparison the artificial stimulus is to the brain's own electrical activity as a bull to a butterfly. Even so it is evident that the limbic brain can manufacture panic or peace. Not only does it elaborate the individual's response to stress, it probably sets the thresholds for emotional reaction.

Andrew Weil, a physician and government drug researcher, described the limbic brain as the realm of the unconscious, just as the neocortex is considered the seat of the conscious mind. Weil suggested that the limbic brain—the unconscious mind—turns against the body only when the conscious mind forces it to.

> Potential circuits exist for conducting unconscious impulses upward, as anyone knows who is aware of his daydreams and intuitions. The sealing of these channels from above forces unbalanced unconscious energies down the autonomic nerves to produce negative physical effects. . . . If we never learn to open the channels by disengaging our minds from ordinary consciousness, we condemn ourselves to sickness.

To Weil the altered states are the end result of "an innate psychological drive arising out of the neurological structure of the human brain." He saw evidence for this drive in such universal behavior as the hyperventilation and the whirling of two- and three-year-olds until they experience vertigo and collapse. He maintained that the individual learns from early childhood to feel guilty about episodes of nonordinary awareness, thus cutting himself off from a natural mechanism for the achievement of emotional equilibrium.

Nor is Weil alone in his view that the altered states are not curiosities but an integral part of our human heritage. A whole new scientific discipline seems to be evolving for the purpose of exploring that exciting possibility.

Charles Tart of the University of California at Davis has proposed the formulation of what he called state-specific sciences. Scientists would conduct their research by entering altered states of consciousness: meditation, psychedelic intoxication, hypnosis, sensory isolation. He emphasized that cumulative reports will confirm the validity of knowledge obtained within such states, just as in normal consciousness we have achieved consensus on certain observable events. Tart pointed out that all knowledge is basically experiential knowledge.

Psychologists are interested in the possibility that there are states of consciousness in which specific knowledge is bound. Roland Fischer, professor of experimental psychology at Ohio State University College of Medicine, cited as an example the millionaire in the Charlie Chaplin movie *City Lights*. Drunk, the millionaire adored the little tramp who had saved his life; sober, he couldn't remember him. Two recent studies support the concept of state-bound experience, Fischer said. In one, forty-eight subjects memorized nonsense syllables while drunk. Sober, they had considerable difficulty recalling the material, but their recollection improved significantly when they were drunk again. In the second study, volunteers were heavily dosed with either an amphetamine or amobarbitol, a barbiturate, and shown a series of geometric configurations. Their recall was later facilitated by the drug under which they had first seen the configurations. Hypnosis can also produce state-bound experiences.

Fischer suggested that instead of one subconscious, we have as many layers of self-awareness as there are levels of arousal. He likened the individual and his states of consciousness to a ship's captain with a girl in every port. Each girl is unaware of the existence of the others, and for him she exists only from visit to visit—that is, state to state. Fischer said that we live from one waking state to another waking state, from one dream to the next. ". . . From one amobarbitol narcoanalysis session to the next; from LSD to LSD; from epileptic aura to epileptic aura . . ."

7

MEDITATION:
"THE EYES SHALL HEAR,
THE EARS SHALL SEE"

An Indian parable tells of a high government official who fell out of favor with his king and was imprisoned in a tower. One moonlit night the prisoner saw his wife far below. She was smearing honey on the antennae of a beetle. After fastening a silken thread to its body, she pointed the insect upward toward the tower window.

Tempted by the smell of honey, the beetle kept crawling up the wall. Finally the prisoner caught it, removed the silken thread, and set the insect free. Pulling on the thread he found that it grew heavier and heavier. Attached to it was a length of sewing cotton and to that a heavy string, which itself was attached to a strong rope by which he escaped.

The German writer, Paul Dessauer, who related the tale in *Natural Meditation,* added:

> The first thing meditation brings in its train is very small—as insignificant as a silken thread drawn slowly up a high, black wall at night by a small weak creature. This is the beginning of meditation. By repeating it, by persevering in repeating it, the silken thread becomes a cotton, then a string, then a cord, and at last a strong rope, which finally is able to bear the full weight of a man.

Alpha training, yoga, Zen, Sufi meditation; psychosynthesis, the Jesus Movement, the Human Potential Movement, the Silva method; ESP, LSD . . . Consciousness expansion seems to be an idea whose time has come. As Peter Mezan observed:

> The millennium is at hand, revelations are back . . . people in saffron robes and ecstasy were chanting Hare Krishna in front of my bank, some stockbrokers I know were playing the market by casting the I Ching (and swearing by it, incidentally), Allen Ginsberg was singing OM MANI PADME HUM in a Chicago courtroom, and my former Harvard roommates were deep in meditation. . . .

Whether the ultimate goal is referred to as grace, unity, *satori, samadhi,* realization, or the peak experience, its essence is liberation. The adherents are seeking freedom: freedom from fear, from ego, from an attachment to things. They believe with the late Abraham Maslow, the father of the Human Potential Movement, that "not having co-religious experiences may be a lower, lesser state . . . a state in which we are not fully functioning, not at our best, not fully human. Experiences of transcendence should in principle be commonplace."

Of all the consciousness-expansion techniques, meditation seems to be gaining the most rapid acceptance, partly because of the recent scientific interest.

A World Conference on Scientific Yoga was convened in New Delhi to formulate plans for an international university to research the meditation methods of many cultures. An International Kundalini Research Foundation has been organized by an eminent group of scientists, among them Carl Friedrich von Weizsacker, director of Germany's Max Planck Institute for Physics and Astrophysics. They hope to discover the scientific basis of the potent phenomena observed in practitioners of the Tibetan meditation system.

Physiologists, psychologists, and their graduate students from Harvard to Stanford to Oxford have been accumulating data on the remarkable effects of transcendental meditation on brain-wave patterns, blood pressure, reaction time, and metabolic efficiency. The field is so new that scientists are now publishing advice on how to design meditation experiments and what controls to employ. Meanwhile transcendental meditation's foremost exponent, Maharishi Mahesh Yogi, has launched his World Plan. By opening teacher-training centers all over the world, including the Communist bloc nations, the Maharishi plans eventually to expose the population of the entire planet to transcendental meditation. The mathematics are so tidy, the ambition so grandiose, that one would be tempted to dismiss the World Plan as blue sky if it were not for the geometric growth of the movement thus far. The campus organization, Students International Meditation Society (SIMS), has been doubling its numbers annually. By 1972 its membership approached 100,000. Because transcendental meditation (popularly known as TM) is uniformly taught and because so many student volunteers are available for research, it is far and away the most thoroughly studied meditation method.

Special populations are also meditating experimentally, among them psychiatric patients, emotionally disturbed adolescents, the mentally retarded, stutterers and aphasics, and secondary-school teachers. SIMS researchers obtained a federal grant to teach meditation to 10,000 high-school juniors to determine its effect on their drug-use habits. The Army and Navy have experimental programs under way. At two American prisons, convicts are learning to meditate. In Germany, factory owners reported increased productivity after they introduced meditation. The Punjab government in India commissioned the meditation training of its civil servants in the hope that it would help to eradicate graft and boondoggling.

Like fire, the meditation phenomenon must have been stumbled upon by man eons ago. Here and there along the journey from the cave, introspective individuals must have noticed that focusing on a single stimulus—a sound, one's breathing— eventually generates a very peculiar type of consciousness.

Word of this effect must have circulated in various cultures. Whole bodies of philosophy, theology, and technique evolved from this altered awareness. For various reasons, the most elaborate disciplines flourished in the Near East. Yoga traveled east to the Orient. At its western fringes, the eastern Christians borrowed its chanting and rosaries. In Islam, Sufi mysticism flowered.

In the 1960s the adherents of meditation in the West were mostly students, arty types, and others not generally considered trustworthy by establishment science. Meditation's greatest impact came after the brainwave biofeedback discovery. Once scientists were forced to admit that brainwave control is possible, they were tempted to take another look at data published by their Indian and Japanese colleagues on altered patterns of electrical activity during meditation.

Joe Kamiya, the psychologist who pioneered in brainwave training, admitted that at first meditation's occult connotations had threatened his "pure lab," as he facetiously put it. "But there was an evolution in our thinking—an evolution in the thinking of large numbers of other scientists. So we asked a few of these meditators to come and try our feedback system. To our great surprise, they were able to increase alpha 'way above baseline right away."

Kamiya and others observed that in meditating subjects alpha activity was sometimes more prominent in the frontal regions and at the top of the head, whereas it is normally found in the occipital area at the back of the head. In more advanced meditators, its appearance in the frontal regions was sometimes accompanied by a slowing to a theta rhythm, which suggested the possibility that a new generator, another source of energy, had been activated in the brain.

By 1972 the direction of brainwave biofeedback research had changed. The eastern disciplines, with their attendant novel EEG patterns, opened broad new areas of investigation. Kamiya predicted that the popular interest in expanded consciousness would "all go to meditation within the next five to ten years."

All meditation techniques are alike in that all involve a focus of attention. The objects of contemplation are numberless: a candle flame, blank wall, crystal, mandala (a concentric geometric design), the rising and falling abdomen, one's breathing, even the sun.* Or one may close the eyes and listen to a sound or phrase repeated mentally. One Zen method centers on an unanswerable question called a *koan*. Repetitive movements can also achieve a trance state. Dervish dances in the Sufi tradition induce a shift in consciousness.

* Reportedly the ancient Egyptians stared at the sun to achieve an altered state. Apparently one looked first through a peephole, then gradually more and more directly until able to gaze at it straight on. Because of the risk of permanently damaging the retina, this technique is not recommended.

The objective of a focus is to narrow the content of awareness to a fine point so that it may eventually break through to a higher, more intense plane—as a narrow passageway might lead up toward an immense, lighted chamber.

Neurologically, the focus stimulates the brain rhythmically. The repetitive quality of the sensory stimulus begins to generate a synchronous brainwave pattern. As is apparent from the flicker experiments in epilepsy research, the brain has an uncanny tendency to respond in kind to rhythmic stimulation, particularly if the tempo is established by its own activity—in this case, the monotonous contemplation of object, sound, or riddle. The brain's stimulation feeds upon itself.

Eventually the focal object changes, even disappears. The psychologist Robert Ornstein relates the meditation phenomenon to the results of an experiment in which a tiny projector was mounted on a contact lens. Wearing the lens allowed the subject to view a completely stabilized visual image, because the projector moved with the retina. Ordinarily, tiny, involuntary eye movements keep the retinal image in continuous motion.

After a few seconds, the image of the projector disappeared and did not return. The results bore out a theory of Donald Hebb, a sensory-deprivation researcher, that varying stimulus is necessary for normal awareness. When the image disappeared, the electrically slow, regular alpha brainwaves appeared—the pattern state typical of meditation.

Ornstein calls attention to a similar phenomenon occurring when a subject stares at a blank visual surface, known in psychology as a ganzfeld (whole field). A ganzfeld can be a whitewashed wall or even, as in some experiments, halves of Ping-Pong balls taped over the eyes.

A very strange thing happens when one stares at a ganzfeld for twenty minutes or so. He finds himself not seeing; that is, he doesn't know whether his eyes are open or not, and he is unable to see. As he goes blank, the EEG usually shows an increased alpha brainwave production.

Ornstein notes that both the stabilized image and the ganzfeld are similar to concentrative meditation. In both there is an unchanging input. Because the stimulus has been traced in the stabilized-image phenomenon, the researchers know that it has transferred between the eyes. Therefore, it got past the retina and *disappeared somewhere in the central nervous system.*

Which brings us to an important and little-understood point. However exotic the chants, contemplation, and dervish dancing may seem, as Ornstein wrote, the techniques "are not deliberately mysterious or exotic but are simply a matter of practical applied psychology." Meditation takes advantage of the structure of the nervous system to produce an altered awareness. The mystery lies not in the methods but in the brain phenomena they exploit.

Although transcendental meditation has become widely known because of the ease with which it is learned and the much publicized laboratory evidence of physiological changes, it is not really an innovation. It is, in fact, a form of mantra yoga, a traditional Indian meditation. A look at transcendental meditation gives one a representative idea of meditation in general, since all such methods are more alike than different in their manipulation of brain processes.

At his initiation, the new meditator is given a mantra, a sound he repeats aloud for a few moments, then silently. The sound is purportedly chosen by the initiator on the basis of the initiate's personality. It is theoretically suited to his nervous system and is to be kept secret. Transcendental meditation is practiced twice a day, twenty to thirty minutes at a time. The meditator may sit in a straight-backed chair or in a lotus position.

Such phenomena as flashing lights, a floating sensation, and euphoria happen frequently for a few meditators, seldom or never for others. Since measurable neurophysiological changes are taking place regardless of whether dazzling bliss is experienced, these phenomena probably depend on the site of stimulation in the nervous system and on the amplitude of the alpha or theta brainwaves.

Age makes some difference. Many elderly, first-time meditators find progress slow. Because anxiety implies low alpha production, extremely tense individuals may feel that they are progressing slowly. Those individuals most susceptible to laboratory techniques for altering consciousness typically show high alpha-wave production.

In the *Journal of Transpersonal Psychology* Charles Tart reported on a year's experience with transcendental meditation. Tart described meditation as a "psychic lubricant." He noticed that material from his past, even from childhood, seemed to surface during the first six months he meditated. The recollections were of experiences that had probably been processed incompletely when they occurred, he thought. After six months there was a leveling off, as if the processing had caught up, and from that point he noticed that material from only one or two days previous surfaced.

Tart observed, as many meditators have observed, that he had lost his tolerance for alcohol. He was more than a little resentful. "If I drank more than half a glass of wine I almost immediately got a headache which lasted for several hours." * He also remarked on a greatly enhanced ability to still his mind, "a general feeling that I am now a much calmer, more relaxed person . . . more sensitive to my inner processes, and [I] generally do not get wound up in my daily activities." He judged himself to be more sensitive to what he was doing than before but less likely to get tense or excited. His resistance to cold struck him as interesting. He felt warm even when nearly nude in a room 50–60 degrees F. As soon as he stopped meditating, even if he didn't move, chilliness would set in. He wondered if the tolerance might be attributed to a dilation of blood vessels.

Increased blood flow is only one of a whole array of physiological correlates of meditation states. It seems that a whole syndrome exists, a state more profoundly relaxed than deep sleep.

The major physiological research on transcendental meditation was pioneered by Robert Keith Wallace, then at UCLA. Wallace's dissertation for his Ph.D. described his measurement of the physiological changes in a number of subjects during transcendental meditation. Herbert Benson of Harvard Medical School had undertaken similar research, and Wallace eventually

---

* In *Nutrition and Your Mind: The Psychochemical Response,* George Watson observed that the truly healthy person cannot tolerate alcohol—that, in fact, a tolerance for it is a barometer of how unhealthy an individual is. As he explained it, alcohol's effect on acetate is the key. A healthy person's cellular acetate breakdown is near maximum, and "any rapid increase, such as would result from a drinking of whiskey, may lead to headaches, sweating, nausea, and vomiting."

joined him in Boston. Their work has since been reported in dozens of scientific journals.

In addition to increased alpha brainwave production in the frontal and central regions of the brain, meditation produces changes in attention as measured on the electroencephalogram. Laboratory tests of normal subjects show that alpha activity is always blocked briefly by a loud click. Each subsequent click produces a smaller change in the EEG pattern until finally there is no reaction at all. Zen meditators and transcendental meditators showed this attention response to each click. There was no habituation. Yogis showed no response to any click. The slow alpha waves (eight or nine cycles per second) were accompanied in many Zen meditators and transcendental meditators by prominent theta waves in the frontal region. Oxygen consumption falls sharply. This is due to a change in metabolism rather than in respiration tempo. Carbon dioxide elimination decreases.

A high galvanic skin resistance (GSR) is an electrical indication of a state of relaxation. After many hours, sleep raises the GSR twofold. Meditation quadruples it within minutes, and the level remains high for some time afterward.

The conviction of meditators that they are much calmer than before was borne out by two studies conducted by David Orme-Johnson, a psychologist at the University of Texas at El Paso. Orme-Johnson determined how quickly his subjects' nervous systems would adapt to noises comparable to the level in a boiler factory. By measurement of the galvanic skin resistance, the meditators stopped reacting physically to the noise after ten to fifteen trials. It took nonmeditators thirty to thirty-five repetitions. The initial reactions of the meditators to the noise were as sensitive as those of the nonmeditators; their adaptation was just faster.

When one is sitting quietly, spontaneous changes in the amplitude of the galvanic skin resistance are indicative of general anxiety level. Orme-Johnson found that the typical subjects produced thirty-five GSR changes in a ten-minute period, compared to fewer than ten produced by the meditators.

If those who take up meditation are not typical of the general population, measured differences between them and nonmeditators could be due to their inherently different personality types. In one of his two studies, Orme-Johnson anticipated this criticism by using as the nonmeditators individuals who were planning to begin transcendental meditation within two weeks. Meditation sharply decreases blood lactate, a product of cell metabolism. Possibly because it binds with calcium, which is essential for transmission throughout the nervous system, a high level of blood lactate has been implicated in anxiety neurosis (free-floating anxiety). Injections of lactate have produced anxiety responses in normal subjects.

In Harvard Medical School tests, meditation caused the lactate concentration in the blood to "decline precipitously." During the first ten minutes of meditation it dropped at a rate four times faster than that shown by subjects resting normally.

The heart rate usually slows during meditation. Overall benefits may accrue, and some clinical studies are now using meditation as a treatment for cardiac arrhythmias and angina pectoris. At UCLA Medical School and Harvard Medical School, studies are under way to determine the effects of meditation on chronic hypertension.

At the University of Texas at Austin, investigators tested the reaction time of meditators and nonmeditators. When the meditators were tested without a preceding meditation period, they reacted 30 percent faster to the cue than nonmeditators. Results after their meditation were even more dramatic. They improved by 15 percent. The nonmeditators, after resting for an equivalent twenty minutes, were 10 percent worse.

Researchers in Düsseldorf and Cologne independently reported that the skin temperature of the throat and forehead, as measured by infrared radiation techniques, increased during meditation. Further experiments should determine whether or not the skin temperature is elevated because of activity in the thyroid and/or pituitary glands.

An increase in visual acuity was reported by scientists studying Zen monks. At the University of Sussex, John Graham tested the frequent observation of transcendental meditators that their senses become more acute. Graham found that twenty minutes of meditation indeed lowered the auditory thresholds for discrimination of frequency and amplitude.

Intense color perception is often said to follow meditation. Also synesthesia, a peculiar blending of senses that may result from atypical neural activity. This phenomenon is not uncommon in altered states. In his *Autobiography of a Yogi,* Paramahansa Yogananda recalled that his guru had promised, "The eyes shall hear, the ears shall see."

Meditation has been suggested for American schoolchildren by a psychiatrist, M. L. Peerbolte.

[Meditation could be used] to ease the overstrained condition of many students who are caught in an increasingly competitive situation. Young people today are challenged by the mysteries of their own consciousness and provoked to experiment. This training, started at an early age, provides a clear and safe opportunity for the individual who is impelled toward the search for consciousness expansion.

Techniques similar to meditation are being taught tens of thousands of children already through such various approaches as Mind Control (the Silva Method), Alpha Dynamics, psychosynthesis, process meditation—even Scientology employs a similar method. Children learning karate and related techniques are routinely instructed in meditation (which is an inherent part of karate). Half a century ago Maria Montessori devised what she called a silence game. It is still used in Montessori schools around the world. The children sit quietly with closed eyes, listening intently to the subtle sounds around them. The teacher, who is across the room, begins to whisper the name of one child. The child silently crosses the room to her and is silently embraced. One by one the children respond to their whispered names.

Most mantras have an interesting common feature. Almost without exception they include *m* or *n* (and frequently *h*), *sounds which seem to resonate through the head even when repeated silently.* A survey of liturgical chants of churches, the sonorous incantations of primitive tribes, and the Sanskrit mantras suggest that mankind has an ancient, intuitive knowledge of the most powerful methods of altering consciousness through auditory stimuli. For practical purposes, *Om mani padme hum, Hari krishna, Dominus vobiscum, Agnus Dei,* and *Om narti narti natapati* * are interchangeable.

Novice practitioners of mantra meditation achieve many of

* A Japanese mantra.

the same physiological phenomena during meditation as do Zen masters of fifteen and twenty years. Possibly it is easier to center on an auditory focus than the objects often contemplated by Zen meditators, such as a blank wall or a *koan*. Distractions might be greater when one's eyes are open. It may also be significant that the region of the brain in which auditory associations are believed to occur is immediately adjacent to the limbic structures.

Even imagining sonorous syllables seems to set up a spreading, vibrating hum in the region of the brain behind the forehead, centering between the eyes. It can be demonstrated that imagined stimuli sometimes involve the same interpretive brain mechanisms as external stimuli. Mentally visualizing an object in minute detail usually blocks alpha production, for example, just as actual visual observation does. And if one tries to hear an imagined sound in a noisy environment, he usually has to "shout" the sound mentally or it will be drowned out by the external racket.

Wallace and Benson, among others, have proposed that meditation creates a fourth state of consciousness, beyond waking, sleeping, and dreaming. They term it a "wakeful hypometabolic state." Because this state is the opposite in every respect to the alarm syndrome, they suggest that it is the body's counterpart —the system for regenerating energy.

> During man's early history the defense alarm reaction may well have had high survival value and thus have become strongly established in his genetic makeup. . . . Although the defense-alarm reaction is generally no longer appropriate, the visceral response is evoked with considerable frequency by the rapid and unsettling changes that are buffeting modern society. . . .
>
> In these circumstances, the hypometabolic state, representing quiescence rather than hyperactivation of the sympathetic nervous system, may indicate a guidepost to better health.

In one survey, individuals reported on health problems apparently cured or much improved after they began meditating. The illnesses mentioned included ulcers, allergies, asthma, epileptic seizures, depression, anxiety, and arthritis. Informal reports mention improved carbohydrate metabolism ("I can eat like a teen-ager again and I don't gain"), more energy, and more intense, prolonged orgasm—changes that imply the involvement of the hypothalamus. One inevitable phenomenon seems to be a higher threshold for stress, which alone could account for the all-round improvement in health.

At the University of Cincinnati, psychologists administered personality tests to two groups. One group was then instructed in transcendental meditation, and both groups were retested after two months. Meditation had apparently had "a salutary influence on a subject's psychological state. . . . Inner-directedness appears augmented. It is as though . . . the meditation permitted the experimental subjects to rely more confidently on their 'psychic gyroscopes.' " The experimental group scored significantly higher in the ability to express feelings in spontaneous action.

Maynard Shelly, professor of psychology at the University of Kansas, questioned 160 transcendental meditators and 145 nonmeditators of similar age and background. From the responses, he concluded that the meditators were happier, more relaxed, developed deeper personal relationships, and had more of what Shelly called personal resources. Both Shelly and the Cincinnati researchers suggested that meditation results in what Abraham Maslow defined as "self-actualized individuals."

Daniel Goleman, who spent a year in India researching meditation for his doctorate at Harvard, proposed that it is a healing force beyond the capabilities and even the ambitions of traditional cures for disease and despair.

I conceptualize meditation as "meta-therapy": a procedure that accomplishes the major goals of conventional therapy and yet has as its end-state a change far beyond the scope of therapies, therapists, and most personality theorists—an altered state of consciousness.

Goleman suggested that meditation may be the main route for a newly emerging fourth force in psychology. (He listed the other three as psychoanalysis, behavior therapy, group encounter.) He compared meditation favorably to systematic desensitization, a popular technique in which the patient confronts his innermost fears while in a state of deep physical relaxation.

Goleman classifies meditation as "natural, global self-desensitization." In a state more profoundly relaxed than even deep sleep, over a gradual period the individual finds his anxieties surfacing for catharsis. Stress may be unkinked with a recollection—or more often with a twitch, shudder, occasionally even weeping. These reactions apparently reflect resolution on an unconscious level and are fairly common to altered states.

Empathy and openness seem to increase in meditation. It appears that one experiences what Gardner Murphy and Sidney Cohen have called "the marrow-shaking breakthrough to the other side of reality" and weeps for no conscious reason. Later the meditator may find himself releasing bottled grief over the long-ago death of a loved one . . . and may even find himself with damp eyes on seeing a fatal wreck on the freeway or on reading a poignant newspaper story.

In his book, *Through an Eastern Window,* the psychologist Jack Huber tells of his experience in a meditation center in Japan.

> And then—it was late in the morning—a white clear screen came before my eyes. In front of the screen passed, or rather, floated, simple images—faces, objects. I have no clear recollection of the images. A rush of feeling came over me. I burst into tears; the tears become quiet sobbing.

Huber debated with himself about the efficacy of meditation compared to an outside agent such as a drug:

> I think there might be great differences between the two effects. The effect on me of what *I* produce may be very different from the effect on me of insights produced by an outside agent. . . . I was the only healer for me. . . .

In *Behavioral Neuropsychiatry,* Stanley Dean made a plea for the investigation of what he called "the ultraconscious mind." The ultraconscious state, he noted, is correlated with a feeling of transcendental love, a realization of the unimportance of material abundance, and a quickening of the intellect. He urged a large-scale integration of western psychotherapy and the healing factors in eastern spirituality. "As practitioners of the healing arts, we cannot afford to dismiss any therapeutic procedure that holds potential promise."

Dean remarked that in the ultraconscious state, "Fear of death seems to fall off like an old cloak . . . *Physical and mental suffering vanish.* This alone should be of particular interest to the physician and psychiatrist."

The virtual elimination of anxiety seems to be the most conspicuous result of regular meditation and peace of mind its ultimate gift. Concluding the parable of the prisoner and the beetle, Paul Dessauer commented that "the strong strange wall and its heights no longer exist for those who have gone out into the land of liberty. . . . Here is the arcane, mysterious basis of meditation. Those who go out into the night can tell no one where they go and can tell no one what it is like to be free."

8

ALPHA—THE PARLOR GAME
OF THE CENTURY

In the course of the centuries, the West will produce its own yoga.

—CARL JUNG

Scene: The second floor of a mid-Manhattan office building. Lying on the floor, thirty New Yorkers of varying ages are listening with closed eyes to a metronome's beat. Then a teacher's voice: "You will continue to listen to my voice; you will continue to follow the instructions at this level, or any other level. . . . This is for your benefit. You desire it and it is so."

Scene: The Hollywood Studio Club. In the auditorium, seventy bodies—some prone, some in lotus posture—are immobile. They wear earphones and electrodes attached to black boxes shared two to a box. Their electrodes are held in place by blue-and-white Indian-style headbands. Through the earphones they hear a pleasant warble, the feedback for alpha brainwave production. Above the sound of the warble, which intensifies as alpha production increases, they listen to the mellow voice of Jack Gariss, head of the Bio-Meditation Society: "The very process of observing your thoughts will slow them down. More space will appear between thoughts. That space is the still mind, the quiet mind of serene reflection. Within that expanding space will flower mystical consciousness. . . ."

Scene: Barbara Brown's laboratory at the VA Hospital in Sepulveda, California—an experiment in telepathic rapport. Two subjects sit in a small room, its walls draped in black velvet to keep out light. They are opposite each other, each facing his own glass screen. For ten minutes each watches a rose-colored throbbing light that appears on the screen as a signal of one subject's alpha production. The brightness of the light varies with the amplitude of the alpha waves.

At the end of ten minutes, only the alpha subject gets light feedback; the receiver is now to press a button when he senses that his partner is in an alpha state. If he is right, a green light flashes. During a final ten-minute period, he again tries to sense his partner's alpha production, but with no green-light feedback.

Scene: A nursery school. A four-year-old is telling the teacher about his imaginary dog. The teacher politely asks him to describe the animal, and he retorts impishly, "Why don't you go into alpha and see?"

It's what one biofeedback manufacturer called "the parlor game of the century."

The alpha boom hit with such impetus that it seemed for a while that it would have to spin silently out of view as hula hoops once did. But subsequent developments point to bigger and better brainwave training. The federal government, which has underwritten most of the laboratory research through grants from the National Institute of Mental Health, will support clinical studies.

Private research will soon develop biofeedback instruments suitable for mass merchandising. Expensive machines are on the market for home use, and dozens of self-improvement courses are advertising that their methods enable the student to enter an alpha state.

What are the alpha brainwaves, and how has something so intangible become a hot commodity? The brain's electrochemical impulses, traveling at from 3 to 400 feet per second, are leadfooted in comparison to household electrical current, which approaches the speed of light.

But there's a critical difference—and therein lies the complexity that makes the most sophisticated electronic computer baby-simple in comparison. The brain is not limited to "wiring," as a telephone exchange or computer is limited. Because each cell is a tiny generator, the possible directions neural activity can travel are incalculable.

The electrical activity of the brain is measured in microvolts or *millionths of a volt*. The activity was first observed via a crude galvanometer devised by an English doctor, Richard Caton, in 1875. The first true EEGs were recorded by Hans Berger, a German psychiatrist, probably in 1924. Berger kept a diary but did not report his findings until almost five years later. He had turned to brain research as a young man because of his interest in a dramatic case of spontaneous telepathy between him and his sister during his army service.

Berger's first subjects were people with congenital openings in the skull. In *Explorers of the Brain,* Leonard Stevens described Berger's first studies:

> His recordings, made by a dancing spot of light on a moving strip of photographic paper, came out as a wavy line which indicated that the tiny cerebral voltages were changing with a regular rhythm of about ten beats per second.

Berger called this regular rhythm, the most prominent of the patterns, alpha. The shorter, smaller waves he called beta. Berger's report, published in 1929, was virtually ignored for five years. Finally two eminent English scientists, Edgar Adrian and B. C. H. Matthews, undertook an investigation because, as they admitted, "We found it difficult to accept the view that such uniform activity could occur throughout the brain in a conscious subject." When they found to their surprise that Berger had been right, they proposed renaming the alpha waves the Berger rhythm, which he opposed.

Asking half a dozen electrodes to tell us what the brain's ten billion cells are up to is tantamount to representing the opinions of two or three people as the results of a national poll. W. Grey Walter, a leading authority on electroencephalography, said in 1949:

> Even now we can probably understand less than one per cent of the total information contained in a record. . . . We are rather in the position of a visitor from Mars who is deaf and dumb and has no conception of the nature of sound but is trying to build up a knowledge of languages by looking at the grooves in a gramophone record.

Even so, Walter and other scientists have found over the years that the EEG patterns are associated with sleep onset, reverie, computation, epileptic seizure, and brain tumor.

The electrodes attached to the head record greatly magnified pulses of electricity that are translated into lines inked on paper feeding through the EEG. The force of each impulse determines the amplitude or height on the chart. Frequency is evident in the number of peaks and valleys drawn each second (cycles per second). The results of several electrodes are interpreted algebraically to determine an overall pattern.

The alpha pattern is markedly regular, the most prominent of the brainwaves in a typical waking EEG. Alpha usually appears only in brief bursts rather than for a sustained period. Alpha conditioning or training refers to the deliberate increase in the percentage of alpha activity in a given period.

Alpha ranges from eight to twelve or thirteen cycles per second and usually is associated with an alert but relaxed state of mind. Most people produce alpha when they close their eyes, but the typical waking, eyes-open EEG shows alpha mixed with the other patterns. Steady alpha is uncommon in one whose eyes are open. It may happen just as one is falling asleep and typically is blocked by a sudden stimulus or by turning one's attention to a specific problem, especially a mathematical problem.

The fast, tight beta pattern ranges from fourteen to thirty cycles per second. It appears in intense concentration and mental agitation.

Delta waves—one-half to three and a half cycles per second—are associated with disease, death, and degeneration according to Walter, who observed that they are appropriately named. Large and slow, they are seen in sleep and may also indicate pathology, such as a brain tumor, when they are conspicuous in an awake subject.

Theta waves, four to seven cycles per second, seem to be involved in emotionality, creative imagery, and computation on a deep level. They are infrequent in the waking EEG.

In the early 1960s, Joe Kamiya asked his subjects at the University of Chicago to tell him, at the sound of a tone, whether they believed their brainwaves were in state A or state B. (A was alpha; B, all nonalpha activity.) His very first subject succeeded in discriminating A from B. Later Kamiya was gratified to find that, within a few hours, most subjects could correctly identify A or B most of the time. Some became 100 percent accurate. They frustrated Kamiya, though, in their inability to say *how* A felt different from B.

After Kamiya went to Langley-Porter Neuropsychiatric Hospital in San Francisco, he wondered if a subject might also learn to sustain or suppress a particular brainwave pattern. Again, his first subject was his star performer. Listening to a tone that hummed steadily during sustained alpha and only bleeped occasionally otherwise, the volunteer managed to increase the percentage time in alpha dramatically.

Kamiya was struck by several observations:

1. Subjects much preferred alpha enhancement to alpha suppression.

2. Subjects with meditation experience were remarkably facile at alpha enhancement, usually mastering the control within the first thirty minutes of training.

3. The reports that meditative states were pleasant but impossible to describe seemed to tally with the volunteers' reports of alpha enhancement.

As other laboratories undertook brainwave biofeedback training, the persistent description of alpha as a desirable state —subjects occasionally compared it to a drug high—began to hit the popular press. Simultaneous accounts linking the alpha-theta production of Zen and yogi meditators to the laboratory phenomenon inspired many newspaper and magazine articles about instant satori and electronic zen.

Although the scientists conscientiously kept cautioning against too optimistic a view of brainwave training, the early clinical results seemed to underscore the potential benefits to mankind.

At the Angie Nall School in Beaumont, Texas, a pilot alpha-training program was so successful that now all the children, most of whom are hyperkinetic, are receiving alpha training. The pilot training program reportedly helped some to sleep, had a calming effect, and seemed to benefit those with learning disabilities.

Psychotherapists are using brainwave biofeedback devices to help their less seriously troubled clients liberate unconscious conflicts. Insomniacs are learning to produce the brainwave patterns typical of sleep onset. Epileptics have been taught to abort the abnormal pattern that precedes seizures.

Alpha training is being investigated for possible therapeutic value among drug abusers. Hypnotherapists are using biofeedback equipment in the hope that steady alpha will facilitate trance induction.

Businesses have inquired into biofeedback training for their employees. Some futurists even envision that coffee breaks will be supplanted by alpha breaks. The possibilities of brainwave training for creativity are being researched in several labs. Before biofeedback training, it had been assumed that visualization blocked alpha production. The imagery reported by volunteers generating abundant alpha or theta brainwaves is of a different nature than ordinary visualization. The images appear spontaneously, move freely, and are likely to be full-blown. The subject has the impression that he is watching them rather than conjuring them up.

Joe Kamiya has said that personality is something of a predictor of success in alpha training. Introspective people do well. Individuals who use words like images, dreams, wants, and feelings are likelier to succeed than those to whom these concepts are vague. Psychotherapists of the kind who are interested in growth techniques and sensitivity training are good candidates. Also:

> People who look you in the eye and feel at ease in close interpersonal relationships, who are good at intuitively sensing the way you feel, are also good at this. Also I notice I generally tend to have more positive liking for the individual who subsequently turns out to learn alpha control more readily.

Hypnotizability and creativity have also been correlated with alpha conditionability. Lester Fehmi, a biofeedback researcher at the State University of New York at Stony Brook, said that musicians, athletes, and artists are adept at learning alpha control. David Rosenboom, a musician, presented a biofeedback concert in New York. His carefully controlled brainwave activity was fed into a computer and an ARP synthesizer. Another musician, Lamonte Young, said that since his mind "is tuned to frequencies and intervals," generating alpha was not difficult.

Do alcohol, caffeine, and various other drugs affect alpha? It all depends. Biofeedback researchers have observed that spaced-out subjects are poor generators of alpha. Marijuana seems to have no consistent effect; in some instances it enhances, sometimes it suppresses.

The effects of coffee and tranquilizers depend entirely on the state of mind of the individual. If he feels low, the coffee might stimulate him enough to enhance the alpha rhythms, but if he were keyed up it would probably just give him coffee nerves. A tranquilizer might bring an anxious person down enough to enhance his alpha activity, but if he were already calm or tired it would only make him drowsy (bad for alpha). The same is true of alcohol.

Tobacco's effects are more predictable. Nearly all heavy smokers show considerable beta activity and very little alpha. Barbara Brown's research showed that the EEGs of heavy smokers were readily distinguishable from those of nonsmokers by a minimal alpha content, even with eyes closed. The alpha that appeared was relatively fast. Her comments:

> The distinctive differences in brainwave patterns between heavy smokers and non-smokers suggest two possible origins: That the effect of heavy smoking is either to produce a persistent and rather intense alerting pattern of the EEG; or, that individuals who have a high frequency (rhythmic) EEG pattern have a significantly greater potential to become habitual smokers.

Since the amplitude of the EEG response to a visual stimulus was no longer than that of the nonsmokers, Brown suggested that the fast EEG patterns of heavy smokers may be related to "diffuse rather than focused attention."

Investigators at the University of Missouri reported that after being deprived of cigarettes for twenty-four hours, seven young males who were heavy smokers showed a significant increase in the slow brainwave frequencies. After they smoked two cigarettes their EEGs showed a return of all frequencies toward their higher levels.

Abraham Black of McMasters University in Hamilton, Ontario, taught dogs to produce long trains of theta rhythms from the limbic brain's hippocampus. Later he successfully taught another group of dogs to produce anything *but* theta. He observed that the brainwave patterns seemed closely correlated with changes in outward movement. Wondering if the brain and body responses might be inextricably linked, he taught another group of dogs to perform the outward skeletal activity he had observed in the theta-trained dogs. And it seemed that the dogs automatically increased their theta percentage. Rats showed the same tandem effect.

Black tried to separate the two responses, but the animals found it all but impossible to produce bursts of theta in the immobile position he had found typical of their non-theta brain-wave activity.

The pairing may have significant implications for human bio-feedback training. It has already been noted that mental states and physiological states seem to be yoked in human beings. The tension-headache sufferers who learned an unusual degree of muscle relaxation at the University of Colorado Medical School also reported decreased anxiety.

At UCLA, anatomist Barry Sterman trained cats to sustain a pattern he calls sensorimotor for a reward of milk. After a time, the pattern itself was so rewarding that the blissful cats would ignore the milk reward and simply continue basking in the pleasures of the sensorimotor pattern.

Even more dramatic evidence of the altered brain activity: Sterman trained a group of cats for several months, then administered a toxic convulsive agent to them and to a group of untrained cats. *The trained cats didn't convulse.*

At the Menninger Research Foundation, Elmer and Alyce Green and Dale Walters are training subjects to sustain theta brainwaves—the slow, four-to-seven-cycles-per-second pattern —in the hope that it will generate creative imagery. Although theta training results in drowsiness for some subjects, others find it full of rich imagery and feeling. Like hypnagogic imagery, the transient phenomena as one is dropping off to sleep, theta material is characterized by vividness, spontaneity, originality, and a tendency to change.

The Menninger researchers hope that "training in the production and control of alpha-and-theta rhythms may make possible an enhancement of creativity in individuals whose potential is yet unrealized."

Another project at Menninger's produced some startling results. Until recently, certain patterns of brain activity had been neatly bracketed; prolonged delta was synonymous with sleep except in pathological EEGs (coma, tumor, epilepsy). Swami Rama, a yogi, told the researchers that he would demonstrate for them an EEG typical of sleep but that he would be aware at the same time. He lay down, closed his eyes, and began to produce prominent delta waves "and a gentle snore." From time to time, Alyce Green remarked on the weather.

> After 25 minutes had passed the Swami roused himself and said that someone with sharp heels had walked on the floor above and made a click, click, click noise during the test, and a door had been slammed somewhere twice in the building, and that Mrs. Green had said—and here he gave her statements, verbatim, except for the last half of the fourth sentence, of which he had the gist correct though not the words.

Asked about his technique, Swami Rama said that he had told his mind to be quiet, not to respond to anything but to record everything, and to remain deeply tranquil until he activated it. He could also produce theta brainwaves on signal (75 percent for five minutes) "by stilling the conscious mind and bringing forward the unconscious." He also gave the investigators an impressive display of alpha activity (70 percent alpha for five minutes) by visualizing an empty sky.

He demonstrated what Green described as "exquisite differential control over arteries in his right hand," causing two areas on the palm of the hand gradually to change temperature in opposite directions until they showed a ten-degree difference. "The left side of his palm . . . looked as if it had been slapped with a ruler a few times, it was rosy red. The right side had turned ashen gray." On another occasion he stopped the blood flow to his heart.

There is alpha, and then there is alpha. The researchers have been puzzled by the regular slow waves generated in the frontal and central brain regions by meditators. The phenomenon is seen in transcendental meditators with as little as two weeks' experience, according to a study at Centre College of Kentucky. A further odd finding is that some subjects, while generating the slow alpha-theta-range rhythms, show the reverse of a normal response. Usually a sudden stimulus blocks alpha. There is the simultaneous appearance of fast beta waves. But individuals in autogenic training and in the Menninger Foundation's

Voluntary Controls Project showed bursts of alpha instead. The Menninger researchers called it "paradoxical alpha."

What does the alpha rhythm signify? The alpha waves clearly result from the synchronous firing, or discharge, of neurons—hence, the regular pattern. Why this pattern should be implicated in a wide array of phenomena is a puzzle, to say the least.

The earliest theories were neat and plausible. Since the pattern appeared when subjects closed their eyes and seemed to be blocked by visual imagery or other attention, it was conjectured that the regularity meant a spontaneous firing of cells not in use, rather as if the brain were an idling engine.

Trying to correlate EEG patterns with mental operations is like playing charades blindfolded. Research in this area is doubly hampered because states of mind are difficult to put into words. Fortunately a few scientists have attempted to remove that blindfold by using themselves as guinea pigs. W. Grey Walter and his colleagues at the Burden Neurological Institute in Bristol, England, experienced for themselves in the late 1940s the peculiar changes in consciousness, the whirling spirals and hallucinated scenes brought on by their flicker device. Walter began pondering the possible brain mechanisms involved.

He expressed the unknown device as x, calculating that x plus alpha produced an image . . . and that flicker plus x produced movement as well. He finally speculated that x must be a scanning mechanism, comparable to the scanning device of a television camera. An American psychiatrist, Warren McCulloch, is said to have hit independently on the scanner theory at the same time.

Walter proposed that *the alpha rhythm signifies that the brain is scanning for pattern.* It ceases when the pattern has been located, he suggested, much as one's eyes scan a page for a certain word, then stop when they find it. In many ways the scanning-for-pattern theory tallies with Donald Hebb's belief, from sensory-deprivation research, that the brain requires varying stimulation for ordinary consciousness. The sustained alpha pattern brings about a state removed from everyday consciousness. And the theory that the brain strives for pattern is supported by the onset of alpha when a monotonous, unvarying stimulus is introduced.

Carrying his television analogy further, Walter suggested that a flickering light in the television studio would interfere with the camera's scanning mechanism. "Blobs of light would dart giddily about the screen. Similar confusion in the brain is seen . . . when the conflict between the two time patterns, the inherent scanning rhythms of the brain, and the flicker, produce a brain storm as wild as any distortion on the television screen."

Unfortunately for the scanning-for-pattern theory, not all images block alpha. Some individuals can perform such tasks as speed reading and even mathematical computation without dropping a stitch in their alpha production. More recently it has been conjectured that the alpha rhythm may represent a timing device necessary for the brain's own complex mathematical interpretation of incoming stimuli.

Why is alpha enhancement associated with such psychological states as serenity, pleasure, altered time perception? Why is the rhythm yoked to physiological relaxation? Why is it associated with enhanced psychic ability? Pain control? As someone once said, "There is hardly any problem, however complicated, which, when looked at in the right way, does not become yet more complicated."

Possibly the spreading slow-wave activity in meditation and autogenic training reflects a wider activation of neurons throughout the brain, which might account for phenomenal recall, color intensity, creative insights.

Since most electrodes are recording from the cortex for the obvious reason that deep brain structures are inaccessible without surgery, we actually know very little of the rhythms deep inside the human brain. In that sense, the early theorists may have been partially right. Perhaps the alpha rhythm reflects what is *not* happening in the cortex. Maybe it is the engine of the new brain that is idling, allowing the limbic brain to regain what Wolfgang Luthe called its "otherwise restricted capacity for self-regulatory normalization."

The no-cortical-interference interpretation of alpha is also reasonable in light of the need to let go in order to enhance alpha. The most successful biofeedback subjects explained that they didn't try, didn't think, just flowed.

The classical advice for altering consciousness was written

by William James long before the invention of the electroencephalogram:

> The way to success is by surrender, passivity, not activity. Relaxation, not intentness, should be now the rule. Give up the feeling of responsibility, let go your hold. . . . It is but giving your private convulsive self a rest, and finding that a greater Self is there. . . .
>
> The regenerative phenomena which ensue on the abandonment of effort remain firm facts of human nature.

Is the alpha pattern then a red herring? If it is significant primarily because it represents a stilling of new-brain activity, we have only deepened the mystery. We then have to shift the blame for the phenomenon to unknown mechanisms in the emotional brain.

Some critics of biofeedback training are afraid that it will produce mindless trippers, passive free riders unwilling to assume responsibilities in society. The fear is unsubstantiated. The alpha pattern is sustained by an alert, poised mind, not a dull one. Some laboratory volunteers have mentioned that their energy levels are higher than before training.

The biofeedback researchers at the Menninger Foundation stated the case well:

> . . . voluntary control of behavior is of primary importance if we hope to establish an ordered society or even maintain a society. Without stretching the imagination, the long-range implications and the effects for society of a population of self-regulating individuals could be of incalculable significance.

One of the commonest accusations of the biofeedback professionals is that the courses advertising alpha training are *not* teaching brainwave control. Granted that the alpha connection is indirect and the ads loose and somewhat hucksterish, it should be said in defense of the courses that they offer some evidence that their techniques enhance alpha production. And the courses vary, of course, with the proficiency of the teacher.

Alpha Dynamics is headed by Louis Rowlett, an executive in Mind Control before he started his own course. Rowlett's approach candidly borrows techniques from autogenic training, although his primary emphasis is on motivation. He also has incorporated biofeedback-research data, hypnosis methods, and meditation techniques.

Alpha Dynamics employs a Toomim Alpha Pacer (a commercial feedback device sold for private and clinical use) for testing, but Rowlett said, "We don't use biofeedback for actual training because we teach our students to accomplish an altered state of consciousness without the use of instruments."

Because of Alpha Dynamics' heavy use of autogenic training methods, alpha enhancement would be a likely result of the techniques.

Mind Control, the widely taught system developed by Jose Silva, obtained EEG corroboration from Trinity University in San Antonio that there is some increase in alpha in the state known in Mind Control as "at level." The Mind Control exercises are an interesting blend of classical autohypnotic techniques, visualization, sensory awareness, and a use of symbols that is probably unique with Silva and a genuinely important contribution to consciousness-expansion methodology.

The conscientious alarm expressed by some scientists over Mind Control and its spin-offs is perhaps disproportionate. Millions of people who have never spent an introspective hour in their lives are suddenly eager to expand consciousness, find inner peace, relate more openly to friends and family, learn self-control. Some graduates report enhanced health, energy, memory. Others claim that they were able to lose weight, quit smoking or drinking, or give up drugs.

One reason for all the warnings from the scientific community may be an anticipation of blame. A biofeedback researcher, Abraham Black, said:

There is a tendency today to condemn scientists who do their research, publish the results, and stop there, without worrying about the consequences of their findings. . . . Such seems to be the case with our work. . . .

One of the characters in Dürrenmatt's play, *The Physicists,* says, "Our knowledge has become a frightening burden. Our researches are perilous, our discoveries are lethal. We have to take back our knowledge, and I have taken it back." This scientist took back his knowledge by pretending to be insane and allowing himself to be incarcerated in an asylum. This did not work for him and a similar strategy will not work for us.

The biofeedback machines marketed for private use represent more of a consumer problem than the courses. Virtually miniature EEG machines, they are expensive (averaging $250). If inaccurate they are worse than useless. Barbara Brown said that she found one user who had been getting feedback for the wrong brainwave pattern and was learning to produce epileptic spikes.

One technical bug plaguing the manufacturers is the elimination of artifacts, the muscle twitches, heartbeat, and other nonbrain activities that may nonetheless be fed through the electrodes.

Since brainwaves are measured in microvolts, millionths of a volt, the machines have to be accurate enough to filter out a grosser energy, the free electricity in the air. Courtesy of the local power company, it averages sixty volts in most urban areas.

No single machine is endorsed by biofeedback research laboratories. Each researcher seems to have found one manufacturer he trusts, one instrument less inaccurate than the others, but there is no agreement as to which product that is. Some manufacturers were experienced in electroencephalography and have worked out bugs in cooperation with research laboratories. Others had a nose for merchandising and a knack for electronics. Some of the more sophisticated instruments have changeable filters (for alpha, theta, and alpha/theta, the borderline range), scoring devices that show the percentage of alpha, artifact inhibitors, and adjustable thresholds so the user can filter out low-amplitude patterns and gradually shape a higher amplitude.

Some manufacturers have added portable electromyelogram devices to their line. The EMG feedback device, if accurate, can train the user to reduce muscle tension to levels far lower than can be achieved by normal relaxation.

Many manufacturers of biofeedback equipment have adopted meditation techniques in training the users of their devices. One meditation group has turned the tables. Now known as the Bio-Meditation Society, the Reseda, California, organization combines traditional meditation methods with the Bioscope, a feedback device with a warble and earphones. A second person can tune in on the warble and guide the meditator by gradually adjusting the threshold upward so that he must generate increasingly higher amplitude waves.

"We seem to have backed into something that the East has known for centuries," Joe Kamiya said. Elmer Green remarked that although the machines were certainly not necessary for attaining altered states of consciousness, they furnish material evidence of the existence of such states for those who need it.

> . . . a semantic trap exists in the frequently used phrase, "training a subject to produce theta waves or low-frequency alpha." In actuality there is no such thing as training in brainwave control; there is training only in the elicitation of certain subjective states that are accompanied by oscillating voltages in the cerebral cortex, detected through the subject's skull and scalp.

The brainwave biofeedback discoveries opened the door to a broad new field, the psychophysiology of altered consciousness.

"With a greatly increased knowledge of meditation, there may be many more feedback-aided exercises in meditation," Kamiya predicted. "Maybe the 'in' thing in 1979 will be the production of theta waves in central or even prefrontal [areas] —because that's what some meditation traditions show among their practitioners."

The following is an account by an individual who became interested in brainwave training after reading in a magazine that most people go in and out of the alpha pattern several times a minute in waking consciousness.

> I closed my eyes and paid attention for a while to the feelings inside my head, which I had never really noticed before. After a while I noticed that there was a brief, delicate, spasmodic sensation that was pleasanter than the rest. I figured that this must be the famous alpha wave.
>
> At first I could only hold the sensation for four or five seconds, but after a day or two I found that I could sustain it for hours, even with my eyes open. I somehow groped around in my head for it; it was like tuning something in. It's pleasant, much like the feeling you get when everything is going swimmingly.
>
> A few weeks after I had started playing with this brain sensation, I got something of a shock. I'd been holding it for a while, and suddenly there was an alarming thing happening, like a million volts going through me. It was paralyzing and delicious at the same time. Not long afterward I noticed a strange thing.

Something happened that would usually have thrown me into a cold panic, but I didn't panic. It's like being on Librium around the clock.

Not realizing that alpha training is based on feedback from the *back* of the head, the do-it-yourselfer had innocently picked up alpha in a less typical region and, as experiments in two biofeedback laboratories later attested, had learned to generate splendid, high-amplitude alpha in the frontal and central areas, the phenomenon usually associated with meditation.

What spectacular gifts might be cached in the patterns of those billions of neurons under our skulls? Perhaps we have been the chained people in Plato's story of the cave, watching flickering shadows on the cave wall and calling them reality.

9

HYPNOSIS AND *ASCID*

*In hypnosis we see how wide and deep is the dominion of the brain
over all other organs and functions.*

—W. GREY WALTER, THE LIVING BRAIN

While biofeedback and meditation have been capturing scientific and popular attention, what of that once-controversial old-timer, hypnosis?

At the Toronto Rehabilitation Center, heart-attack patients were assigned at random to either of two physicians. Terence Kavanagh's patients jogged and did other conventional mild exercises designed to stimulate the vessels in the heart region to develop alternate throughways for circulation. Harvey Doney's patients, on the other hand, were hypnotized and told that they were in a pleasant meadow, breathing deeply of fresh air, feeling the oxygen coursing through their bodies and getting to their hearts.

At the end of a year, rigorous physiological tests showed that the two groups were making "significant progress" at the same rate.

Ronnie-Sue Peek, 28, a lifelong asthmatic, was desperately wheezing in Cottonwood Hospital in Salt Lake City. After three weeks of heavy medication, she was still barely breathing when her mother placed a long-distance call to a doctor who had not seen her since she was a teen-ager.

The doctor telephoned Ronnie-Sue's bedside. After reestablishing their former rapport, he hypnotized her as he had years before. He told her to imagine a situation in which she would feel comfortable, and she envisioned herself in the mountains. Her breathing would become effortless, he said. She was feeling better and better, and when she awoke, the asthma would be gone. When Ronnie-Sue came out of the hypnotic trance, she was breathing easily. Two days later she was discharged from the hospital.

Oscar N. Lucas, a dentist, dreaded extracting teeth from hemophiliac patients so he hypnotized them and told them that they had ice cubes in their mouths. When they awoke they would have no sensation in their mouths, he said, their gums would feel cold, and there would be little or no bleeding.

After forty-nine such extractions, Lucas compared the results to the typical hemophiliac extractions before he began using hypnosis:

> Under conventional extraction techniques, the patients had been hospitalized for an average of six days, had received an average of five pints of blood, and their sockets had taken more than two weeks to heal. With hypnosis, the patients received no blood, were not hospitalized, and gums healed in an average of 4.4 days.

In other experiments, patients were injected with pollen extracts to which they were known to be allergic. They reacted as expected, but after hypnosis showed no reaction at all. Hypnotists have successfully directed subjects to rid themselves of warts on one side of their bodies only.

Hypnosis may be man's priceless practical joke on himself. Suspending his almighty judgment to comply instead with the hypnotist's instructions, he can heal himself, stand immobile on one foot for an hour, recall the names of the children in his kindergarten class—all feats no one with common sense would attempt in his right mind.

Martin Orme, a Philadelphia psychiatrist, told a class of introductory psychology students that, under hypnosis, one's dominant hand becomes cataleptic. When he later hypnotized the students, 55 percent reported that they were unable to move the dominant hand.

Patricia Bowers had found that hypnosis conspicuously enhanced creativity in two well-controlled experiments. Then she conducted a similar study with a group of subjects who pretended to be hypnotized. They did about as well on the creativity tasks as those who had been hypnotized. Bowers speculated that subjects pretending to be hypnotized may have unloosed their powers of originality merely by abandoning responsibility for their typical behavior.

There are no consistent physiological correlates of hypnosis. Although the EEG sometimes records abundant alpha, in most cases it is impossible to distinguish from that of ordinary waking consciousness. Measurements such as blood pressure, heart rate, and skin resistance vary with the suggestion of the hypnotist or are relatively unchanged.

The Kirlian-photography experiments at UCLA and in the Soviet Union indicate changes in hypnosis, but they are not consistent. In fact, Tambiev and his co-workers remarked that the change in "electro-energy" seen in hypnosis can be achieved in unhypnotized states by *effort or emotion.*

Since it is becoming apparent from biofeedback research and experiments with yogis that hypnosis per se is not essential for such phenomena as anesthesia, ESP, self-healing, feats of memory, then why does it work? Apparently its great advantage is the suspension of judgment. In our usual routine, we abide by certain assumptions about what can and can't be done. In hypnosis, we freely disregard these assumptions by focusing on the hypnotist's voice and relinquishing our role as the Doubting Thomas.

Yet all hypnosis is ultimately self-hypnosis; the subject chooses to give up his autonomy, and it is well known that he seldom does anything under hypnosis that is in opposition to his personal code. For several centuries there has been insistent evidence that hypnosis is influenced by expectation. For instance, most people assume that one who is hypnotized does not recall afterward what occurred when he was in trance. If, however, the subject is told before he is hypnotized that people can remember what took place in hypnosis, he remembers. Mesmer's early patients thought they were supposed to convulse, so they did.

When the French Academy was investigating the claims of Mesmer, several members charged that his patients were cured because of their vivid imaginations. One thoughtful scientist said, "Perhaps—but if so, what a marvelous thing is imagination!"

We don't understand imagination or hypnosis, but perhaps the riddle we have already learned to live with is preferable to a fresh riddle. If the hypnotist is not the essential ingredient, what is?

The new approaches have borrowed four ingredients from classical hypnosis: suggestion, visualization, focus, and suspension of judgment. However, the authority of the hypnotist has been transferred to the subject, as in autogenic training. For this reason, the new techniques are successful for many individuals who would find it difficult to surrender themselves to a hypnotist.

The quasi-hypnotic approaches include a number of programs in which inner visualization is employed, not only for creativity but for altering one's physiology. Dancers and athletes are participating in training programs in which they inwardly visualize improved coordination, firmer muscles, more grace. Oddly enough, the results are comparable to actual training.

"Waking imagination" and "simulation" approaches allow the subject to pretend that he can do thus and such, or simulate hypnosis (which allows him to do the sort of thing he thinks a hypnotized person would do). In such circumstances, people have tolerated holding their arms in painfully cold water, distinguished visual patterns on standard tests for color blindness as if they had red-green color blindness. Subjects pretending to be hypnotized showed a sharp increase in creative responses on a test.

In all of the foregoing cases, control groups were also asked to place their arms in icy water or try to see the color-blindness-test pattern or to answer the questions on a test of creativity. The water was unbearably cold, the pattern invisible, the responses to the creativity tests showed no change from one session to another.

Children are notoriously better than adults at biofeedback, almost certainly because they are too ignorant to know that they are attempting the impossible. In the Menninger Foundation biofeedback training programs, children could rapidly learn to raise their hand temperatures. Adult subjects who were told in advance that such control was believed impossible learned with difficulty. Those simply briefed on a technique achieved control in a much shorter period.

Some subjects who had slowly raised the hand temperature with the guidance of a researcher (while watching a needle move to the right) would panic when told they were on their own. The temperature would drop rapidly. Yet they had been responsible for the changes all along. They are like the character in the animated cartoon who walks a dozen steps beyond the precipice, then suddenly realizes that he is in midair—and plunges into the gorge.

At the Suggestology Institute in Sofia, Bulgaria, Georgi Lozanov not only conducts classes in which difficult academic courses (such as foreign languages) are easily mastered in a state of yoga-like serenity and suggestion. Lozanov also has taken suggestology into hospitals, where he urges the patients to relax, suggests that they feel well and have a good appetite. The patients visualize themselves well and happy; reputedly, suggestion effects more rapid cures than would normally be expected.

A practitioner of yoga for twenty-five years, Lozanov believes that yogis accomplish their feats by entering a suggestive state. Certainly the reports of healing phenomena in meditation are similar to hypnotic case histories. The focus of all such techniques tends to crowd out the skeptic who resides in the cerebral cortex.

The psychologist Charles Tart wondered whether the level of hypnosis a subject can reach is really a constant factor (as is usually assumed) or can be deepened. Tart thought that since the quality of rapport is supposed to determine depth, one might increase rapport by having two individuals hypnotize each other and thereby increase the depth of the trance.

His subjects were two graduate students in their twenties, whom he refers to as Anne and Bill. Both had had some experience as hypnotists and were also "moderately hypnotizable." Tart also established his own rapport with his two hypnotists in the event that they, being hypnotized, would be unable to bring each other out at a convenient time.

The two helped deepen each other's trance, after the initial passes and usual induction techniques, by describing aloud the imagery they were experiencing.

Anne described dreaming of the two of them being in a car on the desert, watching the road unwind before them, seeing small lizards run over the sand, then walking along the desert road, feeling hot and sticky, but with an overall feeling of pleasantness.

When asked by Anne, Bill indicated he was dreaming the same dream. From later questioning, both subjects were now completely oblivious to their actual surroundings and totally absorbed in their hallucinatory world(s).

After Anne and Bill appeared deeply entranced, Tart wondered whether they could move about without disrupting their hypnotic state. He asked them to simulate wakefulness.

On signal they both opened their eyes, sat up, lit cigarettes, talked with me and a couple of observers in the room, and claimed they were awake.

However, they were turned off almost automatically when Tart asked them for a report on the depth of their trance. They stopped simulating wakefulness and lapsed into the dreamlike state.

At a second session the subjects wandered deep into a mutually visualized tunnel. They argued at one point about whether or not they could remove anything they found in the tunnel.

Anne wanted to go back into the tunnel and to bring something back, very badly; Bill insisted they could do neither and then forcefully took them out of the tunnel. Anne was very distressed at this. . . .

The tunnel was absolutely real to Anne and Bill. . . . Although it was dark they could "see" its walls in a strange way: Anne said it felt as if she had a "light" coming out from under her eyebrows. . . . Both subjects reported feeling the texture of the rock walls, which ranged from soft and slippery at places where it seemed moss-covered to quite hard where the bare rock was exposed.

In a third session, both subjects undertook deliberately a hypnotic dream. Both their dreams ended similarly, Bill's with a rope ladder and Anne's with a golden rope. Later that session they reported that they found themselves in some sort of heaven. In front of them was water that bubbled like champagne, in which they later swam.

The psychedelic characteristics of mutual hypnosis were evident in the intense internal imagery and sensory enhancement. When the subjects read the transcripts of the three sessions some months later, they were shocked. In the interim they had discussed some of their shared experiences, which they assumed were pure fantasy. Then they realized that there had been no verbal stimuli for many of the shared events and that they had apparently been communicated telepathically. This gave the experience a reality and intimacy they found unsettling, and the experiments stopped.

Tart had observed that they sometimes sat silently for long periods during the mutual hypnosis sessions, and when asked to proceed they reacted with surprise. They seemed to believe that they had been communicating.

Tart warns that mutual hypnosis produces such an intense experience that it can be dangerous with immature or unstable personalities. Two college students who had heard from his subjects about the experiment decided to try it. One of the two could not become dehypnotized until professional help was called in.

Stanley Krippner of the Dream Laboratory at Maimonides Medical Center in Brooklyn studies the effects of various states of consciousness on telepathy and clairvoyance. Dreams, meditation, hypnosis, and a sensory-bombardment device are all used.

In one clairvoyance test, a group of subjects tried to perceive the target objects (art prints in opaque envelopes) in ordinary waking consciousness; a second group attempted the same task while hypnotized. The hypnotized subjects were significantly more successful, but the unhypnotized subjects, who were asked to keep dream diaries for a week, dreamed about the target objects within the next few days. "It's as if hypnosis speeded up the clairvoyance," Krippner said.

In dreaming, as in the other altered states, judgment is suspended.

A number of practical applications for hypnosis are under study. One of these is time distortion, a technique which enables the subject to work out complicated designs, work plans, theses, and the like—all in a matter of seconds. He perceives the time as hours or a full day. I. F. Cooper, a Phoenix, Arizona, psychiatrist, reported that one executive had such a welter of ideas during a few time-distorted seconds that he dictated for three hours afterward, trying to get all his inspirations and insights down on paper.

In one of the earliest experiments, conducted by Linn Cooper and Milton Erickson in 1954, a college student interested in dress designing believed that she was sitting at a table, gazing out a window, thinking, and later sketching. She thought that perhaps an hour had passed. Ten seconds had elapsed. A design was complete in her mind. Typically she had spent several hours per session on four to ten occasions to design a single dress.

Gay Gaer Luce, the science writer, suggested that there may be natural units of time and attention in the nervous system that are available to an individual.

> . . . only future research can tell us whether they approximate the units of our clocks. Studies of time distortion emphasize how limited our cultural view of "time sense" can be, and may offer us ways of enriching the education of the young by compressing more learning into the early school years. A number of scientists have conjectured that any intelligent youngster could have the knowledge of today's college graduate by the age of ten. Children using time-distortion techniques might indeed accelerate their own study. One fact in their favor is a high rate of brain metabolism.

Studies in the 1930s demonstrated that time seems to be passing much more slowly when the body temperature is high, "suggesting that perception of short time intervals may be modulated by a metabolic-chemical pacemaker system in the brain." Possibly a child's higher metabolic rate explains why time seems to move so slowly for him, while it races by for the elderly, whose metabolism is slow.

Jean Houston and R. E. L. Masters have used an unusual method to induce experimental religious experiences. It's ASCID, an Altered State of Consciousness Inducing Device, and the humor is intentional. Houston and Masters have been engaged in a deliberate search for nondrug analogues to psychedelic experience.

They initially developed ASCID to facilitate eidetic imagery. Jean Houston described it:

> It is essentially a metal swing or pendulum in which the subject stands upright, supported by broad bands of canvas and wearing blindfold goggles. The device containing the subject moves in side-to-side, forward-and-backward, and rotating motions generated by the subject's body. Typically, in from two minutes to twenty, an altered state of consciousness or trance state results.

The depth ranges from light to somnambulistic, but the state differs from a typical hypnotic trance in that there is no hypnotist-subject relationship. As Houston and Masters put it, "He goes, if you will, on his own trip." He may or may not do as the experimenter suggests.

Subjects experienced in both hypnotic and ASCID trance insist that these states are distinctly different but the old problem prevails. Language is inadequate to describe the difference.

The Audio-Visual Environment is another method Houston and Masters use for achieving a hypnoid state. Color slides from two projectors dissolve in and out, and the subject listens to "a coordinated taped sound sequence, principally electronic music." The slides—each an abstract oil painting on $2'' \times 2''$ glass—are projected over a semicircular $8' \times 8'$ rear projection screen. The subject feels almost as if he is in the paintings.

The experimenters comment that many of those who work with altered states of consciousness suspect that prolonged television viewing may itself produce a hypnoid state, rendering the viewer vulnerable to propaganda and advertiser suggestion.

Remarking on some of the more profound religious experiences reported by ASCID subjects, the researchers said, "It would probably be more accurate to say that we helped *enable* the experience to occur rather than that we induced it. Each of the individuals in question brought to his session a degree of development and an orientation that made possible the depth and richness of the experience. . . ."

They decided to see what sort of experience might be facilitated in individuals who were not prepared by spiritual growth-seeking or by need. Their design was usually to suggest that the subject, who was entranced by ASCID, would experience his body and all the world breaking down into minute, moving particles. He was instructed to let go of his self-concept, his I, "and to let that also merge with and drift out into the vast and endless sea of being."

They then instructed the subjects to continue in this state for as long as they wished, and then gradually to experience body and ego coalescing. *Whatever the trance depth,* the subjects experienced bliss, a mystical and oceanic ecstasy. The euphoria persisted after the experiment.

In other experiments, the subjects imagined themselves dying and being reborn. The reports of the experiences were stunningly akin to the reports of classical mystical states. One subject spoke of her rebirth:

> There was a tremendous slow-motion kind of explosion and upsurge and outgo of energy all around and from the point where the light disappeared. It was incredible. Then the circle grew and grew to infinite proportions within me, and all the sound was white. It was a silent Beethoven symphony throbbing all over the place. . . . I grew huge and transparent, filled and permeated with the light and the fire. And I thought: My God is a God of Love and he lives within me.

Opening their eyes after the rebirth experience, subjects often report a temporary heightening of perception.

Houston and Masters have said that the induction of religious-type experiences through trance is their effort to achieve access to "the farthest and deepest reaches of the psyche."

Bernard Aaronson also employed trance as a means to induce experiences akin to psychedelic intoxication. His hypnotized subjects were told in a series of lengthy experiments that they were perceiving extreme depth, flatness, blurred vision, or clear vision.

On the occasions of extreme depth (and to a lesser extent, in the clear-vision experiments), the subjects typically experienced euphoria.

> One subject reported that everything was part of a divine order and that he must spend his life serving God. A second subject described the world as ". . . at once a gigantic formal garden and an irrepressible wilderness of joyous space." A third subject titled his account of the session, "And then there was Depth!"

The two subjects with experience [in psychedelic drugs] reported the experience as being like "a pot high."

The subjects typically responded to the no-depth session as if they were schizophrenic. Outside observers who conducted personality tests noted markedly schizoid behavior and test responses. And many schizophrenics also report that everything they see is flat, two-dimensional. But the onset of acute psychosis often is characterized by a heightened perception of detail and color strongly parallel to a good trip. The flatness seems to come during a rebound phase.

When Aaronson suggested that the subjects would see the world as diminished in size or greatly enlarged, their disoriented behavior strongly resembled that of acid-takers on a bad trip.

Interestingly, Aaronson's study included one simulator, who pretended to be hypnotized. He frequently experienced euphoria or schizoid perceptions along with the hypnotized subjects.

Subjects in hypnosis sometimes find themselves observing themselves at another age. Milton Erickson recalled a girl who had identical twin sisters younger than herself. Hypnotized, she found herself to be "a pair of identical twins growing up together but always knowing everything about the other." She seemed to remember nothing about her own twin sisters.

Aldous Huxley, after the psychedelic experiences he reported in *The Doors of Perception* and *Heaven and Hell,* became remarkably adept at a technique resembling self-hypnosis. He called the state he achieved Deep Reflection, and his imagery and powers of recall while entranced impressed Milton Erickson greatly.

After one such two-hour experiment Erickson observed, Huxley came out of his dissociated state with an incredible narrative about how he had found himself on an unfamiliar hillside where he met a small boy six years old. In the fantasy, he was himself at age twenty-six and the small boy was Aldous Huxley at six. He not only could feel the six-year-old from his 26-year-old viewpoint, he even felt the child's hunger for "brown cookies."

He experienced the child's entire life, never knowing what

was coming next, because somehow the 26-year-old Huxley had amnesia for the intervening years. Day after day passed; he followed the child from grade school to high school, the ordeal of deciding whether or not to go to college, what he should study. He felt the anguish, relief, and elation of his observed, changing self.

The breaking apart of ego and the conviction that consciousness has inhabited a strange body are curious components of the altered states.

Amazing as it may seem, the gifted Huxley had been unable to visualize at all before his experiments with psychedelics. The rich imagery he found through hallucinogens and later in his own deep trances were truly remarkable for a man who had had no "mind's eye."

10

PSYCHEDELICS:
THRILLS, TRAUMA, THERAPY

"Booze is what makes people crazy," Don Juan said. *"It blurs the images. Mescalito, on the other hand, sharpens everything. It makes you see so very well."* —CARLOS CASTANEDA,
A SEPARATE REALITY: FURTHER CONVERSATIONS WITH DON JUAN

Never have so many been so high so often. When a Boston research group decided to compare the effects of marijuana on experienced and inexperienced users, it took them two months to line up nine student subjects who had never used marijuana. According to a survey at UCLA, 70 to 80 percent of the medical students were experienced marijuana users. A national survey of 1314 doctors revealed that 25 percent had smoked marijuana at some time; in San Francisco and New York the figures were much higher. One in three American university students has tried marijuana at least once. In California, the rate is higher than that even among high-school students. A 1971 survey in San Mateo County high schools showed that 32 percent of the senior boys had used marijuana fifty or more times in the preceding twelve months. William McGlothlin, a research psychologist at UCLA, estimated in 1972 that 2.1 million Americans were using marijuana three or more times a week and another 5.9 million from one to eight times a month.

The statistics may seem ominously reminiscent of Aldous Huxley's *Brave New World*. Is that the direction psychedelics are taking us?

When marijuana was used primarily by a few jazz musicians, American officialdom had little interest in its properties. Now that its users are legion, crash research programs are under way to discover what marijuana does to the brain and whether any of its effects are permanent. Unfortunately, as one researcher remarked, so much remains to be learned about the brain itself that marijuana's modus operandi may be mysterious for some time to come.

The active ingredient in marijuana is tetrahydrocannabinol (THC). The substance is derived from the Indian hemp plant, whose ground-up leaves and flowering tops are sold as marijuana. The plant's sticky resin is hashish, which is about 20 percent THC. Street-sale marijuana in the United States ranges from 0 percent potency (if it happens to be alfalfa or oregano instead, which is not unlikely) to 0.5 percent. Marijuana grown in Mississippi for federally sanctioned research comes in two strengths, 1.5 percent and 3 percent.

The EEG begins to record a higher percentage of alpha brainwaves as marijuana takes effect. The heart rate increases, the eyes redden, and the mouth goes cotton-dry. Blood pressure, respiration, and blood sugar, however, are unaffected by the drug. Users report euphoria, time distortion, expanded depth perception, and a heightening of sensory impressions.

Memory acquisition and storage are impaired in human beings, but oddly enough marijuana has little effect on the ability to recall information learned before ingestion. The drug apparently interferes with the brain's ability to process new experience. The user finds it difficult to compute or to frame and carry out complex plans. He might be able to count backward from one hundred by fours, but if told to aim for a certain number, he will probably become muddled. Animal studies have also shown impaired learning and memory.

Comparing a marijuana high to alcoholic intoxication, one research group administered the equivalent of six drinks to one group of subjects, and the marijuana subjects smoked until they judged themselves high. A third group received nothing. Then all three groups were tested. The marijuana subjects performed as well as sober ones. The report is often cited by lawyers defending clients who were arrested for driving while stoned. Richard Orkand of UCLA criticized the methodology, saying that it is impossible to determine how much THC the smokers inhaled. Orkand, a participant in a number of marijuana studies in his student days, maintained, "Anyone who has ever been thoroughly stoned knows you're in no condition to drive."

Marijuana enhances the sedation of barbiturates and the stimulating effect of amphetamines. Alone, however, it is nontoxic. Animal experiments have demonstrated that a lethal dose of marijuana is 40,000 times that normally taken by human beings.

Users often develop a curious susceptibility to the drug's effects, a phenomenon known as reverse tolerance. An experienced user typically requires smaller doses for a high than an inexperienced subject. This may be due to cumulative effects, increased sensitivity (as to an allergen), or the acquisition of enzymes that convert THC to a more stable metabolite.* It is also possible that there is a subtle learned ability to exploit or heighten the effect. Experienced users have reported an effect even from placebo cigarettes and injections.

At the University of California Medical School, researcher Reese Jones gave each subject a cigarette containing either marijuana or a placebo; he also gave each subject an intravenous injection of either alcohol or a placebo. The subjects, all experienced pot smokers, were unable to tell the difference between a marijuana high and an alcohol high.

Police in Brasilia in South America answered reports from residents that aggressive rats were picking fights with cats. The investigating officers discovered that the unusually ferocious rats had been nibbling at marijuana that had been seized in an antidrug drive and stored in a city court building.

In most species, however, marijuana is likelier to dampen aggression than increase it. Monkeys become markedly less aggressive, according to several studies, and human beings usually appear more docile than normal. An occasional human user becomes depressed and/or violent, perhaps because marijuana loosens his emotional controls.

Marijuana's relative mildness was recognized as early as the 1940s. When Fiorello La Guardia was mayor of New York City he appointed a commission to study the drug's role in local crime. After investigating the tea pads in Harlem, where marijuana was most prevalent, the commissioners issued a book-length report absolving the drug of any important role in

* In its metabolic processes, the body is continually converting substances into other slightly different substances. These products are known as metabolites.

crime. One study in that era investigated the possibility that marijuana is addictive. Prison immates were given as much marijuana as they wished for a period of weeks. When the supply was withdrawn, there were no problems even though the prisoners had averaged seventeen cigarettes daily.

Although psychosis resulting from marijuana is rare, hashish users in India, using the more potent variety of cannabis, have shown disorientation and grave memory impairment. Fortunately for them, the gross behavioral changes typically disappeared when the accumulated THC was excreted. In Denmark, researchers say they have identified about two thousand cases of a learning impairment they blame on the prevalent use of hashish by high-school students.

Irreversible brain damage and losses of brain protein and DNA have been observed in rats given dosages thirty times higher than the amount tested in human beings. For a valid comparison, a human subject would have to smoke forty to fifty high-graduate marijuana cigarettes daily for years. However ambiguous such studies may seem, the brain-research returns are not yet in. And there is still a very real possibility that subtle brain damage eventually results from cannabis ingestion.

Very few chronic users stick solely to one drug. Amphetamines, barbituarates, tranquilizers, LSD, even antihistamines complicate the investigation of marijuana's role in human brain damage. One university survey indicated that 44 percent of the heavy users had also smoked opium at least once.

The most serious problem resulting from widespread marijuana use is what Louis West, chairman of UCLA's psychiatry department, called "the amotivational syndrome." Social indifference and a lack of motivation have been reported from all parts of the world where cannabis is heavily used. Many psychologists fear that those most eagerly searching for chemical joy are those who can least afford it—the unstable, the escapists, the depressed, the insecure. In an era when psychopharmacology has developed drugs that specifically treat depression, neurosis, and certain types of psychosis, self-medication with pot is questionable therapy.

West pointed out that the learning impairment noted among Danish high-school students using hashish showed up soonest in those from traumatic, deprived backgrounds. The stable, middle-class youngsters could get away with chronic use for a longer period before changes were evident. However, surveys at Wesleyan, Illinois, and UCLA show no correlation thus far between cumulative grade-point averages and marijuana use.

Altered motivation has been observed in some animal studies. Stoned cats observed at the University of Toronto are one example:

> The animals stared into space and often appeared to be following stimuli with their eyes, even though no moving stimulus was discernible to the experimenter. All dosages produced an increase in synchrony [synchronized brainwave activity]. . . .
> All doses produced vomiting and defecation. The animals seemed oblivious to this. In most cases they sat in their excrement, which is very unusual behavior in the cat.

Whatever its adverse behavioral effects, marijuana seems to have therapeutic value as an alternative for problem drinkers. One example is the case history recounted in the *Medical Times* by Tod Mikuiya, director of research at the Gladman Memorial Foundation in Oakland, California. The patient, then forty-nine, had a history of alcoholism dating back to her teens. She exchanged her disabling alcoholism for a mild dependence on marijuana. The slight glow she maintained by periodic puffs on a marijuana cigarette relieved the edge of tension and insecurity she had always experienced when sober, and she was able to rejoin society.

Although virtually all marijuana researchers favor decriminalizing possession, most are reluctant to recommend legalization on the basis of the facts now in hand. Should marijuana be legalized, some scientists recommend that dosages be sold by federal pharmacies similar to the state-run liquor stores in some parts of the country, so that a vast, self-serving industry comparable to the present tobacco industry would not evolve.

Unlike marijuana, many of the major hallucinogens are strikingly similar to the brain's own transmitter substances. *Bufotenin,* obtained from certain toads as well as from a fungus, can also be metabolized from the transmitter serotonin. *Mescaline,* a substance found in the buttons of the peyote cactus used ritually by American Indians, is chemically related to adrenaline and also to a substance found in the urine of schizophrenics. The great promise of LSD has been that it both resembles serotonin and inhibits it. At first there were high hopes that its effects would prove a model psychosis, but other pharmacological agents are now known to inhibit the brain transmitter without producing profound hallucinations. Thousands of papers and millions of research dollars later, neither schizophrenia, LSD, nor serotonin has yielded its fundamental secrets.

Some interesting advances have been made, however, and the psychedelics have been found surprisingly useful therapeutically. Meanwhile, the questions being posed are increasingly provocative.

Under LSD's influence, the EEG reflects a state of high arousal. Several investigators have speculated that this brainwave pattern does not represent a waking state at all but the intense activity of a brain engaged in paradoxical sleep—the so-called REM (rapid-eye-movement) sleep period often associated with bizarre dreams.

As the Swiss researcher Werner Koella pointed out, cats high on LSD appear to be visually hallucinating. They may bat at imaginary flies or appear to be backing off from an imaginary attacker. LSD causes the stimulus to be processed more slowly by the brain's thalamus, but the cortex seems to react in an abnormally short time once the message has been handed on. Koella suggested that in the absence of visual input to the cortex, the more excitable visual cortical networks might be producing their own imagery, independent of what meets the eye. The speculation that the brain is creating an inner world is supported by a U.S. government publication, *LSD-25: A Factual Account.* According to this report, LSD causes impulses to pass through the optic nerve, even when the experimental animal's eye has been disconnected from the optic nerve. Experiments conducted with totally blind human beings have yielded similar results. The authors add, "What is seen is not found in objective reality, but arises from within oneself."

Normally, a repetitive stimulus produces in awake animals a wide variability among the evoked responses. LSD decreases this variability by 75 percent. The psychotomimetic (psychosis-mimicking) action of substances like LSD may be due to their ability to decrease this variability. Koella pointed out that rabbits showed the same effect of greatly reduced variability when given extracts from schizophrenics' plasma protein.

Koella also called attention to the spiders studied in the 1950s. Under the influence of LSD they wove webs with increased regularity of angles. Once again, the phenomenon discussed earlier: altered states of consciousness are repeatedly associated with brain synchrony, regularity, with unvarying stimuli—or, in this case, a drastic reduction in variability to EEG response. Again, there is the suggestion that whoever or whatever lives in the cortex has temporarily changed its address. And there are the common subjective reports of LSD users that they have had out-of-body experiences—known to researchers as OOBEs.

LSD was first synthesized in 1938 by Albert Hoffman, a Swiss chemist who discovered its hallucinogenic properties by accident five years later. One three-millionth of an ounce is adequate for a trip. The drug's incredible potency and the hope that it might solve the mysteries of mental illness inspired research for years before it was bootlegged and glamorized. A near relative in the organic world is the lysergic acid found in some American morning glory seeds.

Although LSD is not addictive, there is an increased tolerance. Users of one hallucinogen often develop cross tolerance for other psychedelics. The substance has raised more questions about brain chemistry than it has answered, but it has been found useful in radical therapy. Because of its powerful, sometimes unpredictable effects, it is used mostly on those who have not responded to conventional treatment.

Victims of what is now usually considered an organic disorder, autistic children live mutely in a world of their own, are unable to learn except in specially designed environments, and engage in endless self-stimulation: head-banging, finger-shaking, rocking. Several psychologists have treated autistic children with hallucinogens—substantial doses daily or weekly over a prolonged period. Somehow the powerful psychedelic has occasionally accomplished a breakthrough where nothing else has worked.

Lauretta Bender, one of the best-known workers with autistic children, has administered LSD to some children daily for as long as a year. She reported improved speech in otherwise mute children, increased emotional responsiveness, mood elevation, and decreases in the classical compulsive behavior.

They appeared flushed, bright eyed and unusually interested in the environment. . . . They participated with increased eagerness in motility play with adults and other children. . . . They seek positive contacts with adults, approaching them with face uplifted and bright eyes, and respond to fondling, affections, etc.

She also reported that the stereotyped whirling and rhythmic behavior were reduced. Some children showed appropriate facial expressions in reaction to situations for the first time in their young lives.

Alcoholism, like autism, is stubbornly resistant to treatment. In 1952 two Saskatchewan doctors, Humphry Osmond and Abram Hoffer, decided to administer LSD to two alcoholic patients in the hope that it might produce a model of delirium tremens. Hitting the bottom, which ex-alcoholics usually said marked their turning point for recovery, was often accompanied by the DTs.

One of the two alcoholics was cured. That 50-percent recovery rate seems to have held true for every major study of LSD therapy for alcoholism since then. Hoffer and Osmond have observed that their alcoholic patients usually have a pleasant experience that gives them insights into their drinking problems. The investigators recommend LSD therapy in conjunction with counseling and primarily as a prelude to joining Alcoholics Anonymous.

To describe the positive, therapeutic effects of LSD treatment of alcoholics, Osmond coined the word psychedelic. He noted that prescreened alcoholic patients were likelier to have a pschedelic trip than a psychotomimetic experience. Hoffer and Osmond advise screening all alcoholics, not only for prepsychotic symptoms, but for what they have called malvaria, or the mauve factor. Malvarians excrete a substance in their urine that stains mauve on a paper chromatogram sprayed with a specific reagent.

"Purple people" are more common than one might guess. Testing two thousand patients, Hoffer and Osmond found the mauve factor in 33 percent of all alcoholics, 27 percent of the neurotics, 10 percent of the physically ill, and 33 percent of close relatives of malvarians or schizophrenics. It also showed up in 75 percent of the acute schizophrenics, 50 percent of the treated-but-still-ill schizophrenics, and none of those who had recovered from schizophrenia.

Osmond and Hoffer exclude malvarian alcoholics from LSD treatment in most instances. Of sixty malvarians whom they treated, they found that few had a true psychedelic reaction, the effects of the drug were prolonged, and not a single malvarian patient achieved sobriety as a result of the LSD experience.

Some human archetypes and myths surface irrepressibly in altered states of consciousness. One of these is apparently the dynamic urge for psychic death and rebirth. The myth of the ego death and transcendent rebirth seems to be the keystone of LSD psychotherapy.

Stanislav Grof, who first became well-known for successful LSD treatment of stubborn psychoses in his native Czechoslovakia, later became chief of psychiatric services at the Maryland State Psychiatric Research Center in Baltimore. The religious symbolism and mythology of his patients fascinated Grof. Despite geographic and cultural differences, there were remarkable similarities in their serial fantasies. Grof's patients seemed to go through four phases during their term of therapy. In each of the phases, religious symbolism is pronounced.

In phase I, they relived their childhood relationship to religious instruction, particularly the conflicts. In phase II, they experienced agony and suffering, usually within a religious framework; they visited hell in whatever context struck them. Judaic and Christian symbols abound. Patients often identified with Christ during phase II, reliving his humiliation, tortures, his collapse under the heavy cross, and the crucifixion.

In phase III there was a glimmering of hope; patients believed they were being purged. Visions of Moses, the Ten Commandments, the burning bush, Sodom and Gomorrah, and the biblical floods were described.

In the fourth and final phase, they experienced salvation, redemption, and liberation, often seeing their ego death and rebirth as Christ's death and resurrection. Grof likened the liberation to the experiences of primitive Christians. The patients felt that a burden of fear and guilt had been lifted and they were radiantly joyful, filled with love and charity.

A wealth of archetypes from Hindu religion and philosophy appeared in phase IV. Grof noted that the parallels are striking. "The important insights into what is meaningful in life and what man really wants, as they repeatedly appear in the LSD sessions, are in full agreement with the Hindu ideas."

One effect of the purgative phase III seemed to be a rejection of material success and a sense of guilt over seeking cheap pleasures. But after the fourth phase, Grof said, the patients see pleasure as an acceptable if trivial goal, and see worldly success as a valid ambition "if pursued at the proper time and to a reasonable degree."

The patients often experienced a union with God, what Grof calls "a melting ecstasy," and expressed a conviction expressed in the ancient Vedic saying, *Tat tvan asi*—literally translated, "Thou art That," meaning "You are God." Grof also said that the general picture of human personality as layered and dynamic, a Hindu concept, fits perfectly with the LSD experiences which reveal one stratum of personality after another.

Other elements of the LSD session are Buddhic, with patients describing a nirvana, a still and exquisite void. Grof observed that this experience is facilitated by 'white noise. A few patients also described a pure inner being, a crystalline core, corresponding to the *jīva* in Jainism. They often went through transitional periods of vegetarianism.

Rarely, an experience akin to the uncoiling of kundalini in Tantric yoga occurs in advanced sessions. Patients totally unfamiliar with the kundalini doctrine have described a power rushing through the spinal cord to the brain. A few patients have also said that whereas before sexual union was a biological act, they see it now as a sacrament—a view expressed in Tantric yoga.

Memories of past lives, whether their own or others', are frequently reported by patients in phase IV, Grof reports— "usually highly charged memories of scenes involving hatred, hostility, jealousy, humiliation, murder, etc." Commonly the events seem to be in past centuries and in foreign countries. The patients are not insistent on a reincarnation rationale, acknowledging that they may be reaching racial memories, parts of the collective unconscious. They do not elaborate delusionally on the memories.

Grof points out that if LSD is administered to well-adjusted subjects instead of psychiatric patients, they often experience the first transpersonal changes in the first session and quickly go on to the "death and rebirth" experiences.

No one knows why LSD therapy sometimes helps neurotic or psychotic patients who were untouched by traditional psychiatry and medication. Perhaps a lasting, unknown neurological change is involved. Or perhaps the impact of the experience is responsible for some kind of personal breakthrough. Grof may well be right when he says that LSD shows the human mind as "a mighty iceberg with elements of individual and collective unconscious as well as ancient phylogenetic memories buried in the depths." He believes that classical and neoclassical Freudian analysis, so-called depth psychology, barely scratches the surface of the iceberg.

The ability of LSD to diminish pain is not its foremost value in the treatment of terminally ill patients. Its psychological benefits have interested several psychiatrists and psychologists.

In Walter Pahnke's study, patients underwent intensive psychotherapy for several days in advance of their LSD session. During the session they listened to classical music on stereo headphones. Their hospital rooms were filled with flowers and with objects meaningful to them. A therapist and psychiatric nurse remained in attendance throughout the day. Then, toward evening, as the effects were wearing off, family members would join the patient.

The most striking result of the therapy was the loss of fear of death. Pahnke reported that after the patient experienced the relinquishment of ego and the mythical transcendence, he became "intensely aware of completely new dimensions of experience which he might never before have imagined possible."

He observed that patients unfamiliar with the writings of William James would paraphrase his view of the brain as a filter of consciousness which transmits only part of a vaster consciousness. In Pahnke's words, they became aware of the brain as "a partially opaque glass allowing through a few rays of super solar blaze. . . ." The death or disintegration of an individual brain does not cause the larger consciousness to cease, the dying patients concluded from their LSD experience. Repeatedly they described the lowering of a threshold that enabled them to experience an eternal now, beyond time and space. They frequently maintained that they subjectively experienced this while "out of the body." A common report was that they had "come home."

The dangers of psychedelic drugs are two: psychosis and possible chromosome damage. The first is very real, the second not at all confirmed. In those already unstable or inherently susceptible to psychosis, a bad trip can be one-way. In addition to the risk of permanent mental illness, there's an immortality syndrome that sometimes results in unintentional suicide by LSD users and schizophrenics. Having experienced what Pahnke described as the larger consciousness, the user may miss some of its subtler aspects and decide that he can safely leap from a high window.

The afterflash is another danger. An actor took LSD under a friend's supervision. Two weeks later, he telephoned for a taxi and was standing at his second-story window. Just as the cab pulled up, someone stepped out of the next apartment building as if to hail it. The indignant actor opened the window and was about to drop twenty feet to the sidewalk when his roommate grabbed him by the shoulders. In that brief moment he had spontaneously experienced the perceptual changes of LSD, and the sidewalk below had appeared only a step away.

The controversy about LSD and possible chromosome breakage is another matter. Scientists have adopted language unique to each field, as all specialists do, and it becomes difficult for them to translate their findings for the press. In March 1967 a report of possible correlation between LSD use and chromosome breakage was reported in *Science*. Although other scientists immediately challenged the report as ambiguous and although even its authors said their material was inconclusive, the press announced within twenty-four hours that LSD caused chromosome breakage. Later *The Saturday Evening Post* published a story titled "The Hidden Evils of LSD" and illustrated it with uncaptioned pictures of horribly deformed babies. One page heading proclaimed, "If you take LSD your children may be born malformed or retarded." Similar horror stories appeared in other general-circulation magazines.

Meanwhile, other scientists were publishing conflicting reports. Chromosome breakage is not yet clearly attributable to LSD for several reasons. (1) It can be caused by temperature changes, changes in oxygen pressure, some viruses or antibiotics, calcium and magnesium deficiencies, chloroform, mercury compounds, or morphine. In one experiment aspirin was demonstrated to cause chromosome breakage at the same rate as LSD. (2) Most experiments have involved chromosomes in laboratory preparations rather than in a living organism. Living organisms can often render substances harmless that are shown to cause damage in a test tube. (3) In the few cases in which badly deformed infants were born to women who had been using LSD, the mothers had also been taking other drugs, including marijuana, barbiturates, and amphetamines. LSD is rarely the only potent drug an individual takes. (4) Some researchers used doses of LSD many times larger than human beings would ingest at a single time. (5) All six abnormal infants reported in the literature were born to women ingesting illicit LSD, which may be contaminated or adulterated in comparison to laboratory LSD. (6) LSD ingested during the first trimester of pregnancy would probably act directly on the growing fetus, as other drugs are known to act, rather than via the chromosomes.

In 1971 *Science,* the journal whose article first triggered the controversy, published a contradictory paper surveying ninety-two reports that had appeared in the intervening years. Norman Dishotsky, Wendell Lipscomb, W. D. Loughman, and Robert Mogar concluded:

> From our own work and from a review of the literature, we believe that pure LSD ingested in moderate doses does not damage chromosomes *in vivo,* does not cause detectable genetic damage, and is not a teratogen or a carcinogen in man. Within these bounds, therefore, we suggest that, other than during pregnancy, there is no present contraindication to the continued controlled experimental use of pure LSD.

A review in the *American Journal of Psychiatry,* covering fifteen studies, came to the same general conclusion. Since those surveys, however, another disquieting report has surfaced. Edward Voss, a microbiologist at the University of Illinois, found that either LSD or one of its metabolic by-products shut off the production of antibodies in spleen and lymph-node cells studied in the laboratory. Earlier there had been informal reports from doctors that LSD users seemed to have difficulty in recovering from infections.

In any event, nearly all clinical applications of LSD involve subjects whose plights warrant some risk—alcoholics, the mentally ill, the terminally ill, autistic children.

In his report on drug abuse to the Ford Foundation and in his book *The Natural Mind,* Andrew Weil suggested that the problem of psychedelic abuse can only be dealt with if we recognize the human hunger for altering consciousness. Pointing out that virtually every culture in history has had its methods for achieving nonordinary awareness, he recommended that society furnish a safe framework for experimentation. Perhaps this would be the ritual administration of mind-altering drugs to adolescents by adults wise enough to guide them through the experience, as in some tribal cultures.

After learning the limitations of drugs, the young people would theoretically then be ready to explore nonchemical techniques for altering consciousness. Weil said:

> One sees many long-time drug users give up drugs for meditation, such as Richard Alpert,* who became Baba Ram Dass, a disciple of a Hindu guru. But one does not see any long-time meditators give up meditation to become acid-heads. This observation supports the contention that the highs obtainable by meditation are better than highs obtainable through drugs—a contention phrased not in moral terms but in simple, practical ones.

Studies at UCLA, Harvard, and in Malmö, Sweden, have shown that transcendental meditation is an astonishingly successful replacement for the drug high. Use of psychedelics, amphetamines, opiates, and alcohol was decimated in the experimental groups. In one study 83 percent of the 143 subjects stopped using drugs completely. The Swedish researchers used subjects

---

* Alpert and Timothy Leary were co-experimenters with LSD when both were young Harvard instructors. Alpert was an advocate of such experimentation for many years.

known clinically as abusers. Ironically, they were able to use their control group for only the first three-month period rather than the six months they had planned because there was so much pressure from control subjects who wanted to learn to meditate.

Eva Brautigan reported that the Malmö experiment supported the statement of Wallace and Benson of Harvard: "Student drug users are, as a group, knowledgeable about the undesirable effects of drug abuse. In general, it is not difficult for most student abusers to stop. The issue is to get them to want to stop."

John Lilly, Richard Alpert, and the anthropologist Carlos Castaneda, all demi-gurus of the psychedelic counterculture, have spoken widely of their own discoveries that drugs offer only an intimation of the richness of expanded consciousness. Castaneda described hallucinatory drugs as deleterious. Recalling his long psychedelic career, Alpert said, "It was a terribly frustrating experience, as if you came into the kingdom of heaven and you saw how it all was and you felt these new states of awareness, and then you got cast out again. . . ."

11

DRUGGING THE BRAIN: THE TROJAN HORSE

I have very poor and unhappy brains for drinking.
—WILLIAM SHAKESPEARE, OTHELLO

The term drug abuse usually brings to mind heroin, LSD, and marijuana. Ironically, the psychedelics and morphine derivatives are not the major culprits in society's drug crisis. Although heroin undeniably plays greatest havoc with an individual's life and contributes most heavily to crime statistics, its users are surprisingly few in number.

Tragedy on a grand scale can be blamed on drugs that can be obtained legally. According to state and federal narcotics authorities, the most abused drugs are amphetamines, barbiturates, and alcohol.

In 1972 barbiturates were the number one drug problem in Los Angeles schools, surpassing both marijuana and alcohol. In a five-year period, state law-enforcement seizures of barbiturates had risen 2000 percent.

And according to a parade of medical witnesses before the House Select Committee on crime, the most widespread, incapacitating, and dangerous addiction problem in the United States is amphetamine abuse. Pep-pill addiction has reached epidemic proportions among white middle- and upper-class young people. The U.S. Justice Department, in a desperate effort to control the illicit traffic, ordered the nation's pharmaceutical houses to cut their 1972 amphetamine production quota *more than 80 percent* from the previous year.*

* Ten billion units had been legally manufactured in 1971. Although technically much of the production is exported, all too often shipments

As amphetamine abuse began edging down slightly, barbiturates picked up. A similar curtailment was imposed on the manufacture and distribution of barbiturates. Meanwhile, a new drug fad hit. Suburban teenagers were buying and selling "sopors," a non-barbiturate sleeping pill (methaqualone—brandname, Quaalude). This time the manufacturers began notifying federal narcotics officers that the drugs were being stolen from the factory.

The impact of psychoactive drugs on brain and body is little-understood, even by those who use them regularly, and many physicians become blasé about the pharmaceuticals they prescribe. Doctors, in fact, are a high-risk group for narcotic addiction. Surprisingly, pharmacists, who have maximum access, are a low-risk group. The explanation among them is that they know too much about drugs to become dangerously involved.

Commenting in *Science* on the hazards of psychoactive drugs, four psychiatric researchers warned:

> In the giving and taking of drugs, one pays for what one gets. The double entries in this ledger are too often ignored. . . . It is part of contemporary medical mythology that drugs somehow do not exact the same price from the user when they are prescribed by a physician.

The psychiatrists reminded their fellow scientists that the body's own self-regulatory functions may be taken over by the drugs used.

This danger is clearly demonstrated by a homely example: the chronic constipation that results from laxative abuse. Eventually natural peristalsis disappears because the drugs have assumed the task of stimulating intestinal contractions.

The body's eventual submission to the intruding agent can be fatal. A sharp increase in the number of deaths from asthma in Great Britain paralleled the introduction of the popular bronchodilators. These inhalers contain substances whose action mimics the body's own sympathetic nervous system. Allergists

---

have been smuggled back into the United States. The drug is also synthesized in black-market laboratories. Whatever the source, in one recent year federal agents seized more than ten million dosage units in the illicit market.

suspect that their use may eventually result in the failure of the natural emergency response. In a critical respiratory situation, no adrenaline pours forth. Of the asthmatics whose deaths were investigated in Great Britain in recent years, 84 percent had been using pressure aerosol bronchodilators prescribed by their physicians.

Paul Ehrlich once anticipated that drugs might be magic bullets, aiming only for a specific organ or virus. Alas, all drugs have side effects. Among those whose primary effect is on the brain are amphetamines, barbiturates, psychedelics, tranquilizers, antidepressants, and the morphine derivatives. Even hormones primarily affect the brain; the Pill, in large, therapeutic doses, caused temporary psychosis in 4 percent of the wives of armed forces personnel being treated for infertility. Drugs with specific ambitions—diuretics, antihistamines—may be indirectly psychoactive.

World War II was fought not only with tanks and bombers but with bennies and dexies. Both sides used brain stimulants for battle fatigue and to keep pilots alert on long missions. Because Japanese munitions factory workers were stoked on amphetamines, the pharmaceutical manufacturers found themselves with great stockpiles at the end of the war. They began pushing amphetamines as energy aids, and by the mid-1950s there were half a million amphetamine addicts in Japan. Fifty-thousand cases of amphetamine psychosis had been reported.

Japan outlawed amphetamines in 1954, and within a few years the epidemic was over. In 1964, in response to a sharp increase in crimes of violence believed linked to addiction, Sweden also banned amphetamines.

The drug was first synthesized in the late 1800s, but the first commercial product, Benzedrine, was not marketed until 1932. In 1938 the first three reports of amphetamine psychosis appeared. All three involved narcoleptics, victims of a puzzling malady in which they may be overcome by sleep in midsentence or while walking down the street. The three had all greatly exceeded the prescribed dosage.

For many years, the euphoric effect of amphetamines was not popular knowledge. The early users were primarily truck drivers, athletes, students cramming for exams, dieting housewives, narcoleptics, and hyperkinetic children. (Paradoxically, amphetamines tend to calm children with certain neurological problems—and, for some reason, the children don't become addicted. Neither do most narcoleptics.)

Solomon Snyder, a Johns Hopkins pharmacologist, traces the first widespread addiction to San Francisco in the mid-1960s when hippies began adding Methedrine to LSD to intensify the effect. Some skipped the LSD and became speed freaks. The speed freak, as Snyder sees it, "often could not tolerate the overwhelming self-revelation induced by LSD and preferred instead to be high, pure and simple."

In capsule form, amphetamines are colloquially called crank, pep pills, cartwheels, copilots, West Coast turnarounds, truck drivers, bennies, dexies, footballs, purple hearts, greenies, coast-to-coasts, black beauties, uppers and ups. Reportedly the term copilot originated from the story of a truck driver on amphetamines who had driven for two days without respite. When he was latter pulled from the wreckage of his truck, he explained to officers that he had decided to crawl into the bunk behind the cab for a nap, while the other driver took over. Unfortunately, his copilot was a figment of the amphetamine; he had been alone all along.

The addict may eventually tolerate a daily dosage one hundred times that prescribed by the manufacturer, and he usually ends up injecting methamphetamine intravenously. As it takes effect he experiences what is known as the flash or the rush, an intensely euphoric moment that has been described as "an orgasm all over your body."

Even the nonaddicted user feels euphoric, confident, and alert on amphetamine, and it is easy to see why this drug is so addictive. The euphoria is not otherworldly, as with the opiates; it is rather an elation, as after good news. The user becomes talkative and excited.

Amphetamines are similar in their structure to adrenaline. They are believed to release the brain's transmitter chemicals at the synapse, the gap between nerve cells. Ordinarily, as soon as the chemicals have done their job in passing the message along to the adjacent cell, they are inactivated; the cell takes up the transmitter again. Amphetamines prevent the re-uptake. The substances continue to excite their neighboring cells. It is as if every light on a switchboard has gone on.

Apparently this prodigal activity eventually exhausts the cells' supply of norepinephrine (NE), one of the transmitters. A sudden letdown may follow a lengthy amphetamine high. Exhausted drivers who press their luck by taking one amphetamine after another may black out at the wheel. The drug has caused profound hypoglycemia in animal experiments, so the blackouts may result from insulin shock.

Prolonged heavy usage inevitably brings on a psychotic episode, a phenomenon many researchers think may lead to a breakthrough in understanding the chemistry of schizophrenia. Amphetamine psychosis is indistinguishable from paranoid schizophrenia. Auditory hallucinations predominate, as in acute paranoid schizophrenia, and the same drug (phenothiazine) is used to treat both. At Vanderbilt University, John Griffin induced psychosis by increasing the amphetamine dosage of four young volunteer addicts. Within two to five days each cracked up. One told the doctors that he was the target of "rays from a giant oscillator," and another confided that his wife was planning to murder him.

Later interviews determined that in each case the subject's first paranoid thinking had preceded overt psychotic symptoms by about eight hours. Psychotic symptoms disappeared within eight hours of drug withdrawal in three of the four subjects. The fourth was not clear of symptoms for another three days.

Snyder and his co-workers, observing that amphetamines affect the brain's pathways for two transmitters, dopamine and norepinephrine, believe that the drugs provide vital clues to schizophrenia. The speed freak exhibits not only hyperactivity but bizarre, repetitive behavior. He may fold and refold a handkerchief, may thump a table leg for twenty minutes. Snyder suggests that dopamine stimulation probably accounts for the repetitive behavior and that NE stimulation is responsible for the euphoria, appetite suppression, and hyperactivity. (NE tracts ascend through a pleasure center in the forebrain and also probe the hypothalamus, where they may affect not only pleasure regions but also the satiety center.)

Snyder conjectures that the peculiar behavior and feelings

brought on by the relentless dopamine stimulation puzzle the addict. Because the NE stimulation has alerted him, he begins scanning the environment for an explanation of what is happening to him. That is when the paranoid ideation surfaces. Investigators are now searching for a drug that stimulates only the dopamine systems. Snyder believes that such a drug might well produce pure schizophrenia rather than the paranoid type seen in amphetamine addicts.

Although cocaine is officially listed as a narcotic in federal annals, it is actually a brain stimulant. First isolated from the coca leaf in 1859, cocaine was known to be addictive by 1890 but has never approached the present popularity of amphetamines. Known colloquially as coke and snow, the drug is usually sniffed. Overdoses of both cocaine and amphetamine can be toxic.

Some barbiturate addicts take amphetamines simultaneously to counteract the drowsiness produced by the downers. They like the barbiturate intoxication but they don't want to pass out.

Nowhere is the magic bullet myth more melancholy than in man's search for a harmless sedative. Alcohol has been abused for thousands of years. In the nineteenth century, chloral hydrate and paraldehyde were introduced as sedatives, and then abused. First marketed in 1903, barbiturates were expected to supplant the earlier drugs safely. When barbiturate addiction became a social problem, new sedatives and hypnotics—and then tranquilizers—were introduced and in turn became widely abused. Ironically, it was a search for a safe sedative that brought about the thalidomide tragedy in which thousands of European babies were damaged prenatally. Unlike barbiturates, thalidomide could be taken in enormous amounts without toxic effect—on the user.

Barbiturates interfere with the brain's oxygen supply and its ability, therefore, to integrate stimuli. Other effects are pupil contraction, slurred speech, muscular incoordination. Because of impaired intellectual function, the confused user may commit involuntary suicide by fatally overestimating the time elapsed since his last barbiturates. By depressing the respiratory centers, barbiturates can produce coma or death. Although heavy users develop a tolerance for the desired effect and must continually increase their dosages, they do not develop corresponding tolerance for the lethal effects. Joseph Busch, Los Angeles County district attorney, told Senate investigators in 1972 that during the preceding year only alcohol had contributed to more deaths in the county than barbiturates. Barbiturate overdose had killed 971 compared to 242 deaths from hard narcotics.

In many urban areas, even elementary-school children can obtain barbiturates from a young pusher if not from the family medicine chest. Busch told of one eight-year-old who had been "dropping a red" every day after school because, he said, he enjoyed the feeling it gave him. (Barbiturates are also known as barbs, goofballs, yellow-jackets, downs, downers.)

The barbiturate addict's liver has developed the enzyme capacity to detoxify the abusive doses quickly. A state of hyperactivity and excitement precedes the down feeling. Like amphetamines, barbiturates can produce violence and derangement. Unlike amphetamine withdrawal, sudden barbiturate withdrawal can kill a full-fledged addict. The drug should be withdrawn gradually in a hospital environment.

Most drugs interfere with rapid-eye-movement sleep periods, and barbiturates virtually eliminate them. An individual who has been using sleeping pills over a long period and then withdraws will go through days or weeks of REM sleep, as if the brain is urgently trying to compensate for the long dry spell. Unfortunately, the accompanying nightmares often drive the user back to barbiturates.

The effect on REM sleep may be one of the gravest side effects of many drugs. Because these periods seem to serve an array of restorative, vital functions, even the individual who takes only one legal Seconal each night may be doing slow but sure damage to his overall health.

During an eight-month period, Washington Hospital Center in the District of Columbia treated thirty-six patients for what could have been either acute schizophrenia—or toxic psychosis caused by an over-the-counter sleeping medication. Such products as Sominex, Sleep-Eze, and Compoz contain scopolamine, an alkaloid. Many cold compounds and antihistamine capsules also contain scopolamine.

"Antihistamines scare me to death," said Richard Orkand of

UCLA. Orkand maintains that antihistamines should never have been made available over the counter. The drowsiness caused by Compoz and Nitol is due to an antihistamine, incidentally. Orkand remarked that a California law makes it an offense to drive while under their influence.

The mental dulling may be due to the reduced amount of histamine which functions as a brain transmitter.

Alcohol's action on the brain has not yet been spelled out, but some interesting theories have been put forth. Gerald Cohen of Columbia University's College of Physicians and Surgeons and Michael Collins, New York State Psychiatric Institute, announced that a metabolite of alcohol combines with epinephrine (adrenaline) and norepinephrine to form alkaloids similar to those found in the peyote cacti. Virginia Davis, a VA researcher in Houston, and Michael Walsh of Baylor suggested that the metabolic disposition of the transmitter dopamine may be modified by alcohol to form a morphine-like substance. A morphine-like metabolite could certainly explain the addiction.

The brain's reaction to alcohol is complex. Although the drug is technically a depressant, in small amounts it may act as a stimulant by releasing inhibitions. For many years it was believed that alcohol's action was to affect one brain center after another. More recently researchers have related its effects to changes in the brain's reticular formation, the center of sleep and attention mechanisms. Progressive intoxication is believed to cause a progressive shutdown of the arousal machinery, beginning with diminished alertness and ending in relative unconsciousness. Alcohol may interfere with the transmission of impulses at the synapse. It clearly affects the oxygen available to the brain.

Even a small amount of alcohol slows the brain's ability to process and integrate information. In a study at UCLA, Herbert Moskowitz gave the subjects each a single drink containing four ounces of vodka in orange juice. Their information-processing ability lagged by 11.5 percent.

The common subjective feeling that a little alcohol lubricates the mind is largely an illusion. German scientists designed a simple experiment in which the subject had to respond with his right hand to a tap on the left knee, and vice versa. The taps came at irregular intervals. An electrical measurement showed that alcohol shortened the subjects' reaction time over their sober performance but also greatly increased the errors.

Sixty-four medical students at Yale were measurably better at solving problems in symbolic logic when they had had a small dose of alcohol. Apparently it curbed their self-doubts and reduced tension enough to facilitate the mental functions in some individuals. Heavier doses resulted in a worse-than-sober performance.

Researchers blame coagulation caused by alcohol for the death of brain cells. Alcohol creates a clumping effect in red blood cells which then block capillaries. The brain cells fed by those capillaries are then starved for oxygen. Because brain cells are unable to regenerate, the damage is permanent.

Whether or not coagulation is a grave factor, alcoholism causes brain damage gross enough to be seen without the aid of a microscope. The pathologist may see brain lesions, varicose veins, a damage to the hippocampus. The last probably accounts for the memory deficiency seen in some alcoholics.

After several attacks of delirium tremens, the alcoholic may develop a chronic, incurable, and sometimes fatal condition known as wet brain. Confusion becomes chronic, the functions of the central nervous system are impaired, and if the victim doesn't die he will be permanently institutionalized. In the Wernicke-Korsakoff syndrome the patient has no recent memory. He tells lies, unaware that he is lying. The brain damage evident in postmortems is similar to that produced in animals by deprivation of thiamine (vitamin B_1). Megavitamin therapy has been effective in the treatment of alcoholics, but by the time this syndrome is seen nothing seems to help.

Cyril Courville, director of the neuropathology laboratory of Los Angeles County Hospital, believes that alcohol acts directly on the cell membrane and protoplasm. "While one must recognize that each individual alcoholic insult to the vulnerable brain is not marked by any recognizable change in the individual nerve cells, slowly and imperceptibly these elements are undergoing punishment that many of them cannot withstand forever."

Eleanor Jacobs and her research team at the VA Hospital in Buffalo found that they could reverse transient memory loss in some elderly patients by giving them powerful oxygen treatments. Of the failures, half were alcoholics. Strangely, the oxygen treatment seemed to intensify their memory loss.

Alcohol suppresses REM sleep. Laboratory records show that when an alcoholic withdraws, he spends 100 percent of his sleep time in REM for several nights preceding his first round of DTs. Some alcohol investigators believe that delirium tremens hallucinations are dreams breaking into the waking state because of the tremendous pressure built up for REM activity.

Genetic predisposition plays a role in alcoholism. According to a study conducted by Washington University (St. Louis) researchers, alcoholics' sons reared in foster homes by nonalcoholics show a much higher rate of alcoholism as adults than do men whose own biological parents were not alcoholic but who were reared by an alcoholic foster parent.

Racial differences in physiological response to alcohol have been observed. Japanese, Taiwanese, and Koreans, even in infancy, are more sensitive to alcohol than Caucasians. (The responses measured included flushing and optical changes.) Scientists have hypothesized that the intolerance of the Tarahumara Indians of northwestern Mexico for alcohol may be due to an inherited metabolic trait that is also responsible for their astonishing physical endurance.

Gender differences in alcohol metabolism may destroy an old myth. On a pound-for-pound basis, women may be able to hold their liquor better than men. In mice, whose metabolic processes are surprisingly similar to those of human beings, females metabolize and excrete alcohol's intermediate product acetaldehyde more quickly than males.

Therapeutic uses for alcohol are being explored. It appears to enhance the moods of elderly nursing-home residents. In one, an old-fashioned beer tavern was set up for the patients. And in England, alcohol has been given freely to terminally ill patients in the hope that they might suffer less from pain and anxiety.

Nicotine is a habituating drug, not an addictive one. Although smokers would probably disagree, scientists say that there are no significant physiological withdrawal symptoms when one quits smoking. Nicotine's well-known arousal effect

—heightened blood pressure, increased heart rate, increased respiratory activity—probably involves the brain's hippocampus. Its effect on appetite, sometimes blamed on a gradual dulling of the taste buds, is thought to be due to its action on appetite centers in the hypothalamus.

In experiments with both human and animal subjects, large doses of nicotine have produced tremors and even convulsions. Brainwave changes are clear-cut, as are differences between the EEGs of smokers and nonsmokers. Italian researchers reported an 80-percent drop in EEG voltage and a speeding up of the alpha rhythm during smoking. The EEG changes may be due to increased adrenaline or to lowered cerebral oxygen caused by a combination of carbon monoxide and nicotine. This may account for the fact that smokers show a noticeably smaller amount of alpha than nonsmokers and that the alpha they do have is usually of a higher frequency. Withdrawal from nicotine for twenty-four hours has been shown to slow the alpha frequencies.

The psychological aspects may also be important. In a study of healthy young adults, an increase in the dominant alpha frequency was observed not only with nicotine ingestion but also in some subjects who were puffing on placebos.

No reasonable observer would deny the positive role of psychoactive drugs in mankind's armamentarium against disease. Amphetamines, dangerous as they are when abused, have enabled thousands of neurologically handicapped children to function normally during their critical learning years. Even barbiturates serve a useful purpose when they provide respite for those who desperately need it. Lithium therapy has given a new lease on life to untold numbers of former manic-depressives. The major and minor tranquilizers, used cautiously, serve a therapeutic purpose.

But alas, we have assigned to drugs a savior role they can't play. Tens of millions of prescriptions for tranquilizers, barbiturates, and stimulants are filled annually, and these drugs become part of the life-style of tens of millions of our citizens. This point was made in the *Science* article quoted earlier:

Changing the human environment is a monumental undertaking. While seeking to change cognitive shapes through chemical means is more convenient and economical, the drug solution has already become another technological Trojan horse.

Drug action is complicated not only by the user's mental state (i.e., phase of brain activity) but also by the time of day. Gay Gaer Luce warns of the inadequacy of our present drug-testing procedures, which don't take into account the oscillations of the body's own chemistry over a 24-hour period. Doses of amphetamine high enough to kill 6 percent of laboratory mice at 6 A.M. killed 77.6 percent of the same strain of mice at midnight. Even alcohol has wildly fluctuating effects. Mice were injected with alcohol the equivalent of one quart of vodka consumed by a human being. The group injected at their period of awakening had a 60-percent mortality rate. Mortality was 12 percent in those given the alcohol at the beginning of their rest period.

Drugs as Trojan horse might be exemplified by the history of the hard narcotics. When morphine was introduced to the medical world of the West, it appeared that the harmless pain-killer had at last been found. Addiction became a major problem. When heroin was first synthesized from morphine, it was hoped that it was less dangerous. By 1914 there were 200,000 addicts in the United States, according to one estimate, and probably many times more who were never counted.

Authorities estimate that today there are only 60,000, nearly half in New York City alone. Seventy-five percent of the addicts are in the ten largest cities. Surprisingly enough, fewer Vietnam veterans are addicted than nonveterans. Still, because heroin addiction is more deadly than any other drug abuse, great effort has been poured into programs to get the addict off H. Heroin addicts are being converted to Methadone addicts. Methadone is cheaper, safer, and allows the user to live a relatively normal life. However, a number of deaths from Methadone overdose have been reported, and it is now known that babies born to Methadone addicts become addicted prenatally. One study reported that twenty-three such babies had suffered for up to ninety days after birth from such Methadone-withdrawal symptoms as irritability, violent twitching, and cold sweats.

Even our most refined psychoactive drugs are indescribably crude compared to the system they act upon. It is as if we were attempting to repair a delicate watch with a large screwdriver and a pair of dime-store pliers.

SLEEP CONSCIOUSNESS:
THE DREAMING BRAIN

The dream is its own interpretation.

—THE TALMUD, QUOTED BY CARL JUNG

Experimenters, curious about whether animals would hallucinate in sensory isolation as human beings do, devised a training procedure in which rhesus monkeys were placed in restraining chairs and trained to press a bar rapidly every time a faint image appeared on a screen. If they failed they were given a shock.

After the monkeys were thoroughly trained, they were fitted with corneal contact lenses which gave them a monotonous visual field and placed in isolation. Like human beings in similar dull environments, the monkeys fell asleep. Whenever they would enter the rapid-eye-movement or REM stage of sleep, associated with intense visual imagery in human beings, the monkeys would begin bar-pressing frantically.

Sleep and dream research has grown more rapidly than any other aspect of brain research during the past two decades, yet the findings are little known to the public. For example, although evidence has been accumulating since the early 1960s that dreaming, fragments of dreams, and random thoughts are continuous throughout sleep, books and magazine articles still tend to speak of REM periods and dreaming as if they were synonymous.

Sleep has become an all-but-useless term. There is no unitive sleep state, but at least two types of sleep arising from two overlapping brain systems. Nor is sleep a quiescent state. Many populations of brain cells are more active than in the waking state. Furthermore, the mind maintains constant awareness of its surroundings and is able to respond at times even from the deepest slumber. Laboratory volunteers have demonstrated that they can awaken within a few minutes of an assigned time. And now there is evidence that not even chemically induced unconsciousness is true oblivion.

Because mental activity is apparently unceasing, researchers are struggling for consensus on what constitutes a dream. David Foulkes of the University of Wyoming, one of the first workers to emphasize the problem of definition, has devised a dream fantasy scale ranging from one through seven. Fragmentary, pedestrian thoughts would score one; a bizarre, thoroughly plotted nightmare would rate the top score, seven.

As the brain drifts toward sleep, its electrical patterns change. Volleys of slow, large-amplitude alpha appear, and imagery may surface—fragmentary images with little emotional impact. This is the hypnagogic stage, neither sleep nor waking.

After a few minutes another downward shift is marked by mixed EEG frequencies. This is Stage 1 and lasts from one to seven minutes. Sleep spindles (loose, jagged patterns) begin to appear on the graph, signifying the onset of Stage 2. Individuals awakened from either of these stages may insist that they have not really been asleep. Mental activity in these segments could best be described as reverie.

The EEG then begins to trace great peaks and valleys many times the voltage of waking alpha activity. Stage 3 is typified by a slowdown of vital activity: heart rate, blood pressure, temperature. An observer would describe the subject as sound asleep.

As the subject's slumber deepens into Stage 4, the EEG shows an even greater amount of the bold script of the slow waves. This is a curious altered state. Drawing a subject out of it is difficult. By the time he is awake he has very likely lost any recollection of dreams or thought fragments—yet mental activity has clearly taken place. So-called night terrors, sleep talking, and sleepwalking all take place during Stage 4. The somnambulist may move about the sleep laboratory with his eyes open. He walks around obstacles and may even make cryptic remarks, yet he is blind and deaf to his questioners. If awakened, he recalls nothing of the episode nor of his dream's subject matter. Night terrors are marked by a panicky awakening, perhaps screaming, but no recollection of what was so frightening.

Every ninety minutes or so the sleeper ascends from the deeper stages to the strange world sometimes known as Stage REM (rapid-eye-movement) or paradoxical sleep (because the brainwave pattern is so similar to that of waking).

If we were to liken Stages 1 through 4 to a graceful ballet, paradoxical sleep (Stage REM) would come on like a horde of dervish dancers. The backdrop, too, would change. Against a background of the fast EEG activity, loss of muscle tone, doubled blood volume in the brain, there are also intermittent, almost convulsive changes during paradoxical sleep. Researchers refer to the changes of the overall state as *tonic,* the periodic phenomena as *phasic.*

The body's sympathetic nervous system puts on a spectacular show of alarm. The heart rate surges, slows, surges again wildly. Body temperature rises, blood pressure becomes erratic. Stress hormones increase; so do levels of fatty acids. Respiration becomes more rapid. Under the closed lids, the eyes begin darting frantically at speeds not seen in waking consciousness.

Paradoxical sleep can be fraught with risk: Duodenal ulcer patients may experience an enormous increase in gastric acid. An intense paradoxical sleep period may bring on a fatal stroke or coronary, in which case dying in one's sleep is hardly a tranquil end. Statistically, heart attacks occur most commonly during the nocturnal hours of greatest REM frequency. There is even speculation that the sudden-death syndrome in infants happens during this paradoxical sleep.

In males of all ages, testosterone levels rise prior to paradoxical-sleep periods, and a penile erection occurs. These changes seem to be unrelated to erotic dream content.

With the violent paradoxical phase of sleep, the transmitter chemical norepinephrine either increases or becomes more available. That may explain why some manic-depressives go to bed depressed and wake up manic. Intense cellular activity has been observed during these phases; protein synthesis seems to be stepped up.

Mental activity shifts into the bizarre format we have come to think of as dreaming. A relative paralysis caused by a sudden lack of muscle tone keeps the dreamer from acting out his dream (and may account for the terrifying inability to scream or run in nightmares). Very likely REM dreams are more vivid and more easily recollected because of this dynamic arousal. They are also more fantastic than the dreams of slow-wave sleep.

As night wears on, the mental imagery in all sleep stages becomes more intense and dreamlike. Longer interludes of paradoxical sleep and more frequent autonomic storms are observed. A sleeper allowed to awaken spontaneously usually awakens from paradoxical sleep.

Sleep is not oblivion. For reasons we can only guess at, higher mammals have evolved this peculiar tandem of altered states, and some element therein is crucial to life. Sleep may mend the body, regenerate unknown vital substances, perhaps detoxify unknown poisons.

The enigma that most fascinates sleep theorists is paradoxical sleep. Why has it evolved? What triggers it, and what turns it off? Drug use has made it especially imperative to answer these questions because most psychoactive drugs interfere with paradoxical sleep. We need to know how serious the deprivation is.

Rapid eye movements in paradoxical sleep are measured in unborn children, in the congenitally blind, and even in human and animal subjects without a cerebral cortex. Very few researchers now believe REMs to be synonymous with actual visual scanning of dream images, although there may occasionally be a correspondence. Ralph Berger, a sleep researcher at the University of California at Santa Cruz, has pointed out that some people have characteristic eye-movement patterns in paradoxical sleep—vertical, horizontal—that change slowly over their lives. The rapid eye movements may also play some role in the renewing of binocularity in the eyes.

Paradoxical sleep may involve activity more basic to survival than early investigators guessed. Frederick Snyder, National Institute of Mental Health, commented that "the sheer universality, regularity, and lawfulness of this phenomenon smack of a basic biological process." Snyder suggested that dreaming has become integrated with this older mechanism much as human speech makes use of the ancient biological mechanism of respiration.

Barry Sterman of UCLA noted that Nathaniel Kleitman,

coauthor of the first report of the REM phenomenon in 1952, had originally suggested that the phase might correspond to waking cycles. "But the researchers took off down a dream-REM correspondence path. They forgot that he kept saying it was part of a permanent cycle."

Researchers now speak of the biological hour, the basic rest and activity cycle. These periods of 90–120 minutes mark off our waking activity in a way that corresponds to the sleeping REMs.

One much-cited example is the timing of the typical work-day, which seems to assume a need for rest and restoration every ninety minutes or so: nine-o'clock starting hour, break at 10:30, work resumed until noon . . . and so on, around the clock. The crest of these waves would be the paradoxical sleep phase or its waking counterpart, a burst of energy and efficiency.

The deprivation of paradoxical sleep results in mild behavioral changes such as heightened sexual tension and increased appetite. Depriving a subject of this sleep is all but impossible after a time because the instant he is asleep he enters REM. Subjects have been awakened thirty or more times per night in an attempt to prevent REM activity.

Human beings and animals who have been deprived of REM time show a great rebound of that phase when they are allowed to sleep spontaneously again. Even so, the effects seem to level off after a prolonged period of deprivation.

Paradoxical sleep has inspired countless theories, many of them complementary. Any, all, or none may be valid. The periodic arousal may serve to protect a creature from environmental threats. Ian Oswald, whose work at the University of Edinburgh has contributed much to sleep science, believes that paradoxical sleep is a period of cellular repair. Others think that the phenomenon is a source of sensory stimulation for the nervous system, perhaps essential to its maturation. Another theory suggests that REM sleep reflects intense discharges that are gradually depressed as an infant's forebrain matures.

Building on Giuseppe Moruzzi's concept of two types of activity in paradoxical sleep, William Dement and his associates at Stanford have looked closely at a neural discharge that apparently involves an interaction of brain structures. These discharges—PGO * spikes—occur most heavily, but not exclusively, during paradoxical sleep. These bursts may bring on the intense visual imagery associated with REM sleep, and, during the interburst lulls, the brain as playwright links these elements together with dramatic unity.

Dement's team, by a series of intricate experiments, demonstrated that the PGO spikes, not the REM sleep, are the critical element. They even managed to deprive cats of paradoxical sleep without interfering with the spike production, and none of the usual REM rebound followed this deprivation.

If animals were deprived of sleep altogether, the PGO spikes began to appear in waking consciousness. The cats seemed to be hallucinating and became enraged, ravenously hungry, and hypersexual. The researchers saw previously indifferent male cats "stalk a raging, clawing, highly resistant tom and persevere until the quarry is finally backed into a corner where a mount can be executed."

Dement suggests that it is not the lack of paradoxical sleep per se that causes the mysterious buildup resulting in a rebound, but rather that it is an accumulation of undischarged phasic activities. He postulates a sort of power pack in the brain, a neural system that provides energy for certain "more or less preprogrammed behavioral reflexes." Such a hypothetical system would accumulate metabolic energy without leakage. To accommodate sudden demands; the brain would have to maintain a reservoir. The organism could then expend energy furiously in an emergency.

Obviously, the power pack would have to discharge some of its energy from time to time as a regulatory device. According to this theory, paradoxical sleep is the safety valve by which the excess energy is discharged. Because the motor centers are virtually paralyzed, the brain can set off storms of neural activity "without behavioral consequence." Dement conjectures that nerve cells sensitive to the transmitter serotonin regulate this powerful drive system.

One puzzling finding in earlier research had been the ceiling on REM rebounds. After deprivation there would be a rebound but only up to a certain point. The power-pack theory would

* Pontine-geniculo-occipital spikes.

account for it: Once the reservoir of energy has been depleted, there would be no further drive to discharge.

This accumulation would be like the force building inside a pressure cooker. As long as small amounts of steam are discharged, a relatively stable state is maintained. *Without* this periodic discharge, enough pressure could build up to blow off the cooker's petcock—and send a steady jet of steam through the vent. Eventually, however, the accumulated pressure would be relieved. The uncontrolled discharge would end.

Schizophrenic patients, if deprived of paradoxical sleep, showed no rebound. This strongly hints that they are discharging phasic activity (PGO spikes) while awake. "This has far-reaching implications for understanding the bizarre abnormalities of behavior that accompany this illness," Dement said.

Indeed, if the acute schizophrenic is experiencing waking PGO bursts, they may seem to him to be externally caused. Animals behaved as if they thought the effects were caused from outside themselves. If so, one can understand the common complaint of schizophrenics that they are being "shot through with rays," that "electricity is falling from the sky" or being directed at them through air vents or radiators.

The apparent tie between sleep disturbance and mental illness is striking. Paranoid schizophrenia, sleep-deprivation psychosis, and amphetamine psychosis are first cousins. There is some evidence that acute schizophrenia may sometimes be the product of prolonged insomnia rather than its cause. The manipulations of brain chemistry that produce experimental insomnia are similar to the chemical abnormalities noted in schizophrenics. Sleep therapy often brings about remission in acute schizophrenics, and various EEG studies of mental patients have shown that their improvement is often preceded by an increase in REM sleep.

Psychotically depressed patients also show reduced REM sleep and lower total time asleep. One study suggests an abnormality in the mechanism that produces PGO spikes. As the depression begins to lift, the pattern becomes more normal.

Sleep-deprivation studies are usually conducted with paid volunteers in carefully controlled settings. Even so, a subject may, by the fourth day, begin to accuse the sleep researchers of conspiring against him. He may see them as agents of some foreign power and decide that he was tricked into the project for some sinister motive.

The Navy researcher LaVerne Johnson has listed some of the dramatic, incapacitating changes seen in sleep-deprived subjects: feelings of persecution, inability to concentrate, disorientation, illusions, and hallucinations (mostly tactile and visual). Some investigators have observed that the periods of most intense hallucination seem to come at intervals of 90–120 minutes, just as REM periods would. Johnson noted that the deprived subject rallies from time to time. The waxing and waning closely follow the increased and decreased presence of alpha activity.

In the sleep-deprived subjects, the low point for both alpha and strength was 3 A.M. One is reminded of the famous passage from *The Crack-Up,* F. Scott Fitzgerald's poignant essay on insomnia:

> At three o'clock in the morning, a forgotten package has the same tragic importance as a death sentence . . . and in a real dark night of the soul, it is always three o'clock in the morning, day after day.

An intuitive observation. It does appear that for those who are deeply disturbed, the clock has indeed stopped at 3 A.M.

After about 115 hours of sleep loss, not even closing the eyes generates alpha. Johnson, Dement, and J. J. Ross observed Randy Gardner, a seventeen-year-old San Diego high-school student who stayed awake for a record-breaking 264 hours without the aid of coffee or other stimulants. Perhaps because of his youth and the fact that he was in his own home, attended by his family physician, Gardner's psychological disturbances were relatively mild. However, after 249 hours of sleep loss his EEG was no longer responsive to eye opening and closing. External stimuli had no effect on the brainwave pattern.

Peter Tripp, then a 32-year-old New York disc jockey, launched a wakathon for charity. Tripp's symptoms were in the classic tradition. He saw cobwebs in his shoes, a tweed suit appeared to become furry worms, and a dresser drawer seemed to be ablaze. Most frightening to Tripp was a growing conviction that he was not really himself. By now his brainwave pattern was that of a man asleep, although he was still functioning. His paranoia at two hundred hours had become so intense that he ran from examining doctors because he believed one of them to be an undertaker and thought he was to be buried alive. Thirteen hours of sleep restored his sanity, but Tripp showed the symptoms of depression for several months.

No one knows how long a human being can survive before he dies of exhaustion. Adult dogs died in from nine to seventeen days. In other studies, puppies were kept awake for from four to six days, and many of them died. Postmortems showed significant brain damage. It is a tribute to the brain's adaptability that some animals have survived such experiments by engaging in microsleep—brief moments of sleep not evident to the observer but recorded by the EEG. In one study, cats were placed on a treadmill. If they didn't keep moving, the treadmill would dump them into a vat of water. The cats learned to run quickly to one end of the treadmill, lie down and sleep as the conveyor belt carried them toward the water. At water's edge they would jump up, scurry back to the end and take another micro-nap on the conveyor belt.

Wilse Webb of the University of Florida placed rats on a mesh wheel partially submerged in water. Very young rats could keep moving atop the wheel for as long as twenty-seven days before tumbling off. Like the cats, they rode the apparatus for just long enough to catch a few seconds' nap. Soldiers can apparently micro-sleep while marching. A sailor who was washed off his ship in midocean and rescued the following day reported that he must have been swimming continuously . . . and he had, in fact, awakened at one point to find himself doing the breaststroke.

Nocturnal sleep can be affected by naps during the preceding day. Male medical students who napped in the morning showed predominantly paradoxical sleep, and their nocturnal sleep was not affected. Afternoon nappers spent much of their siesta in Stage 4, and that stage was reduced markedly during the night's sleep. (Nap dreams are less aggressive and less fantastic than night dream reports, which probably means that they are from non-REM sleep.)

No one knows how much sleep is optimal for human beings. Individuals who regularly sleep three hours per night have been studied by researchers who say that they are healthy and productive specimens. In Boston, Ernest Hartmann compared the performance, health, and personalities of thirty short-sleepers and thirty long-sleepers. The individuals who slept five hours or less nightly tended to be efficient, organized, and solid citizens. Physiologically and emotionally, they seemed not to have suffered from their short sleep. They performed better on tests than the subjects who regularly slept more than nine and a half hours nightly.

The long-sleeper tended to be more ethereal, working at a more creative job than the short-sleeper (if he held a job at all), and there were more disturbed personalities among the long-sleepers.

Stage 4 seems to be the most critically needed sleep period, and after sleep deprivation the greatest rebound is Stage 4. Wilse Webb remarked, "Short-sleepers are known to compress their sleep into a pattern that results in no deprivation of Stage 4 and REM, the two states shown to have 'need' characteristics." Three studies of preschoolers had shown that the bright children slept somewhat less than their age-mates of average intelligence. On the other hand, Lewis Terman reported in his monumental study of gifted children that they slept more than their average age-mates.

One problem, as Allan Rechtschaffen pointed out, is that we do not yet know what sleep does. "Without knowing what it is that sleep accomplishes, how can we say when we have had enough of it?"

Insomniacs awaken more frequently and their sleep seems to be less restful. Their heartbeat is faster, they toss and turn, and their rectal temperature is higher. Rechtschaffen believes that these physiological differences indicate a more aroused state. Insomniacs have lower-than-normal REM time and a higher incidence of personality disturbance.

Rechtschaffen sees their plight as something of a whodunit, a "causal webb" . . . a matrix of the four variables: poor sleep, lowered REM time, physiological arousal, and personality disturbance. All four could be caused by the same unknown factor. Or one of the four could cause the other three. "Or there could be a reverberating, reciprocally enhancing effect of the variables on each other."

For whatever reason, their sleep is not complete and restorative, and insomniacs are apparently justified in their insistence that they have not slept well. Night workers and shift workers show a great variability of phases from one sleep session to another, unlike most sleepers who develop something of a regular pattern.

Although infants and children spend a large percentage of their time in Stage 4, its volume decreases, and the elderly spend almost none. Their reports of insomnia are supported by the research. The typical elderly subject awakens an average of seven times per night, possibly because the brain's regulatory mechanisms have degenerated. (Frequent awakening is one of the chronic manifestations of a serious senile disorder, the so-called chronic brain syndrome.)

A significant correlation has been reported between the density of paradoxical sleep time and IQ, and some theorists wonder if the REM period is associated with memory consolidation. In any event, most mental retardates have little REM sleep. The Czech researcher Olga Petre-Quadens has documented the sleep patterns of infants and young children. Because mongoloid (Down's syndrome) infants usually show abnormally low REM sleep, she experimentally administered oral doses of a substance converted by the body to serotonin; a major brain transmitter, serotonin is suspected of playing a vital role in REM production.

The babies' sleep indeed showed an improved REM density, and they developed normally during the first year. Observers commented that there was markedly less tongue protrusion and a healthier muscle tone than are usually seen in mongoloid babies. After one year the dose had to be increased from time to time. It seemed that some sort of habituation was taking place. Significantly, one child began to exhibit autistic behavior on the higher dosage; unusually high blood serotonin levels have been reported in autistic children.

Prenatally, normal fetuses show two apparent paradoxical-sleep cycles—their own and the one influenced by their mother's hormones. Sex hormones seem to be intricately involved in sleep chemistry. They are concentrated in the brain region where sleep mechanisms are postulated. Testosterone production is closely tied to the paradoxical-sleep cycles. Progesterone in concentration can produce sleep, anesthesia, even convulsions, and the elevated levels of progesterone are blamed for the overpowering sleepiness of early pregnancy. REM time increases in pregnancy, especially as the time for delivery nears, and it remains high in women who breast-feed their babies, declining in those who don't.

REM time also varies with the shifting hormones of the menstrual cycle. Estrogen seems to suppress it. Enovid, a contraceptive combining estrogen and progesterone, has been shown to erase the REM segment female rabbits usually experience after coitus.

Whether the sex steroids have a direct or indirect role in triggering sleep isn't known. Unfortunately no comprehensive theory of sleep chemistry has been formulated. As sleep scientists all over the world report their findings, more questions than answers are forthcoming. But at least the questions are increasingly sophisticated.

Paradoxical sleep and slow-wave sleep (Stages 1–4) apparently involve two interrelated but somewhat autonomous brain systems. Either kind of sleep can be eliminated by surgical interference. Controlling structures for paradoxical sleep are apparently in the dorsal region of the pons. Removing all other brain structures does not affect paradoxical sleep if the pons is intact. Chemical activity there gives rise to spontaneous discharges into the visual region, which almost certainly explains the pronounced imagery of this state.

Michel Jouvet of the University of Lyon reports that the braking mechanism that inhibits motor activity is probably controlled by a brain structure called the locus coeruleus. If this structure is damaged, lab animals seem to act out their dreams.

Various brain chemicals are implicated in the phenomena of sleep. Jouvet dosed rats, rabbits, and cats with PCPA * to deplete the brain's serotonin. For the first twenty-four hours no change was observed. From the thirtieth to the sixtieth hour there was total insomnia in the laboratory cats, and after the sixtieth hour sleep recovery began. By about the hundredth hour it had resumed its normal patterns. However, if Jouvet's team administered a substance to restore the serotonin, they could terminate the insomnia earlier. Apparently serotonin was

* Parachloralphenalamine.

vital for sleep chemistry. A region of the brainstem known as the raphe system is rich in clusters of cells containing serotonin. Lethal insomnia usually resulted when Jouvet surgically excised these cells in cats.

Jouvet believes that there are three key chemicals involved in paradoxical sleep. Serotonin, norepinephrine, and acetylcholine have to act, each on its separate brain site and in a specific sequence—"Like a fail-safe system," Jouvet put it. He believes that the fail-safe device usually prevents the hallucinatory processes from breaking through into the waking state.

His findings seem to dovetail with Dement's suggestion that PGO spikes breaking through may be responsible for grave thought disorders. Dement has said that perhaps in schizophrenics the brain's equivalent of a fail-safe system has broken down.

An area at the base of the forebrain plays a part in sleep. Stimulating animals there has produced sleep within twenty seconds. Damage produces insomnia for a month or two. More serious lesions have caused fatal insomnia. Barry Sterman and his associates have stimulated the site in cats who were toying with a just-captured rat. The cat typically drops the rat as if it has lost interest . . . and falls asleep shortly thereafter. In similar experiments in other labs, stimulation has sometimes caused sleep so instantaneous that animals who were eating have slumped forward, their heads in their dishes.

With a biofeedback technique, Sterman trained cats to produce a brain rhythm typical of a motionless state. He thought that perhaps the altered EEG would facilitate sleep; results suggest that the animals sleep more efficiently after the training, showing less motor disturbance and an increased number of sleep spindles. The technique is now being used experimentally on human insomniacs to see if they can learn to produce a more restful sleep physiology. Preliminary results are encouraging.

Electrosleep machines, first used by the Russians, deliver mild pulses of electrical current to the brain. This technique seems to relax some anxious patients. Normal volunteers reported a euphoria that one young woman compared to a happy pill. American volunteers said that they seemed disinclined to worry after an electrosleep treatment.

At the Brain Research Institute at UCLA experimenters sounded bell tones while they stimulated sleep regions in animals' brains. The animals eventually would drop off to sleep just upon hearing the bell tone. For many human beings, bedtime rituals may perform a similar Pavlovian conditioning.

Awareness during sleep and chemically induced unconsciousness is apparently unceasing. As early as 1927 researchers were reporting that laboratory subjects could awaken from sleep at a randomly chosen target time or within ten minutes in either direction. A number of studies have substantiated the early findings.

When the sleepers awaken they are disoriented, don't know how they awoke, and can't recall any dream content that triggered the awakening. "The process by which the subjects were able to perform this task is completely unknown," W. M. Zung and William Wilson reported in *Biological Psychiatry*. All environmental clues were eliminated. This target awakening can take place during any stage of sleep, however deep.

Sleep awareness has been demonstrated for every sense, but tactile and auditory perception seem most sensitive. The brain can make interesting distinctions from the depths of sleep. In one experiment, sleep-deprived subjects had to press a microswitch periodically to avoid a nasty shock. Soon they were able to perform without showing any arousal on the EEG.

The brain may choose to ignore gibberish, even loud noises, while still responding to relevant stimuli. While volunteers slept, a series of names was repeated on a tape recording, but some of the names had been recorded backward. K-complexes (a brainwave pattern of arousal but not awakening) appeared for the meaningful names more often then for the nonsensical ones.

A sleeping subject may snore through a sudden din, yet awaken to his whispered name or a key phrase. Names that are emotionally meaningful to him may be incorporated into his dream content . . . sometimes after editing. The name Robert may inspire the dreamer to give his friend a role in the dream, or he may transform the name into a dream rabbit.

Sleep learning varies from one stage of sleep to another and with the time of night. At the University of Florida, the average recall for five nights of material presented during deep sleep was 13 percent. During light sleep, the retention ranged from 10 percent (first three nights) to 17 percent (last two nights). Taped material heard during light sleep late at night was better remembered. Scores averaged as high as 30 percent. Possibly the greater REM frequency toward morning is responsible for more efficient processing. The experimenters, Michael Levy and Wilse Webb, say that sleep learning appears to improve with training.

David Cheek, a gynecologist at Children's Hospital in San Francisco, believes that all operating rooms should post a sign: "Shhh . . . the patient may be listening." Cheek and Bernard Levinson of Johannesburg have published case histories of patients who recall under postsurgical hypnosis just what was said during their surgery.

Cheek maintains that the hearing sense "is maintained to depths of chemical intoxication beyond that at which all other perceptions are suppressed." He cites a case report by a colleague in which a patient was in sudden crisis. When the surgeon lifted out her stomach as planned, her breathing and heartbeat stopped.

> Before cutting down on the heart for massage, the surgeon asked that the husband be notified of the emergency. Nobody knew where the husband could be found. At this point the patient aroused and whispered around the endotracheal tube, "John's in the lobby."

One of Cheek's surgical patients reported under hypnosis that she had become frightened during her surgery the preceding week. She recalled almost verbatim the anesthesiologist's casual remark to the surgeon, "Oh, Dave, that unit of blood is all ready any time she needs it." Cheek had quickly said something reassuring for the patient's benefit (and a little absurd to the medical personnel, who considered her unconscious). She added, "I·. . . I didn't know I might have to get some blood and I thought something more than you had told me must be wrong." She said that she had been reassured by his reply.

In one study fifteen hundred patients were given therapeutic suggestion near the close of their operations while they were still deeply anesthetized. The typical patient would be given a calm, optimistic report about the success of his surgery and told that there would be no discomfort in the area of the operation. The suggestions worked for around 50 percent of the patients, who were an unselected group. Not a single pediatric patient reported any pain, nausea, or vomiting after the surgery.

In a double-blind experiment, earphones were placed on eighty-one surgical patients. Each patient listened to one of the four master tapes: (1) five minutes of music, then blank; (2) all music; (3) mild suggestions about relaxation and diminishing pain; (4) strongly worded suggestions about relaxation, healing.

The results were striking. The patients who had heard either of the two suggestion tapes stayed in the hospital an average of 8.63 days. Those who heard only music or blank tapes stayed 11.05 days.

Both Cheek and Levinson report that deeply anesthetized patients seem to hear only significant remarks or ominous silences. Trivial conversation is seldom recalled under later hypnosis, but patients can repeat intact such phrases, as, "Good gracious! It may not be a cyst at all. It may be a cancer. . . ." (That was a Levinson case.) Some doctors are now wondering how many inexplicable deaths on the operating table or shortly after surgery might be attributable to the patient's eavesdropping.

Evidence suggests that dreaming is a secondary rather than a primary biological process. Dreaming seems to be subject to the changing neural activity of the various sleep stages. Mental activity shifts gears as the EEG patterns change. Mind, being infinitely flexible, seems to exploit this rich altered state of consciousness to surprising advantage.

In the equatorial rain forest of the Malay Peninsula live the Senoi tribesmen, a preliterate people. The sophistication of the Senoi dream culture has been compared to our level of attainment in nuclear physics.

The Senoi child discusses his dreams with the family over breakfast, and they help him to interpret the dreams and any fear that might have been engendered. If a Senoi dreams that he has hurt someone, he must apologize, perform a favor, or give the person a gift. If he dreams that he was mistreated, he tells the guilty party, who attempts to compensate with a gift or friendly act.

Throughout life the Senoi seeks community counsel on cryptic dreams. The male population assembles daily after the family dream clinics to discuss further the dreams of the older children and all the men. Precognitive dreams are considered particularly valuable, and if one is warned of danger by another's dream, he is again obligated to thank him and perhaps offer a gift.

The late Kilton Stewart, a research psychologist who studied the Senoi society for fifteen years, said that the tribe believes that "any human being, with the aid of his fellows, can outface, master, and actually utilize all beings and forces in the dream universe."

Should the Senoi child report a falling dream, his parents would congratulate him. "That's a wonderful dream, one of the best you can have!" They ask him where he fell to and what he found.

The child might answer that the dream had not been splendid at all, but rather frightening and that he awoke before landing. The adult then explains that all dreams have a purpose. The next time he has a falling dream he must relax and have fun because such dreams mean that the spiritual world wants to bestow its powers on him.

"The astonishing thing," said Stewart, "is that over a period of time . . . the dream which starts out with the fear of falling changes into the joy of flying. This happens to everyone in the Senoi society."

The Senoi have no war, no violent crime, and astonishing mental health. Stewart believed that all men might profit by studying them. "In the West the thinking we do while asleep usually remains on a muddled, childish, or psychotic level because we do not respond to dreams as socially important and include dreaming in the educative process."

The Senoi have become the objects of such intense interest on the part of anthropologists and psychologists that one wonders if they still have time to dream. Several colleges now offer courses in Senoi-inspired dream therapy, and one group of American students lived for eighteen months in a dream-based communal society patterned after the Senoi community. Some psychologists have begun using Senoi techniques in group therapy. The Senoi movement, like the burgeoning interest in eastern techniques for altering awareness, seems to reflect the West's growing absorption with the mind technology of other cultures.

There are certainly many clues that sleep mentation has rhyme and reason. Montague Ullman, chairman of the department of psychiatry at Brooklyn's Maimonides Hospital, believes that day residue precipitates the dream subject matter, acting as "a faint beam of light playing upon a shadowy, unknown, and sometimes rather frightening territory." He suggests that the dreamer builds his abstraction from concrete blocks: scraps of experience from the preceding day. These incidents become dream analogies, "metaphors in motion."

Ullman deplores the view of dreaming as infantile wish-fulfillment. He sees it rather as "truer and more inclusive aspects of the dreamer's own existence as partially exposed by a recent event in his life." The dreamer is asking himself, *What is happening to me? What can I do about it?* He is actively trying to work through some aspect of his life.

One example Ullman cites is the dream of an architect who had closeted himself in his study for four successive Sundays so that he could meet a deadline. As he worked he was vaguely aware that his wife was sharply scolding the children from time to time.

He napped for a few minutes. In his dream he called the weather bureau and asked if a hurricane was expected to hit the city that afternoon. He later told Ullman, "As I was asking the question I began to feel embarrassed and guilty." He had grown increasingly uneasy about the burden he was placing on his wife but had decided that nothing could be done about it. Asleep he was forced to confront an unresolved problem: the storm that was brewing.

Like Stewart, Ullman regrets our society's historic disregard of dream life. He maintains that the dream analogy forces the dreamer to risk saying something new about himself, but "to the extent that a metaphor dies . . . unread and unappreciated, its power to enhance self-awareness is dissipated."

David Foulkes reported that a recent episode renewed his interest in a dream theory put forth by a Viennese physician,

Otto Poetzl, in 1917. Poetzl believed that visual experiences incompletely realized during the day are incorporated into the night's dreaming. Poetzl's subjects were exposed to a series of unfamiliar color slides exposed at rapid rates. Then they recorded all that they could remember seeing.

They were asked to pay careful attention to their dreams. When they returned to the lab the next day, they sketched what they could recall of the dream fragments. Oddly enough, the sketches seemed to follow a law of exclusion. None of the material they had perceived the previous day was included in the dream sketches . . . *only those elements that they had not consciously remembered seeing.*

Most experiments trying to replicate the Poetzl phenomenon have been poorly designed, Foulkes said; he suggests that sleep-onset studies might reveal the complementary nature of dreaming. While studying sleep-onset imagery, Foulkes and Gerald Vogel recorded one dream report about an abstract painting of blue shoes. On the following morning the dreamer was at work in a large office. She happened to glance at an abstract calendar painting she had seen many times but had never understood . . . and she did a double take. She asked a co-worker what he saw in the painting, and he assured her that it represented, as she had just realized, two pairs of crossed ballet slippers. One pair of slippers was blue.

Another complementary effect may be the finding of dream psychologists that strong, well-adjusted people are less likely to have bizarre, emotional dreams than are average subjects. Dream intensity seems to correlate with waking insecurity and inhibitions.

Dreams can even fulfill a need for companionship. When volunteers are isolated during their waking hours, according to one study, they tend to socialize a great deal in their dreams. Sleep mentation can be surprisingly efficient at meeting the individual's needs.

"Most investigators," said Ralph Berger, "now believe that mental activity does not totally cease at any time during sleep." There is now ample evidence of slow-wave, or non-REM (NREM), thinking, usually called mentation rather than dreaming, to distinguish it from the bizarre activity of fast-wave sleep.

David Foulkes, probably the leading investigator of NREM mentation, compares it to the background thought in waking life, "those fragments of experience that pass along the borders of consciousness. . . ."

Gerald Vogel observed that NREM dream reports sometimes repeat and sometimes anticipate the content of other NREM and REM reports collected on the same night. He sees the more intense REM-period dreams as "the most vivid and memorable part of a larger fabric of interwoven mental activity during sleep."

If Vogel, Foulkes, and several others are right, REM mental activity would represent only a stormy, supercharged interlude in a night-long reverie.

The limits of the depths and heights of sleep consciousness have not been explored. Sleep awareness has been described as the lucid dream by Frederik Van Eeden, a British researcher who amassed a wealth of subjective dream observations beginning in 1896. In a lucid dream one dreams that he awakens into normal consciousness, yet he knows that he is asleep and experiences the dream world from this dual point of view. Yogis, being connoisseurs of altered states of consciousness, have naturally evolved certain techniques for controlling consciousness during sleep. Various schools of meditation offer methods for maintaining a continuous lucid dream. The euphoric effect was piquantly described by one individual as "like vanilla ice cream in your head all night."

Charles Tart has defined a layer of sleep consciousness he calls the high dream. Although it resembles an LSD trip, Tart said that he hesitated to call it a psychedelic dream because that adjective has been so loosely used. "The primary shift in this dream is the great intensification of sensory qualities and the dropping out of ordinary intellectual activity, to the point where the dreamer no longer experiences the usual split between the knower and the known. The dreamer often feels ecstatic even after awakening."

Dreams have yielded mystical experiences strikingly like the insights reported from other altered states of consciousness. An example is recounted in J. B. Priestley's *Rain Upon Godshill*. Priestley dreams that he was standing atop a very high tower, alone, looking down on a "vast aerial river of birds." Tens of thousands of birds of every kind were flying past. Then time seemed to speed up, and before his eyes the birds began to shrivel, weaken, bleed, and disintegrate. He was overwhelmed with sadness at what seemed the absurdity of living and dying.

I stood on my tower, still alone, desperately unhappy. But now the gear was changed again and time went faster still, and it was rushing by at such a rate that the birds could not show any movement but were like an enormous plain sown with feathers. But along this plain, flickering through the bodies themselves, there now passed a sort of white flame, trembling, dancing, then hurrying on; and as soon as I saw it I knew that this flame was life itself, the very quintessence of being; and then it came to me, in a rocket-burst of ecstasy, that nothing mattered, nothing could ever matter, because nothing else was real but this quivering and hurrying lambency of being. . . . What I had thought was tragedy was mere emptiness or a shadow show; for now all real feeling was caught and purified and danced on ecstatically with the white flame of life.

In common with the other altered states, sleep consciousness seems to enhance psychic phenomena. Scientific research into dream telepathy and clairvoyance has yielded statistically impressive data. At the Maimonides Dream Laboratory, Montague Ullman, Stanley Krippner, and Charles Honorton have designed many carefully controlled experiments involving dreams and the possible occurrence of psi.

Freud and Jung wrote of telepathic phenomena in dreams. Carl Meier, a Swiss psychiatrist, recently said:

You may call me superstitious or unscientific, but I am convinced that these things happen frequently, more frequently than we think or perceive them, and in rare cases we can determine almost irrefutably that these incidents cannot be just coincidental, particularly when the likeness of the two coinciding phenomena is photographic to the minute details. . . .

He asks his fellow researchers if the world of dreams could be the place where the two realities of psyche and soma coincide—if perhaps the dream state is "the strange elusive something which through the ages has been called 'the subtle body.' "

III.

the vulnerable brain

Man's most transcendental accomplishment would be the conquering of his own brain. —SANTIAGO RAMON Y CAJAL

13

HURT BRAINS: WHO IS NORMAL?

In 1966 in Austin, Texas, a bright, good-looking young man named Charles Whitman shot and killed his wife and mother before going to the landmark tower of the University of Texas, where he killed the receptionist. From atop the tower he carefully picked off victims; his rifle killed fourteen and wounded twenty-four. Because Whitman was killed, he couldn't explain why he had initiated the massacre.

Psychologists, curbstone psychologists, and the media began tossing out possibilities. He had grieved over his parents' separation. He felt pressured by studies. He had been conditioned to violence, having owned guns since he was a small boy. *Life* magazine depicted two-year-old Charles proudly posing with his father's rifle in the family's backyard.

But Whitman had kept a personal diary in which he had noted for several months that something strange was happening to him. He had complained of headaches and told a campus psychiatrist that he found himself becoming so angry that he could "go to the top of that university tower and start shooting at people."

A blue-ribbon postmortem examination of Whitman's brain revealed "a highly malignant type of primary infiltrating tumor of the brain called a glioblastoma multiforme." Although Whitman's head had been torn apart by the gunfire that ended his life, William Sweet, one of the examining neurosurgeons, expressed a belief that the tumor had been located in one temporal lobe, a site where brain damage is often found in connection with violent behavior.

It is a hard blow to one's self-image to realize how fragile is our claim to normalcy. One-fourth of the population is supposedly carrying a genetic predisposition to schizophrenia. One-fourth is prone to flicker fits; more than one-half of us can be driven to seizures under certain circumstances; perhaps a million of us are undiagnosed temporal-lobe epileptics; millions more are alcoholic . . . or hyperkinetic . . . or senile. One-tenth have dysrhythmic EEGs. We might paraphrase the old saying: "All the world is mad—including thee and me."

Commissions to investigate unprovoked violence usually inquire into such obvious factors as television programming, poverty, and the appalling availability of weapons. Social factors are obviously important in the prevention of senseless violence, but the impulsiveness and aggression of millions of our citizens may be due to brain abnormalities.

In our wars on crime, early diagnosis and treatment of these problems may hold greater promise than juvenile-court and prison counseling. A psychiatrist, Frank Ervin, and his neurologist colleagues at Massachusetts General and Boston General have urged that counselors, psychiatrists, judges, prison officials, and guards should all be trained to detect possible evidence of brain pathology in the culture's hotheads. Even traffic policemen could be made aware that repeated dangerous driving often is symptomatic of an uncontrollably violent personality.

The Boston team reported, for example, the case of a brilliant 34-year-old inventor who was quiet and kind except for recurrent episodes of violent behavior that had begun ten years earlier. Typically he would brood over a mild disagreement with his wife for thirty minutes or so until he had worked himself into a storm of brutality during which he might beat his wife and children or burn them with a lighted cigarette.

For seven years he had undergone psychiatric treatment with no success. Luckily, his observant third psychiatrist happened to notice the subtle symptoms of temporal-lobe epilepsy: The inventor stared blankly, smacked his lips, and repeated an irrelevant phrase. Anticonvulsive medication didn't help the patient, but electronic stimulation did. Stimulation of the amygdala at one point gave the patient pain and the feeling that he was losing control, about to attack. A point only four millimeters away from it turned on a euphoric hyperrelaxation. The inventor said that it felt like Demerol. "The room is getting larger and brighter. . . . I feel like I'm floating on a cloud."

The euphoria lasted thirty-six hours. His doctors began a schedule of electronic stimulation that prevented attack behavior for three months. Since the need for treatment seemed to persist, they destroyed a small amount of brain tissue in the appropriate area. They reported that in the ensuing two years there had been no episodes of rage. A patient with similar symptoms was rage-free with stimulation alone for a year, then relapsed. The doctors implanted electrodes and inserted a small built-in stimulator under the skin so that when he felt an attack coming on he could abort it by stimulating the positive brain regions.

One grim example of undiagnosed brain malfunction was Gloria, a teen-ager, the daughter of chronic alcoholics. Her foster parents, who reared her, said that she was a model child until age thirteen, when she became "moody and uncommunicative." When they objected on one occasion to the loud playing of records, she smashed up her room, tore her curtains, and partially destroyed her bedroom door with a heavy object. Police subdued her. Thereafter, according to her case history, her behavior altered between "angelic" and "devilish." Then, on May 11, 1967, she became "tired and angry" with a screaming 26-month-old foster brother and suffocated him with a plastic bag.

At a state mental hospital she attempted suicide and also attacked a younger child. Learning that her 23-year-old brother was confined for epileptic violence, a psychiatrist suspected organic brain disease and referred her to Massachusetts General for neurological testing. All the usual tests were normal, and the investigators located abnormal hippocampal discharges almost by accident.

By then Gloria had admitted to them that she had once suffocated another of her foster siblings, who was thought by its parents to have died of pneumonia. The doctors fitted her with electrodes to measure activity from the suspect area and began talking to her quietly. As the EEG scribbled its record, normal up to that time, the sound of a crying baby came from a tape recording. Within seconds her hippocampal brainwave activity built into a seizure pattern. Abnormal EEG patterns appeared at once, growing more exaggerated over the next minute. When the tape was switched off, her EEG returned to normal.

Observers don't always find it easy to separate purely psychological causes for uncontrollable temper from symptoms of organic brain dysfunction. Psychological causes are nearly always overlaid on the pathological ones, for one thing; individuals with explosive tempers are likely to be socially ostracized to some extent, and are also troubled by guilt. Too, the organic symptoms can be vague, such as headache, dizziness, forgetfulness. Ervin and his co-workers have listed a number of clues to possible brain disorder:

History of birth trauma, meningitis, and other high childhood fevers may mean that such sensitive brain regions as the hippocampus were damaged by lack of oxygen. Head injuries may have caused temporal-lobe epilepsy, which is often associated with episodic dyscontrol. Long periods of unconsciousness, as after an automobile accident, are of interest. Since violent persons are likely to engage in many fights, the case history has to differentiate between head injuries prior to the dyscontrol and those resulting from it. Also, the high frequency of temporal-lobe epilepsy among alcoholics is believed partly due to the many falls a drunk takes.

One patient at Massachusetts General was a 27-year-old murder suspect who later hanged himself in jail. While undergoing psychiatric examination, he explained that he had been shot in the head at sixteen. He complained of blackout spells, periods of confusion, occasional visual hallucinations of animals like buffalo and squirrels. He had a history of episodic violence that culminated in the murder charge.

After the patient's jail suicide, neuropathologists found that the bullet which had ripped through his head eleven years before had cut off arteries supplying vital oxygen to the limbic brain, resulting in extensive damage in the region where impulse control is believed to reside.

Pathological intoxication,* a state in which an individual commits acts of which he has no sober recollection, suggests a possible focal epilepsy. The Boston team believes that such blackouts are temporal-lobe epileptic attacks.

They are over and over again ignored, neglected, or not even seen. For example, we have admitted patients to the hospital who everybody agreed had no symptoms of epilepsy. Yet simply by observing them on the ward for eight hours, we could recognize clearly classic epilepsy of one kind or another. This is particularly true of the focal epileptic. What most American physicians do not seem to realize is that focal epilepsies are the most common kind of epilepsy, commoner than either grand mal or petit mal.

A triad said to be predictive of criminal behavior includes fire-setting, cruelty to animals, and bed-wetting. Obviously most bedwetters don't become violent criminals, but in combination with pyromania and torturing of pets, prolonged enuresis is apparently a clue.

Dangerous driving often reflects a tendency to episodic violence. Case histories often include incidents where patients angrily drove their cars into other cars. One individual became so enraged when another driver cut in front of him that he chased him for two blocks. Others have driven their own cars into walls and trees; when an urge to destruction comes on, the individual may injure himself if no one else is available.

According to one study, half of those with episodic dyscontrol own weapons; for those who don't, the automobile can be an effective weapon.

Confused sexual identity and abnormal sexual behavior are seen in a striking percentage of violent patients. Many are homosexual or admit to a deep fear of homosexuality which sometimes results in their stabbing or beating any man who strikes up a conversation in a bar. Some individuals with the dyscontrol syndrome complain of impotence and say that they become violent toward women with whom they are impotent.

Diagnosis is not easy. The EEG is still a crude, limited tool

---

* When they feel tension and destructive impulses building, these individuals often attempt self-medication with alcohol; the effect, of course, is to worsen their impulsiveness.

when it comes to locating and defining injured regions deep within the limbic brain. Robert Young, a neurologist and electroencephalographer, said, "It is entirely possible to have a patient being recorded during an actual focal seizure and yet have no abnormality show up on the scalp tracing." Detecting the abnormal discharge might require surgical implanting of depth electrodes. Vernon Mark, director of neurosurgical service at Boston City Hospital, has said that no one knows for sure what constitutes normal functioning of the limbic brain and that the region remains "silent to clinical examinations." Diagnosis is also complicated by the patients' violence. Hospital employees and even examining doctors are understandably wary of the patients, reluctant to be within arm's reach while suspect brain regions are being stimulated. Telemetry equipment now makes it possible for the exploratory stimulation in some hospitals to take place from a distance.

Low blood sugar can trigger an attack in temporal-lobe epileptics. Alcohol seems to precipitate attacks. The drug Dilantin reduces the incidence of seizures. Librium, a tranquilizer, raises the threshold for seizure in the limbic system. Antidepressants —mood elevators—sometimes heighten aggression. In hyperkinetic children and some adolescents, amphetamines are calming, but their abuse can result in violent behavior. Psychedelics, oddly enough, seem to mitigate against violence and may even play a therapeutic role someday. Hormones may be involved in the violence syndrome. Since the syndrome is much more prevalent among males, testosterone—known to produce fierce aggression in experimental animals—may well play a part.

Although there is no criminal brain per se, abnormalities may make some individuals more susceptible to such psychological stresses as childhood beatings, sexual assault by parents, extreme poverty, broken home, low self-image, quarrels with spouse or friends, and the responsibility of supporting or caring for a family. Psychological events may set off the vulnerable brain.

Chromosomal abnormalities have been found in prisoners at from twenty to fifty times the rate in the general population. One study found EEG abnormalities in as many as 50 percent of a criminal population. In one study of one hundred criminals, thirty-three showed clearly abnormal EEGs; fully 77 percent of their case histories included such organic clues as convulsions, head injuries, blackouts, and uncontrollable outbursts of violence.

Treatment of individuals with the dyscontrol syndrome is bitterly controversial. Anthony Burgess' novel, *The Clockwork Orange,* fantasized one approach (made particularly melodramatic in the movie), and the popular press has sounded the alarm. Can neurosurgeons create conformity with a scalpel? Is it ethical to alter another's brain if it means preventing potential murder? How do current surgical techniques differ from the lobotomies that left patients peaceful zombies? Can implantation of electrodes allow one to be controlled from a distance, like a robot?

Psychologists have noted with amusement and some relief that electronic stimulation in lab animals does not necessarily interfere with their good sense. A cat wired for violence will seldom strike out in blind rage at a bigger cat. A monkey will seldom challenge a cagemate who has dominated him in the past.

Monkeys, like many homicidal criminals, can learn to direct their electronically stimulated violent impulses, integrating the urge with higher brain activities. For instance, they will learn to open doors and perform stunts in order to get to an object they can assault, such as a stuffed animal, rather than blindly battering the nearest wall.

Yes, an individual could be electronically stimulated to fear, anger, or euphoria from a distance. However, the procedure is complicated, not always accurate, and far too tedious and expensive as a method for taking over control of the world. As some wag has observed, it's easier for a would-be tyrant to use such time-honored methods as the politician's traditional mass hypnosis.

Controversy in California centered on psychosurgery performed on prisoners who had requested it or who had submitted voluntarily. The three in Vacaville's Maximum Psychiatric Diagnostic Unit underwent surgery in which lesions were placed in specific structures in the limbic brain, for the control of violent seizures. Results were mixed.

The greatest problem in neurosurgery, as in electronic brain stimulation, is our relative ignorance of the limbic brain. If moving the electrode a few millimeters can make the difference between heaven and hell, precision is of the utmost importance —and we're not quite there.

In animal experiments it was found that "attack behavior elicited by limbic system stimulation can be prevented by lesions made 'downstream.'" Removal of the amygdala tames such ferocious creatures as the lynx and bobcat temporarily. Removal of a section of the temporal lobe sometimes leaves a human patient with impaired memory and with behavioral eccentricities, particularly sexual problems, so lobectomies are a last resort. If neither drug control nor electronic stimulation of the brain is effective, tiny portions of the amygdala may be destroyed by radio waves directed through depth electrodes. Such operations, called amygdalotomies, have had mildly encouraging results in Denmark, Japan, and the United States.

A more socially acceptable approach might grow out of a program under way at the Veterans Hospital in Sepulveda, California: brainwave biofeedback training of epileptics. Because cats that had learned to produce a certain brainwave pattern did not convulse even when given convulsant drugs, Barry Sterman began training human epileptics to produce a similar pattern. When they feel a grand mal seizure coming on, they voluntarily shift their brainwave activity to the sensorimotor pattern, thus aborting the fit.

A young woman with an eight-year history of epilepsy went from two or three seizures per month (in spite of anticonvulsant medication) to only three seizures in six months. She reported a dramatic positive personality change, too. She said that she fell asleep more rapidly, slept more restfully, and awoke more easily. This interested Sterman, because it correlates with the more efficient sleep patterns of the trained cats.

The prelude to a temporal-lobe seizure may be less apparent to the sufferer than a grand mal aura would be. Nonetheless, biofeedback training has already made subjects aware of even more subtle changes—from alpha to beta, for instance, and the training is a promising tool for the control of episodic violence triggered by electrical abnormalities in the brain.

The epileptic aura is a much-discussed phenomenon that, of course, can only be defined subjectively. Epileptics tell of flashing lights, colors, humming or singing noises, a swimming sen-

sation or dizziness, a feeling that one's hands or feet are elsewhere than where they appear to be, tingling, *déjà vu,* and
sometimes peculiar odors or tastes.

> Suddenly, in the midst of sadness, spiritual darkness and oppres-
> sion, there seemed at moments a flash of light in his brain, and
> with extraordinary impetus all his vital forces suddenly began
> working at their highest tension. . . . His mind and heart were
> flooded with extraordinary light; all his uneasiness, all his doubts,
> all his anxieties were relieved at once. . . . But these moments,
> these flashes, were only the prelude of that final second (it was
> never more than a second) with which the fit began. That second
> was, of course, unendurable. —Fyodor Dostoevsky, *The Idiot*

The falling sickness, also known as the sacred disease, is not
as rare as might be supposed. Some authorities estimate that as
many as one in ten persons in the general population have a
dysrhythmic EEG and probably have some unrecognized seizures. According to studies at the Burden Neurological Institute, more than 50 percent of normal adults will experience par-
oxysmal discharges similar to the type seen in epileptics, if
they are exposed to a light whose flash is fired by the brain's
own rhythms.

A surprising number of people are susceptible even when the
flicker rate is automatically set. In one study in France scientists tested a group of crack airline pilots who had shown rapid
reflexes and an ability to perform skillfully in a crisis. The pilots were twice as sensitive as the general population to flicker
fits.

Samuel Livingston, an authority on epilepsy, lists among the
triggers: a fine mesh pattern in the visual field, music, startling
sensations (like a sudden noise), and lights. Emotional disturbances, premenstrual hormonal changes, overbreathing, fever,
allergies, alcohol, and certain drugs can precipitate a fit. There
is even a subcategory known as reading epilepsy. One nine-
year-old American-Jewish boy had to drop his Hebrew lessons
because reading from right to left caused a seizure. A Lon-
doner reportedly has seizures every time Big Ben strikes.

As many as one person in four may carry the hereditary trait
for photosensitivity, with or without obvious symptoms. An erratic fluorescent light or psychedelic light show may provoke an

attack or a peculiar feeling. Freeway divider posts flashing past can set off a minor storm even in nonepileptics—what *Medical World News* called "environmental epilepsy." Individuals with no history of a disorder have lost their equilibrium or become unaccountably dazed while walking past a long row of pillars or driving along a poplar-lined street. Rotating helicopter blades are particularly likely to cause flicker fits. A flickering television set provoked a temporal-lobe seizure in one teen-age boy who began attacking family members with a baseball bat. Some individuals are particularly susceptible to red and are helped by wearing glasses that filter out the red wavelengths. For some reason, females are more susceptible than males to flicker fits.

The key to the phenomenon is the evenness of the stimuli, particularly at around ten cycles per second—near the alpha rhythm. The brain does eerie things when hit by unvarying stimuli. As W. Grey Walter said, "Even the normal brain may not enjoy a wide margin of operating stability." He believes that the epileptically inclined may have a lower-than-normal resistance to the alpha rhythm.

The possible prevalence of seizure susceptibility could well be taken into account in freeway design. Many one-car fatalities might be due to the driver's being flicker-dazed rather than falling asleep at the wheel. In one accident-plagued freeway section near Los Angeles, state highway engineers installed a solid concrete divider rather than the usual posts. Its purpose is to prevent cars from plunging through the divider into the path of oncoming traffic.

During the next six-month period, traffic fatalities dropped to zero. True, cars could no longer crash through the barrier, but perhaps it was also significant that divider-post flicker was eliminated.

When there is an organic epileptic focus on one side of the brain, a mirror focus often appears in the other half. Surgical excision of the original injury has no effect on the mirror focus. Apparently that hemisphere has "learned" to create that activity.

The interaction between the brain's hemispheres has brought about a spectacular research breakthrough. In a handful of desperate cases, violent epileptic storms have involved this interaction. Neurosurgeons have excised the connecting region of the brain, the corpus callosum, also known as the great commissure. One such patient had had fifty seizures within the previous three days and was in a coma when surgery was scheduled. After the operation she was free of seizures, and after a few months there were few apparent effects on her coordination. She could swim, tie her shoes, ride a bicycle.

But specially designed tests showed that she and the other split-brain patients now had two apparently autonomous centers of consciousness, one in each hemisphere. If the left hand felt an object behind a screen—a toothbrush, for example—the patient couldn't identify it verbally. But the left hand, asked to find the object again, could identify it from among several items. The left hand could feel the shape of a three-dimensional number and correctly signal what it was by raising the correct number of fingers, but the patient could not say the number and appeared not to know.

In most individuals, speech resides primarily in the left hemisphere, which is in touch with what happens to the right hand only. (The half containing the primary speech faculties is referred to as the major hemisphere.)

Literally, in a split-brain patient the left hand does not know what the right hand is doing. Roger Sperry of California Institute of Technology, who studied the split-brain patients extensively, said that if the articulate left hemisphere doesn't know the answer, it will make one up. "If one hemisphere hears the other give the wrong answer, it seems to get very frustrated. The mute right hemisphere may be shaking the head while the left hemisphere gives a wrong answer verbally. Sometimes the subject says, 'Why the heck was my head shaking?' "

The left hemisphere tends to analyze the whole into its parts, while the right sees the whole. For whatever reason, the right hemisphere is superior at spatial reasoning. In one film the researchers made, a male subject was attempting to arrange a group of wooden forms to match a given design. So long as he used only his right hand (left hemisphere), he couldn't form the pattern. He had to *sit* on his left hand to keep it from trying to get into the act. Finally the experimenters let him use both hands to assemble the design—and the spatially oriented left hand *had to knock the right hand aside* several times in order to complete the pattern correctly.

Asked why the patients don't become schizoid, Sperry answered, "Perhaps they do. The right half of the brain might be very unhappy, but we have no way of finding out since it's mute."

Because both hemispheres usually receive simultaneous input through eyes and ears, usually they have no serious problems of coordination. During the weeks and months after the surgery, patients may have difficulty writing their names, but eventually they recover most functions. The motor centers apparently learn to work together as they adjust to their cleft state. Sperry speculates that the minor hemisphere, which receives the greatest surgical trauma, may be in a state of shock for some time after the operation.

A few rare individuals are born without a corpus callosum. They have a congenitally split brain. Most of the cases have been discovered during autopsies. But when a nineteen-year-old coed from the University of Southern California appeared at a clinic complaining of headaches, a routine neurological examination revealed a hole where the corpus callosum should have been. Sperry and his associates took advantage of the rare opportunity to study a living example of agenesis of the corpus callosum.

The brain, ever flexible, had developed redundant functions in each hemisphere. "This is a tribute to the plasticity of the brain," Sperry said, "but apparently the necessary crowding of functions into each hemisphere was not achieved in this person without paying a price. When we went on to test for complex mental tasks, she performed subnormally in some areas. In verbal ability she was above normal, but she did poorly in such nonverbal areas as math, map tests, spatial relationships in general."

In a few rare cases, the major hemisphere of the brain has been removed because of a malignancy. Usually the patients are mute—except, oddly enough, for singing and swearing! Sometimes they can sing a response that they could not articulate in regular speech. Since the minor hemisphere seems to include the center for musical comprehension, perhaps it also retains, as a distinct function, the ability to verbalize in song.

The critical nature of speech centers is suggested by another case. The patient was undergoing brain surgery for a different problem entirely when the surgeon noticed that each hemisphere seemed to have developed a speech center. Knowing that the patient had a bad stammer, the surgeon "scooped out" the speech center in the minor hemisphere. The patient never stuttered again.

Age is important in recovery from split-brain surgery. An eighteen-year-old had far fewer aftereffects than the older patients, and he can now identify verbally the unseen objects held in his left hand. He can feel three-dimensional numerals in his left hand and signify the number by raising the fingers of his right hand.

Although animals have symmetrical brain hemispheres, in human beings handedness is evident even in stillborn infants. According to one recent report, dominance may be partially determined by the blood supply to the two hemispheres. Handedness seems to be a familial trait. Females seem to have more thoroughly integrated hemispheres than males, which may account, to some extent, for the greater prevalence of reading and other perceptual problems in male children.

Hemisphere dominance may affect personality and mental processes to some extent. Purportedly those with right-hemisphere dominance (the left-handed) are more hypnotizable and produce more alpha. A psychologist, Paul Bakan, suggested that the right hemisphere might be important in the altered states of consciousness. Associated with euphoria, usually characterized by ineffability, these states indeed belong to the minor half of the brain.

Bakan believes cerebral dominance can be ascertained by posing a question that requires reflection. The left-hemisphere-dominant individual will gaze toward the right as he ponders. Activation of the right hemisphere causes him to look to the left. Bakan says that "right-movers" tend to be higher in scholastic aptitudes, left-movers in verbal; left-movers are more fluent in writing, right-movers likelier to be scientists. Rights have more tics and twitches, sleep less, prefer cool colors, and make career choices earlier. Left movers tend to have more vivid imagery, are more sociable, and are likelier to be alcoholic, musical, and religious. Asthma is commoner in left-movers, headaches (especially migraines) in right-movers.

A study by Marcel Kinsbourne, a neurologist at Duke University Medical Center, expands on the relationship between reflection and gaze. According to his extensive study, the direction of the gaze is determined by the nature of the problem and the left- or right-handedness of the subject. An individual may gaze in one direction while pondering a spatial puzzle, the other direction if involved in a linguistic problem.

Tourette's syndrome is a relatively rare disorder of the central nervous system; its victims suffer from compulsive fits of grunts, swearing, tics, and twitches. The compulsive swearing, called coprolalia, may cause the individual to be ejected from theaters, churches, department stores. Gilles de la Tourette described the syndrome as seen in eight French patients, including the Marquise Dampierre, who died at ninety after seventy years of total seclusion because of the humiliating fits.

Arthur Shapiro of New York's Payne Whitney Clinic has diagnosed and treated forty-five cases. Most respond to a major tranquilizer, haloperidol (Haldol). One patient remarked that for the first time in his life he didn't have to worry about whether his windows were open. When Shapiro had first seen him, he had been about to undergo a lobotomy—a final desperate gesture after decades of the traumatic illness.

Faruk Abuzzahab of the University of Minnesota, a psychiatrist, said, "The disease isn't as rare as we once thought, and it is missed by many pediatricians, psychologists, and neurologists." Haldol is about 95 percent effective. Individuals whose seizures are not completely controlled sometimes learn to mutter clean phrases, one authority said, in place of the usual swearing. Others can suppress the oncoming fit long enough to get to a public rest room where they can pour forth the animal-like sounds or obscenities. One young man was diagnosed after his family had spent $50,000 on fruitless medical and psychiatric treatment. With drug therapy, he now is an accomplished musician and hardworking college student, but as his parents said, "You have some emotional scars after being called crazy for most of your life."

The sociopath is an entirely different animal from the person suffering episodic dyscontrol. Many uncontrollably violent individuals go voluntarily to hospital emergency rooms to ask for help because they fear they may hurt someone. The sociopath —known as a psychopath in England—couldn't care less. He is forever remorseless. Unable to experience empathetically, unable to foresee what results his acts will have, he is supremely dangerous. Like the little girl in *The Bad Seed,* many sociopaths killed as children, perhaps murdering playmates over a disputed toy or honor. Surprisingly often the deaths are believed to be accidents. Who would suppose that a child would push his brother off a precipice or pier? And they become a matter of record only when the sociopath casually mentions the event to a prison psychiatrist.

No one knows whether the sociopath is born defective or if his chilling selfishness develops because of an environmental lack. Often he has normal brothers and sisters, which would argue against the environmental influences. On the other hand, an early institutional upbringing seems to produce a disproportionate number of psychopathic personalities.

Psychotherapy is wasted on sociopaths. Recent experiments in EEG labs around the world offer a possible explanation for the relative hopelessness of rehabilitating the psychopath. In 1964 W. Grey Walter discovered a distinctive brainwave pattern that appears in a normal subject's EEG when he knows that something is about to happen—that a tone will sound, a light will flash momentarily. This anticipatory pattern Walter called the contingency negative variation (CNV).

All normal persons show the CNV just before an expected event. In schizophrenics the response is variable, in manic-depressives it's small. Repeated tests on sociopaths show *no CNV at all.* They simply don't relate what has happened to what might happen—a failure in logic that may explain why they are not deterred from crime by the thought of punishment, much less the victim's suffering. Nor do they learn from punishment. In one study subjects had to choose between receiving a painful shock immediately or waiting for ten seconds. Normals and nonsociopathic criminals usually asked for the shock immediately, but the sociopaths preferred to wait. As J. E. Orme of Sheffield, England, put it, "Non-psychopaths find that waiting for an unpleasant event to occur is so distressing that they prefer to get it over with. Psychopaths tend to avoid immediate discomfort, as the future consequences of their behavior have little emotional significance for them."

W. Grey Walter suspects from the exaggerated heart, pupil, and pain-threshold responses of sociopaths that incoming stimuli might be reduced or otherwise distorted, causing them to make "faulty and impulsive responses." Their autonomic nervous system overreacts, and their thresholds for detecting stimuli are high. This is the mirror image of the physiological changes resulting from meditation, in which the autonomic responses (heart, breathing, galvanic skin response) become more stable and sensory perception becomes keener.

LSD has been used experimentally in treating psychopaths. In one study, the drug was given to twenty psychiatric patients, nine of them psychopaths. The investigators designated them as responders or nonresponders during the LSD session, depending on whether or not they experienced early memories, viewed relationships differently than they had, connected memories and insights to present problems, and resolved to change. Of the eight patients judged responders, seven were psychopathic personalities. At the end of six months, the LSD responder group showed the greatest improvement of the patients studied. They were still somewhat improved after one year, but several had begun to show signs of relapse. The researchers suggest that a single treatment might be less valuable than a series of LSD sessions.

As Julian Silverman pointed out in his report on LSD therapy, the autistic child's nonsocialized behavior is far different from the sociopath's antisocial behavior. Still, there are parallels. In both types LSD has reportedly facilitated a breakthrough—an almost normal relationship to others—that lasts only briefly. Both autistics and psychopaths may be afflicted by a distortion of input and a failure of the brain to integrate. In both situations, emotional attachment to others is weak or nonexistent.

For years autism was attributed to environmental factors, and the parents of autistic children were described as "emotional refrigerators." Now scientists say that autism can sometimes be diagnosed at birth by an abnormal substance in the urine. Whether its origin is genetic or prenatal isn't known, however. James Simmons, psychiatry chief at UCLA's Chidren's Inpatient Services, believes that the disease stems from a genetic deficiency. Bernard Rimland, head of the Institute for Child Behavior Research in San Diego, himself the father of an autistic child, attributes it to a biochemical malfunction, possibly an inability to use certain vitamins.

Although autism is often referred to as childhood schizophrenia, the two are not the same. Childhood schizophrenics may have developed normally up until their illness, and they can often be cured. Thus far, autism—literally, involvement with oneself—is innate and incurable. Training can, however, improve the child's social behavior and his ability to learn.

In infancy the symptoms may not be too alarming. Many normal · children appear uncommunicative, bang their heads against the crib railing, or seem to be obsessed with a single plaything. The autistic child is unresponsive, so he may seem a little dull. The usual adult horseplay may not elicit any sign of amusement, nor does the typical autistic baby smile at familiar faces.

He may be precocious in his motor development, walking earlier than his siblings. His speech is slow to develop and usually consists of parroted phrases and television slogans. Thinking in the abstract and generalizing seem all but impossible for the autistic child. He may say, "Do you want a cookie?", repeating his mother's standard question rather than asking, "May I have a cookie?" The autistic child has great difficulty in using "I" in its proper context.

Autistic children spend hours rocking themselves, spinning, or watching their own whirling hands. This self-stimulation seems to give them great pleasure. An autistic child may be transfixed by anything he sees whirling, even the water spinning down a just-flushed toilet. Such behavior is reminiscent of the gestures of epileptic children and adolescents, who whirl their hands before the sun or an artificial light to trigger photic seizures because they enjoy the aura preceding the fit.

Rimland has compared the autistic child to a traveler on a narrow path illuminated only by the narrow beam of a flashlight. The child, he said, "is grossly impaired in a function basic to all cognition—the ability to relate new stimuli to remembered experience."

One grave problem is that the child's repetitive, bizarre, destructive behavior often provokes his frustrated parents into responses that reinforce his autism. His mother may anticipate his needs to prevent possible disruption, thereby smothering whatever feeble instincts to communicate he might have had. Most of the successful work with the autistic involves tough but patient behavioral conditioning. The children learn that they get no reward unless they perform in a desirable way—for instance, by meeting the therapist eye to eye, or by saying, "I want" such and such. Destructive behavior is unrewarded. Some therapists even resort to paddling a misbehaving autistic child on the theory that only drastic stimulation will get through the child's apparent perceptual cloud.

One therapeutic approach involves behavioral conditioning but no punishment or negative stimuli. In experimental projects set up by the Central Midwestern Regional Education Laboratories, therapists simply "terminate exchanges that reinforce autistic patterns and set up exchanges that reinforce normal patterns." The children live in the Greater St. Louis area and are brought to the lab for daily sessions lasting anywhere from twenty minutes to three hours. They also spend some time in classrooms in groups of four or five. Their mothers are trained to be assistant therapists both at home and in the laboratory.

The staff believes that most autistic children play the game, "Look at me, I'm stupid," or "Look at me, I'm bizarre." Adults react, reinforcing the behavior. As an example they tell of Larry, who had been diagnosed earlier as a mental retardate of perhaps 30 IQ. Because of his gaze aversion, the staff suspected that he was an autistic child feigning stupidity to get what he wanted from adults. Larry "began to tip his hand," as they put it, as he started responding to exchanges. His mother, who was being trained as an assistant therapist, told Larry that as soon as he strung some beads he could get gum from a machine across the room.

For about ten minutes he fumbled, he whined, all the time crying, saying, "I can't." Finally, he threw the beads at his mother. Eventually the mother had the good sense to leave the room, saying, "As soon as you string those beads, you can have your gum." With his mother out of the room, according to our observers, he sat right down and in less than 30 seconds filled a string with beads with no apparent trouble.

Although completely normal behavior is rarely if ever achieved, the autistic child can be helped dramatically. As the CEMREL psychologists and educators said in a report on the autistic project, "Watching these children as they go peacefully and productively about their lessons toward the end of each experimental series is both an exhilarating and humbling experience. It is almost impossible to believe that so many had been written off as 'uneducable' by professionals, that without this therapy and training—or something similar—most would have had dark and hopeless futures."

One new approach to training autistic children was discovered almost accidentally. When a $40,000 talking typewriter was bought for the small, private Clinic for Reading and Educational Advancement in El Cajon, California, the director, Lloyd Smith, planned to use it for his regular load of neurologically handicapped students. "I had no intention of using it on autistic children," he later said. "But along the way we accepted five children who had been diagnosed as either autistic or aphasic.* And they all responded."

A soundproof booth houses the talking typewriter, formally known as the Edison Responsive Environment. It includes a multicolored letter keyboard, two video screens, a speaker system, and a tape recorder. The child is asked by a voice coming over the speaker to strike a certain letter or repeat the spelling of a word on the screen. When he makes a correct response, a chime or voice congratulates him. When he spells aloud, his answer is tape-recorded and played back to him. To some adults, the whole concept might sound like *1984,* but it unquestionably works for children with reading and perceptual disabilities,

* Incapable of using speech and perhaps incapable of understanding it.

even for many once believed hopeless. Omar K. Moore, who was instrumental in developing the talking typewriter, said, "Learning to read is learning to learn."

The Responsive Environment has inspired meaningful speech and taught reading to the five children who had been diagnosed autistic and/or aphasic. Even more remarkable, a five-year-old mongoloid boy has learned to recognize and type the letters of the alphabet, can count clearly to twenty, and, according to his parents, has expanded his vocabulary explosively since his exposure to the typewriter. Earlier his IQ had been estimated at 40.

Smith said, "Our good luck with the typewriter may run out one of these days. Maybe all the so-called autistic or aphasic children we've had have been improperly diagnosed to start with. Maybe we won't be able to reach the next one we try to help. But I think that too often we fit children into some category or other—autistic, aphasic, mongoloid, whatever—and then treat them that way from there on, without trying to help them advance any further."

One of Smith's clients was brought in at age seven with a diagnosis of profound retardation. An optometrist designed a visual-motor program for her perceptual problems, which included strabismus, poor coordination of the eyeball muscles. She was also found to be highly allergic. After treatment for her physical disabilities and six years at the reading clinic, she entered a regular classroom. On a standard psychological test her IQ was measured at 114, somewhat higher than average, and later she was named the outstanding all-round student at her school. She continues to spend two hours a week on perceptual training.

At the Institutes for the Achievement of Human Potential in Philadelphia, Glenn Doman and Carl Delacato have been unhampered by preconceived ideas since the day in the 1950s when a severely damaged four-year-old named Tommy Lunski showed them that he could read. His father had told them so but they had been unwilling to believe him; Tommy had been described as a hopeless vegetable. When they realized that he really had learned to read fluently, they began teaching other brain-injured children. They found that three-year-olds, even two-year-olds, took to the printed word with great enthusiasm. The institute has now taught several thousand brain-injured tots to read, and their coordination, hyperactivity, and emotional problems seemed to improve as a result.

There are an estimated six million retarded persons in the United States. A potentially retarded child is born every four minutes. Ironically, most retardates have not suffered a known organic disability, such as Down's syndrome, but are at least partly the products of their environment. Experience changes the brain, a tremendously significant finding of recent research. Early intervention offers the best hope for stimulating development in not only congenitally damaged children, but also those whose sterile environment contributes to poor brain development. These children are not mentally defective at birth but simply fail to advance. Functional retardation is tragically evident in children reared in institutions. At one Tehran orphanage, children who had spent their lives in cribs, staring at a blank ceiling, were unable to walk without support at age three.

The promise and perils of environmental influence are evident in the astounding results of a long-range program conducted by Rick Heber, a psychologist at the University of Wisconsin. A careful survey and testing of Milwaukee slum families indicated that grave functional retardation might be due to the retarded parent residing in the slum, rather than the slum itself.

Heber and his associates located forty newborns whose mothers had an IQ of 70 or less—feebleminded by traditional standards. Half the children were given intensive stimulation over the next four years. From infancy they were picked up each morning by their teachers and transported to a center where they spent most of each day. At first they were tutored on a one-to-one basis. At two years they were playing and learning in groups of five; at three, in groups of eight. By four, they shared three teachers with ten classmates.

These children developed so phenomenally that even Heber was stunned. By age four these offspring of retarded mothers had a mean IQ of 130, in the so-called gifted range of intelligence.

Furthermore, the scores showed a steady advance, climbing from test period to test period. The control children at the same age scored in the 80s, a mean expected for their circumstances.

If the usual pattern holds true, these children will steadily lose IQ points over the next few years until their measurable level of intelligence resembles that of their mothers.

Premature babies have a much higher retardation rate than full-term babies. Lewis Lipsitt, professor of psychology and director of the Child Study Center at Brown University, said, "Premature children contribute heavily to the populations of nonreaders, to the populations that require treatment in child-guidance clinics, and to the population of school deficient children." Although it has been widely believed that such children were defective at birth, there may be another explanation.

"In a typical good premature nursery, the baby exists in an environment largely devoid of variable stimulation," Lipsitt said. The infant lies in an incubator, surrounded by white. A plastic dome diffuses the light. The only sound he hears is the monotonous roar of the incubator motor. "Thus, during the crucial weeks or months of his life, the child is subjected to a deprived environment."

At Providence Lying-in Hospital, a colleague of Lipsitt's, E. R. Siqueland, separated the premature babies into two groups. Those in the control group received standard care and treatment. They were picked up only to be changed.

Infants in the experimental group were rocked, sung to, patted or stroked, given all the stimulation and affection normal full-term babies would have received. When all the babies were later taught to illuminate a screen by sucking on a nipple, the stimulated infants were distinctly better learners. Among the several sets of identical twins who had been included in the test, the sibling who received the stimulation learned more quickly.

Lipsitt believes that preemies may be further deprived because their mothers are afraid to relate to them and handle them when they get them home. He suggests that the mothers should be allowed to touch and talk to the babies while they're still in the hospital.

Millions of children are troubled by hyperkinesis—frenetic, uncontrollable activity, usually accompanied by poor sleep. Scientists suspect that hyperkinesis is the result of a failure of transmission within the brain. The hyperkinetic child's brainwave response to stimulation resembles that of much younger children.

This syndrome crosses all ability levels, from the severely retarded to the obviously bright. Although hyperactivity is not nearly so grave a problem as autism, the sufferers are seriously impaired in a learning situation because they have difficulty in concentrating. Their low tolerance for frustration is also an educational handicap.

The most common effective treatment thus far is paradoxical: Stimulant drugs, such as amphetamines, calm about 70 percent of the children diagnosed as hyperkinetic. Perhaps by freeing the brain transmitters, amphetamines tend to normalize attention and aggression. In one experiment, hyperkinetic children were shown to perform remarkably better on intelligence tests after they received their medication. In another study, dextroamphetamine was shown to decrease the "photic driving responses" in hyperkinetic children—that is, their susceptibility to light-induced EEG abnormalities.

Such calming techniques as meditation, brainwave training, and psychosynthesis have also been used successfully to help hyperkinetic children. Diet may also make a difference. Many have low blood sugar. A few suffer from dysinsulinism, a disorder in which the pancreas responds very sluggishly to blood sugar, allowing it to build to dangerously high levels, then overreacts, producing such a flood of insulin that the sugar drops to a hypoglycemic low. In either blood-sugar problem, the Harris diet for hypoglycemia can help graphically.

The citizens of El Paso, Texas, have, on the average, extraordinary mental health. According to John Dawson, a biochemist at the University of Texas, "They have hardly any admissions to neuropsychiatric hospitals at all." Dawson attributes their well-being to the water. El Paso's well water contains a high level of lithium. Dawson said that he found a mathematically proven relationship between lithium compound levels in the drinking water and mental hospital admissions in dozens of Texas cities.

Lithium compounds control the mania in a large percentage of manic-depressives, and the patients' depressive symptoms are treated as a separate entity. Excited depressions are controlled by one drug family, repressed depressions by other drug therapy or electroshock therapy. The excited depressed state is marked by loss of appetite, insomnia, and anxiety, the repressed type by overweight and fatigue.

Manic-depressive psychosis often has a 48-hour rhythm, with days of mania and depression alternating for years.

Pollution may damage the brain. A pilot study of Hawaiian agricultural workers exposed to pesticides showed neurological changes, including conspicuous abnormalities in the EEGs. The workers also suffered from a high incidence of hypoglycemia, muscle weakness, "and a surprising ability to fall asleep." The researchers fear that their long-term study may show that as many as 45 percent of poison-exposed workers have brain abnormalities.

Brain damage may even vary according to the type of pollutant. In one test, pregnant mice were exposed to low dosages of either DDT or sulfur. The offspring of the DDT-exposed mice were less aggressive than normal mice, but the sulfur-contaminated animals were more aggressive than normal.

Must the brain grow old? Why do some individuals grow senile in their sixties, while others are alert into their nineties? Intellectual stimulation plays an important role, of course. So do several more tangible factors: diet, exercise, the amount of oxygen available to the brain.

Free radicals—molecular fragments that attack one's cells from birth on—help form a fibrous protein that is found in the brain blood vessels in ever-increasing amounts with the passing years. This protein is a constituent in the degenerated brain tissue found in senile patients. Denham Harman of the University of Nebraska School of Medicine believes that free radicals are the agents of senility, by their action on brain cells and blood vessels over a lifetime. By adding antioxidant chemicals—BHT, vitamin E—to the diets of mice, Harman has increased their natural life span by 25 to 30 percent. He believes that the antioxidants counter the damage caused by free radicals.

Nucleic-acid therapy has been tried by Ewen Cameron, director of the Allen Memorial Institute of Psychiatry at McGill University, and a New York M.D., Benjamin Frank. Both report hopeful results. Cameron gave RNA (ribonucleic acid) to senile patients, whose memory improved noticeably, but only for the duration of treatment. RNA and DNA are critical in the body's regeneration code and messenger system. Cameron also did some of the first human experiments with the drug magnesium pemoline, known under the trade name Cylert. This drug had apparently improved the recovery of memory in rats that had undergone electroshock. Cameron reported that the double-blind test on twenty-four senile patients showed positive improvement. Some patients resumed activities, such as bridge-playing, they had long since given up. Unfortunately, further tests of Cylert have been inconclusive, and the drug is not yet marketed in the United States.

If oxygen is all-important to the brain, seriously high blood pressure should theoretically worsen intellectual deterioration. It does. At Duke University eighty-seven volunteers, who were in their sixties when the study began, were examined periodically over a ten-year period. Every thirty months they received a battery of tests—psychological and physiological, including a measurement of blood pressure. During the ten-year course of the study, those with hypertension underwent a marked intellectual loss. Those with normal blood pressure showed no decline.

Two treatments daily for fifteen days in an oxygen chamber can reverse transient memory loss or senility in most patients. The oxygenation has remarkable effects. At the Veterans Hospital in Buffalo, Eleanor Jacobs and her associates treated eighty elderly patients. Of these, seventy were declared successful; as noted earlier, five of the ten failures were chronic alcoholics whose brains had probably received more abuse than could be attributed to mere old age.

For one study, five elderly patients received pure oxygen in the chamber and the other five only normal air. The results were judged blind, but it was clear who had received the pure oxygen. The treated patients were more active, asked for reading material, began sprucing up—and four were so improved they were sent home!

Most of us take for granted a measure of self-determination. We are, at least to some extent, masters of our fate and perhaps even captains of our souls. But it's worth remembering that a few clumps of brain cells may make the difference between responsibility and degeneracy.

SCHIZOPHRENIA AND SURVIVAL

Life is more than permutations in the DNA molecule as the Fifth Symphony is more than vibrating air. And mental illness is more than an aggregate of errors in body physics and chemistry. It is a universal human experience which has a vital function in maintaining the vital balance. —KARL MENNINGER

The new psychiatry, if we might term it that, is suggesting that labels are inadequate . . . that even in pathology there may be hope. Perhaps, for many, schizophrenia really is a benign fever, burning out the old and making way for real self-discovery. Madness, in its way, illustrates in living color the creative technology of the brain and body.

Research is attempting to track down the elusive biochemical causes of the schizophrenic episode. Investigators are studying the limbic brain structures that may be involved, analyzing genetic factors, and cataloging an incredible array of physical and sensory abnormalities that accompany schizophrenia.

Schizophrenics have abnormally high or low copper levels and blood histamine levels. In the early stages of acute schizophrenia, patients are able to detect stimuli too subtle for normal senses. Many psychiatrists report that schizophrenics seem to have enhanced telepathic ability. Their sleep patterns are abnormal, their time estimation inconsistent, their brainwave responses atypical.

Psychiatrists sometimes examine nail-fold capillaries and palmar creases because there are certain patterns sometimes predictive of childhood schizophrenia. Low blood sugar is common in schizophrenics, but diabetes is only one-thirtieth as prevalent as in the general population. Seventy percent of schizophrenic children, according to one monumental study, had adverse circumstances of birth, complications during pregnancy or delivery.

Many exotic substances, some of them unidentified, have been found in schizophrenics' urine or plasma. Three such substances are hallucinogenic when administered to normal subjects. A deficiency of B_{12} has also been observed.

Autoimmunity has been blamed. Some theorists suspect an antibody reaction in the brain following encephalitis or rheumatic fever. Sexual hormones play some role. The hormone circulated in the mother's blood by a male fetus reportedly may forestall her schizophrenia until after delivery. Some schizophrenic women are greatly improved when taken off contraceptive pills.

However bewildering, the findings make a critical point. Whatever schizophrenia is, psychotherapy isn't likely to affect it. As the professional committee of the Schizophrenia Foundation put it, "You might just as well try to cure a patient of diabetes by psychotherapy."

There is strong evidence for a genetic predisposition to schizophrenia. For example, there is the case of Paul and Esther, siblings reared apart (one with each parent). Their mother was said to be a pathological liar and to have lived in a world of her own. Their father had been given a psychiatric discharge from the Army. Although Paul was a bright student, progressive confusion and depression afflicted him when he was seventeen. At twenty-three he was hospitalized with a diagnosis of schizophrenia.

Esther was equally studious. At seventeen she began suffering the first symptoms of mental disturbance, and at twenty-three she entered an institution where she was diagnosed as schizophrenic.

These cases were reported in the *American Journal of Psychiatry*. Psychiatric literature has many similar reports that indicate a genetic basis for schizophrenia. Schizophrenic quadruplets have been treated. A long-term California study followed schizophrenics' children who had been placed in foster homes before the age of one year. Several times as many of these children became schizophrenic as should have occurred in a normal population. If one identical twin is schizophrenic, there is reportedly an 85-percent chance that the other will also become ill. In one particularly strange case, identical twin brothers reared apart in Texas were admitted to the same state hospital during the same month. Each was diagnosed as a paranoid schizophrenic. Each believed that he was being poisoned.*

The genetic susceptibility can probably be traced to the failure of an important enzyme. It is not clear which enzyme, but monoamine oxidase (MAO), a substance important in the functioning of the nervous system, has been implicated. A team of U.S. government psychiatrists reported that less active than normal MAO was found not only in schizophrenics but in their identical twins. The significantly lower MAO activity in *both* twins was an important finding because up to that point scientists thought that the lazy enzyme might be attributed to medication, dietary differences, or the effects of hospitalization.

The legendary Zelda, wife of Scott Fitzgerald, showed evidence of periodic thought disorders while still a teen-ager, but her schizophrenia didn't enter its florid stage until her late twenties. From then until her death in a sanatorium fire twenty years later, she was periodically ill.

Fitzgerald explored every possible medical avenue, including famous Swiss psychiatric clinics. He, Zelda, and their relatives and friends blamed each other endlessly for the tragic state of affairs. Out of the Freudian theories of Zelda's doctors, Fitzgerald created one of his most admired novels, *Tender is the Night*. Even so, he had an irrepressible suspicion that there was some other explanation. Once, on an impulse, Fitzgerald wrote to Zelda's Swiss doctors. Apologizing for what he felt must sound like a layman's crackpot notion, he suggested that "some uneliminated poison attacks the nerves. . . . I can't help clinging to the idea that some essential physical thing, like salt or iron or semen or some unguessed-at holy water, is either missing or is present in too-great quantity."

Ironically, Freud himself had once urged a favorite disciple, Schiler, to study schizophrenic behavior quickly because science was surely on the verge of discovering its chemistry and it would become as rare as the American Indian. Jung also be-

---

* This particular case, cited by John Pfeiffer in *The Human Brain*, showed such striking similarity in the delusions that telepathy might be a likelier explanation. Identical twins are said by parapsychologists to have an unusually high degree of telepathic rapport.

lieved that a biochemical basis for the psychoses would be found; psychoanalytic techniques were a holding action at best.

When it was observed that as many as 50 percent of heart-transplant patients had become briefly psychotic, one psychiatrist announced to the press that these patients were no doubt upset over having a stranger's heart. Yet postcardiotomy delirium has since been described as a definite syndrome among open-heart surgery patients, regardless of whether they receive a transplant. As many as 20 percent become psychotic in from three to five days after surgery. According to Ernest Hartmann, Tufts School of Medicine, the disorder usually lasts from twenty-four to forty-eight hours and is marked by hallucinations, paranoid thought, and general confusion.

Hartmann compared the symptoms to sleep-deprivation psychosis and sensory isolation phenomena. Because anesthesia and the low body temperatures of open-heart surgery can alter the blood-brain barrier, there may be an increase in the serotonin available to the brain. Too, platelets breaking down may increase the blood serotonin. And "patients are not allowed much opportunity to sleep, both because of their anxiety and because of various technical procedures in the period before and after open-heart surgery."

Schizophrenia—literally, a cleaved mind—disables more of our citizenry than any other ailment. *One-fourth of all hospital beds are occupied by schizophrenics.* The two million diagnosed cases, 1 percent of the population, probably represent only a fraction of the total number of sufferers. Mild schizophrenia is often misdiagnosed as neurosis.

Schizophrenics' suicide rate is twenty times that of the general population and their reproduction rate only 70 percent that of the general population. Why, then, has the disease persisted from generation to generation? Random mutations could not account for it. Biologists and geneticists have suggested that a major dominant gene—sometimes called SC—has a 25-percent penetrance in the general population. Schizophrenia has some unaccountable beneficial side effects that may compensate for the statistical risks such as suicide. Some observers believe that schizophrenics are oddly resistant to virus infections. A monumental study of mortality statistics in Russia, Greece, Scotland,

Wales, and England disclosed that psychiatric patients are afflicted by cancer at less than one-third the rate of the general population. Schizophrenics are especially resistant to cancer. The long-awaited breakthrough may have come. One of thousands of body chemicals, a substance called alpha-2 globulin, is present in everyone, but there are unusually high concentrations in many schizophrenics. More significantly, a high percentage of the alpha-2 globulin molecules in schizophrenics are defective. Rather than randomly shaped, they are spiral. Injected into rats, the defective form produces confused, disoriented behavior.

Charles Frohman, a biochemist at Detroit's Lafayette Clinic, and Edward Domino of the University of Michigan maintain that the formation of defective alpha-2 globulin results from the failure of an enzyme they call "anti-S" (S for schizophrenia). Theoretically this enzyme, which can be obtained from beef brains, should clear up the disordered thinking of schizophrenics apparently by unkinking the defective molecules.

John Berger, a physiologist at the Worcester Foundation, has begun studies on the effect of anti-S on the behavior of monkeys. Since defective alpha-2 globulin produces distinctive brainwave patterns, anti-S may restore the EEG to normalcy.

Alpha-2 globulin controls the concentration of tryptophan, a chemical that produces another substance vital to transmission. Tryptophan in schizophrenics may be 50 percent above normal, which may account to some extent for the sensory flooding. Another tryptophan derivative is DMT,* a hallucinogen. Normal individuals have only a tiny amount of DMT. Three times as much has been detected in schizophrenics.

The onset of acute schizophrenia is characterized by overstimulation, sleeplessness, and sometimes a euphoric, psychedelic perception. The individual is supernormally sensitive to stimuli and integrates them rapidly. This early stage is virtually identical to the creative bursts that have produced some of our greatest music, mathematical formulae, and art. In fact, Joan Fitzherbert, an English psychiatrist, found that in the period immediately preceding a psychotic break, schizophrenic chil-

* Dimethyltryptophan.

dren scored twenty or more points higher on IQ tests than their healthy norm. They were untestable while ill, but dropped to the lower score after recovery. Another researcher said, "There is evidence to suggest that genes involved in schizophrenia affect the arousal level of the brain and that, apart from their potential for causing psychosis, they may be conducive to giftedness and creativity."

In the early phase the schizophrenic, like the artist or mystic, may feel at one with the universe, newly awakened. He may say that everything clicks, makes sense, for the first time in his life. He makes new connections, reads fresh meanings into everyday language, like a poet finding metaphors. He may suddenly begin to place literal interpretations on common phrases and figures of speech. A friend who says, "I'm darning socks," may seem to the schizophrenic to be literally darning or condemning menial household chores.

If the schizophrenic receives sleep therapy at this point, the pathological breakdown may not come. Usually, though, the insomnia worsens and the excitement increases. The dizzying, vibrant external stimuli become unbearable. The schizophrenic frequently says that he has somehow been charged, electrified, energized. If he blames outside factors he evolves a schema that may be paranoid, in which case his illness takes a slightly different turn from that of the nonparanoid. He may decide that if he is worth persecuting, he must be important; perhaps he is Christ or an astronaut.

Most hallucinations are auditory. Some schizophrenics see changes in the visual field comparable to LSD-induced hallucinations—a face may seem to change form, a wall to move—but these are less common. In full-blown schizophrenia, the heightened perception is no longer a joy but a hideous assault. Most of the major anti-psychotic drugs sedate the brain and raise the supersensitive arousal threshold. It is not unusual for patients to regret, after they are well, that the world has become drab and unattractive again in comparison to its vibrancy during the early stages of their illness. Their sentiments parallel Wordsworth's sorrow that childhood's glorious perceptions pass and one lives thereafter in "the light of common day."

Some suicides of schizophrenics can be blamed on the early euphoria, others on the depression and confusion of later stages. Frequently, because of what seem to be insights into immortality, the schizophrenic believes that he can safely leap from a tower or stop an onrushing train. The curious literalness may also take its toll. One man considered ingesting a toxic toilet-bowl cleaner, Vanish, because he wanted to disappear.

The intensity often rebounds into a deep depression, perhaps because the brain amines are exhausted. One-third of all acute cases clear up spontaneously; the body chemistry seems to regain its equilibrium somehow.

The human biochemical factory has a remarkable capacity for manufacturing psychedelics. As noted earlier, even normal individuals have small amounts of DMT in their bloodstream, having converted it from tryptamine. Dopamine can be methylated to create mescaline. Adrenaline can be converted to adrenochrome, a mild hallucinogen. Serotonin can be chemically altered to bufotenin, a psychedelic. Bufotenin was found in twenty-five of twenty-six hallucinating schizophrenics in one survey. The body may also change alcohol into substances resembling both peyote and morphine.

Finding a galloping psychedelic in the body doesn't answer the basic question of how its interaction with the brain causes thought disorder. If the failure of a basic protective enzyme is proved, the various biochemical theories might well be integrated.

The role of sex hormones is unclear. Testosterone therapy is surprisingly successful in treating some female schizophrenics. Reportedly some women recover spontaneously after the menopause. Abnormal hormone activity is blamed for postpartum psychosis, a disorder that for many years was attributed to the patient's fear of motherhood, sense of inadequacy, or the emotional anticlimax of delivery. The Schizophrenia Foundation of New Jersey reported the case of a woman who had postpartum psychosis after her fifth, sixth, seventh, and eighth children.

Sex hormones play a part in some cyclical psychoses. Many women report overt symptoms only at the time of menstruation, and a few men seem to become mentally aberrant on a similarly lunar schedule. Some schizophrenics report that a suddenly increased libido is one of the first signs of an impending break. Puberty, with its rush of hormonal activity, triggers a high percentage of cases; in fact, the old name for schizophrenia was dementia praecox, insanity of youth.

Trace minerals are important both in hormonal activity and histamine production. Carl Pfeiffer and his associates at Princeton noted that many schizophrenics had abnormal levels of copper. Copper activates an enzyme that removes histamine. Treated with a copper antagonist, the patients' thought disorders seemed to lessen as their histamine levels rose to normal.

Histamine is another brain transmitter that can be methylated to produce a stimulating compound. The Princeton group had earlier determined that there were two schizophrenic types, high-histamine and low-histamine. The low-histamine patients, termed *histapenic,* were hyperactive, had a high tolerance for pain and a poor attention span. They seldom showed allergic symptoms or any sign of a head cold. The other group, the *histadelics,* had high histamine levels. They were inclined to be suicidal and complained of a blank mind. Although more than half the histadelics diagnosed were female, the Schizophrenia Foundation cautioned that the statistics may reflect "the greater efficiency of the male patient in his suicide procedures."

The Princeton group reported also that female patients showed a marked difference in trace metal levels during the premenstrual period, a time commonly associated with anxiety and depression. Some schizophrenics taking the Pill had high copper levels and improved rapidly when taken off the contraceptives. The electrical activity of the minerals plays a vital role in the body's busy metabolism (five thousand known enzymes, over two million reactions per minute).

Some researchers are studying the effects of trace metals on the brain's EEG activity. A zinc compound decreases the amplitude of brainwaves in the cortex and lowers their variance of amplitude in the hippocampus. The zinc compound may act as an antidepressant. In the 1930s a French scientist, M. L. Robinet, reported that suicides correlated statistically with the levels of magnesium content in the soil in various locales. He said, "The use of magnesium permits one to support adversity with serenity." A San Francisco psychiatrist, Richard Kunin, checks his patients' trace mineral levels by analyzing a lock of hair. Abnormal levels of zinc, copper, magnesium, manganese, and potassium are common in disturbed patients, and normalizing the trace minerals often restores mental health. Other studies have shown that zinc and manganese sedate some schizophrenics, changing brainwave activity into calmer patterns.

Robert Heath of Tulane has suggested that an autoimmune response, a sensitivity to one's own brain, may trigger the manufacture of a psychedelic protein he calls Taraxein. Injecting a small dose of histamine into the septal area of a monkey's brain produces schizophrenic symptoms. Brainwave activity from that region of a schizophrenic's brain sometimes shows epileptic-like spikes.

Hypoglycemia has been found in a high percentage of mental patients. When the brain is low on sugar, confusion, excitement, depression, dizziness, and erratic thinking are among the symptoms. The high incidence of hypoglycemia among the mentally ill has made the once-popular insulin-shock therapy inadvisable. Insulin could push the hypoglycemic into a brain-damaging, perhaps fatal, coma.

Schizophrenics have some mildly characteristic brainwave responses, particularly to flashing lights. Schizophrenic subjects in one study had a more variable individual response to tones. Remarking on the subjects whose EEGs he had studied, W. Grey Walter said, "Some of these patients have mentioned how they find difficulty in concentrating on the trivial stimuli [of the test situation] while they are considering the scintillating events in their own minds."

Research has drawn a fine sketch of the schizophrenic aboard his strange carousel. Bombarded by stimuli to which he is hypersensitive, the nonparanoid may drop a curtain between himself and the environment. He turns inward. The paranoid increases his vigilance, missing no trivial details in the environment but oblivious to direct questions and loud noises.

Brainwave studies of catatonic schizophrenics, as well as their own recollections, indicate that while the catatonic may appear stone-still, he is struggling in a furious inner saga. He maintains his outward rigidity to control the seething world within.

Schizophrenics have an abnormally sensitive autonomic reaction to stress and a strangely rapid recovery. Their galvanic skin response to a clanging noise, for example, is much greater than that of normals, and they also fail to habituate to the sound, responding each time as if for the first time. But after each response, the skin returns to its base level instantaneously, rather than fading gradually as in normals.

This phenomenon was observed by the Danish researcher Sarnoff Mednick, who collected data on more than 9000 consecutive births at a Copenhagen hospital. He then undertook a long-term study of the 207 children born to schizophrenic mothers and 104 low-risk children with no known genetic susceptibility. Seven years after he began the study, 20 of the high-risk children were disturbed, 13 of these hospitalized.

He then compared the sick children to a group of high-risk children who had not yet developed mental problems. He found that *70 percent of the sick children had suffered from serious prenatal and birth complications,* compared to 6 percent of the well high-risk children. Mednick speculates that these children, who showed the characteristic stress reaction, may have been brain-injured during pregnancy or birth. The hippocampus is particularly vulnerable to oxygen deprivation. If damaged it would not adequately perform its function of monitoring the delicate balance of stress hormones produced by the pituitary and adrenals.* Rats with hippocampal injuries behave in a test situation very much like the sick Danish children. They overreact, fail to habituate, and learn an avoidance response very quickly. Unlearning comes hard.

Under the auspices of the World Health Organization, Mednick is undertaking a study on the island of Mauritius in the Indian Ocean. Because the island population is stable and easy to keep track of, a long-term study should be fruitful. Mednick will determine the high-risk children on the basis of birth and pregnancy complications, then will locate those three-year-olds who already exhibit ominous physiological and psychological symptoms. In a nursery-school environment, the psychologist and his team will try to teach the children to deal with stress positively rather than by avoidance. He said, "The nursery school may be the preventive treatment center of the future."

For patients who recover, schizophrenia is sometimes a valuable experience, providing insights similar to those in psychedelic therapy and mystical experience, or those that result from many years of costly analysis. One psychiatrist compared the

---

* The stress hormone derivatives, such as cortisone, have caused psychotic symptoms in arthritics. Stress also markedly affects the histamine levels.

illness to an earthquake that "by convulsing the upper strata of our globe, throws upon its surface precious and splendid fossils. . . ."

Karl Menninger emphasized that many persons transcend their illness, "an extraordinary and little realized truth." A patient recovering from a rather long illness may improve past the point of his former normal state of existence.

> He not only gets well, to use the vernacular; he gets as well as he was, and then he continues to improve still further. He increases his productivity, he expands his life and its horizons. He develops new talents, new powers, new effectiveness. He becomes, one might say, "weller than well."

Admitting that this doesn't always happen, Menninger maintained that psychiatry should be alert to such possibilities, much as "the bobbing lid of his mother's teakettle caught Watts's attention and curiosity."

As examples he cited such famous figures as Abraham Lincoln, William James, and John Stuart Mill, all of whom went through a period of psychotic depression before the brilliant years of achievement. He quoted his collaborator and colleague Martin Mayer, who said that "inner unrest, even turmoil, need not signify only illness; it may often signal incipient change for the better." Mayer suggested that, even among the healthy, what seems to be wasteful inner strife may be positive striving.

The psychiatrist Julian Silverman, research specialist with the California Department of Mental Hygiene, emphasizes that schizophrenia may help many individuals if well-meaning doctors don't chemically abort the journey.

"There are forms of schizophrenic experience that can be positively and creatively constructive. . . . There is mounting evidence that some of the most profound schizophrenic disorganizations are preludes to impressive reorganization and personality growth—not so much breakdown as breakthrough."

Silverman believes that schizophrenia sometimes becomes the answer when all of one's usual problem-solving techniques fail in the face of a crisis. The patient most likely to benefit from his schizophrenia is one whose illness was sudden, probably precipitated by an event. Slow-developing schizophrenias are less likely to be helpful.

Silverman, R. D. Laing, and a number of other psychiatrists

have proposed that many of the mentally ill should be given sanctuary rather than treatment. These practitioners compare the psychotic experience to the religious experiences that are socially acceptable, even prized, in other cultures.

Dr. Humphry Osmond of Saskatchewan reminded his colleagues that drug-induced psychotic experiences should prove to the sane that the schizophrenic is neither imagining or fantasizing when he says that the world has changed.

> We should listen seriously to mad people, for, in phrases that are usually clumsy, ill-constructed, and even banal, they try to tell us of voyages of the human soul that make the wanderings of Odysseus seem no more than a Sunday's outing. They tell us of a purgatory from which none return unscathed. They tell us of another world than this; but mostly we don't hear, because we are talking at them to assure them that they are mistaken. The least we can do for these far voyagers is to hear them courteously and try to do them no harm.

Psychotic experience can be viewed in much the same light as dream experience: Whatever its biochemistry, it is rich in symbols and fresh self-knowledge, and sometimes it even furnishes answers.

Comparing mysticism and schizophrenia, the psychologist Kenneth Wapnick cited as examples St. Teresa and Lara Jefferson, a woman who wrote of the liberating influence of her schizophrenia. The schizophrenic, Wapnick said, is thrust into his seething inner world without preparation. By moving gradually and deliberately inward, the mystic develops what Wapnick calls the "muscle" to withstand the powerful experience. Some schizophrenics are virtually reborn, however. During the course of their trip, they discard their old, limiting, fearful personae and experience a birth, the liberation of a richer, more authentic self. As Lara Jefferson put it, "Remember, when a soul sails out on that unmarked sea called Madness [it has] gained release." The person born during her schizophrenic illness became the surviving Lara.

Many psychiatrists and psychologists have suggested that their proper roles might be as guides, much as one leads a subject through an LSD trip, helping him explore the symbols he sees, talking him down if he should panic.

Treatments that have proved useful for schizophrenia include drug therapy, megavitamin therapy, and shock therapy. By lessening the hyperarousal of the schizophrenic, the major tranquilizers calm the buzzing, blinding confusion that so torments his perception. Some of the side effects of the antipsychotic drugs include muscle contractions, tremor, restlessness, decreased red or white blood cells, jaundice, depression, convulsions, sensitivity of the skin to sunlight, increase in appetite and body weight. The psychiatric depression that sometimes results at least gives the therapist something new to work on!

Megavitamin therapy has been highly successful alone and in combination with drug treatment. Large doses of niacin (B_3) and sometimes B_6, C, and E are administered. (Another form of B_3, niacinamide, is often given to schizophrenic children but seems to cause depression in adults.) Nutritional problems alone can cause bizarre mental disturbances. Pellagra, solely a deficiency of B_3, filled madhouses all over the world before its origin was discovered. Magnesium and calcium deficiencies have caused symptoms, including suicidal depression; violent derangement has been seen in hypoglycemics and can be corrected by diet.

Among the disorders once lumped with schizophrenia are syphilitic psychosis; porphyria, caused by an identified chemical abnormality; myxedematous madness, severe thyroid deficiency; amphetamine psychosis; homocysteinuria, an enzyme abnormality that can be treated by diet; and B_{12} (cyanocobalamine) and folic acid deficiency. In 1970 London hospitals reported an epidemic of the latter. Most of the patients were Vegans, members of a vegetarian cult opposed even to eggs and milk. Old people who develop a first-time psychosis are commonly B_{12}-deficient.

Add to the list postpartum psychosis, postcardiotomy delirium, temporal-lobe epilepsy, and barbiturate psychosis, and it becomes apparent that diagnosis is no easy matter. Brain tumors and concussions can cause schizophrenic symptoms.

In one case a young husband and father complained for months of headaches, disorientation, and anxiety. Psychotherapy didn't seem to help. One day he called his wife from a service station miles from their Miami home, explaining that he was hopelessly lost. On his doctor's advice, the wife committed him to a psychiatric ward. As he lay in his room, a neurologist stopped in for a routine examination—and immediately diagnosed an abscess in the sinus cavity. Too late; the patient was dead within the hour.

In its early stages, acute schizophrenia bears a strong family resemblance to the less pathological altered states, and, like the others, it has been associated with enhanced psi abilities.

Even in 1948, when such admissions were unpopular, 23 percent of psychiatrists surveyed reported that they had observed what seemed to be extrasensory awareness in their patients. The British psychiatrist L. J. Bendit reported that many mental patients displayed ESP; he convinced them that some of the phenomena were paranormal rather than irrational, a possibility they found less threatening. Carroll Nash of St. Joseph's College in Philadelphia, who has surveyed medical parapsychology on a worldwide basis, tells of some Brazilian hospitals in which patients disturbed by voices or visions are trained to hear and see them more clearly. This approach seems to improve their mental health.

Some theorists blame the frequency of psi on the schizophrenic's regression: Alienated by his illness, perhaps he falls back on more primitive channels of communication. Another school maintains that the channels are available and in order all the time, but they are attended to only rarely—as in psychosis.

Jan Ehrenwald, a New York psychiatrist, has suggested that the paranoid individual may be telepathically sensitive to the repressed sadistic-aggressive tendencies in others' unconscious minds. He believes that much of what the patient finds uncanny is due to telepathy.

Ehrenwald, Jule Eisenbud, and Montague Ullman are among the prominent psychiatrists who first became interested in parapsychology because of telepathic interaction with patients. One of the earliest instances Ullman recalls involved a patient's dream sequence about a cat, alcohol, and cream. On the night of the dream, Ullman and his wife had viewed a colleague's movies of a laboratory cat that had been experimentally transformed into an alcoholic. The animal preferred alcohol to cream.

As early as 1949, Ullman remarked on such phenomena:

Very ill individuals teetering on the brink but not yet over on the psychotic side often indicate remarkable psi ability in the course of analysis. . . . Once psychosis, or the complete absence of effective relationships with other people, sets in, the psi functioning is not remarkable. . . .

Of course, the full-fledged psychotic is a poor experimental subject. First of all, as the EEG researchers have found, he is not motivated. Like Alice in Wonderland, he is absorbed in a world vastly more compelling and real than the one outside.

With some psychiatric patients it is hard to determine which came first, the psi or the psychosis. Thelma Moss reported that in the course of one year the Neuropsychiatric Institute at UCLA treated three individuals who had dabbled in automatic writing. Two had to be hospitalized. The writing had become so obsessive that it now took over if they tried to type a memo or jot down a grocery list.

Asserting that the various mind-training courses have resulted in a number of psychotic breaks, Elmer Green said, "A lot of people are being catapulted off into altered states of consciousness, and they're not all prepared for the psychic phenomena they may encounter."

Any technique that facilitates a sudden unleashing of unconscious forces is inherently risky, of course. A number of psychiatric journals have devoted issues to the paranormal during the past few years, and practitioners are more openly discussing clinical aspects of the problem. Speaking to the Academy of Psychoanalysis in 1971, Montague Ullman sounded a warning:

> Those of us who have taken a public position espousing the reality of psi events are aware of a lost battalion of people who are in distress and wish to seek psychiatric help but who hold back out of fear of rebuff. They are people who have had psi experiences they consider to be both genuine and either central to their problem or related to it. They fear exposing themselves to an entrenched bias. . . . [They fear that] no credence is to be expected and that what they have experienced . . . couldn't be anything but pathological. Caught in this kind of bind, many such individuals ultimately gravitate toward fringe groups in search of the support they need.

15

BRAIN FOOD: OBESITY AND MALNUTRITION

Obesity is a uniquely human problem. Blame the brain . . . not because of mysterious psychological reasons, although these may play a part, but because the new brain—the neocortex—has overruled the appetite and satiety centers in the old brain for so long that they no longer signal the body's needs.

By insisting on three substantial meals a day rather than the frequent small meals of our ancestors and of infant human beings, the neocortex overrules the hypothalamus. The neocortex takes an esthetic interest in food, hungry or not. When incipient hunger or satiation warnings from the old brain come at an inconvenient time, the neocortex ignores them. Little by little, the signals come faintly or not at all.

In the obese and in the millions who are fighting encroaching overweight, the desire to eat apparently originates in the visual cortex rather than in the primitive hunger centers. For example, French researchers found that obese subjects who had been loaded with glucose still found the sweet taste of sucrose pleasant. Normally, the sweet taste would become sickening. Somehow the natural satiation mechanism has been subverted in the obese.

The brain supervises the body's nutrient needs ceaselessly. It measures the difference between the glucose in the arteries and the glucose in the veins. It also measures blood volume, and a slight drop signals thirst.

Electrical stimulation of the brain's hunger center will produce a raging appetite, even if the subject has just stuffed down an enormous meal. Stimulation in the satiety center generates a sensation of overpowering fullness, even in a half-starved subject. Thirst, too, can be stimulated artificially.

If the experimenters damage the rat's hunger center, he will starve himself to death unless force-fed. If his satiety mechanism is damaged, he gorges until he has doubled or tripled his weight. But strangely enough, the gluttonous rat is finicky. If the laboratory chow is stale he only picks at it, and if it is given a slightly unpleasant flavor, he won't eat at all. If he has to press a lever or perform a trick for his food, chances are he won't bother.

Human beings are much the same. In studies of obese and lean subjects, researchers found that lean subjects would eat at regular intervals, even if the only nutrient available was Metrecal. The obese would skip eating altogether. On the other hand, when a plate of roast beef sandwiches was offered, the lean subject would typically eat one . . . and the obese person would lick the platter clean.

Nibbling may indeed be our innate eating pattern. Lower mammals certainly seem to be nibblers, as do young human beings. At the University of Virginia Medical School, one group of rats was given access to food all day long. Another group was allowed to eat during a two-hour period only. The latter group soon learned to gorge enough for the day's requirements, then began eating more than their nibbling counterparts. At the conclusion of the study, they weighed one-third more than the nibblers.

In another experiment, rats fed once daily were found to have acquired twice the fat in their carcasses as that accumulated by the free feeders.

"When you eat a great deal in a very short period," said Jay Tepperman, professor of experimental medicine at Upstate Medical Center in Syracuse, "you sort of train your fat-forming apparatus to form more fat."

P. Fabry, a Czech researcher, studied four hundred men between the ages of sixty and sixty-four. One group ate three or fewer meals daily; the other group ate five times or oftener. Far fewer of the nibblers became overweight, and they were dramatically healthier in glucose tolerance. Even their cholesterol was lower.

The responses of the obese body are like a slow-motion movie. Normally, starvation stimulates the tissue to release stored fat. In a 27-day fasting study of obese and lean subjects, three-quarters of the obese displayed a pronounced lag before their bodies finally began releasing stored fat.

The so-called fat doctors, MDs specializing in obesity cases, often put their patients on a 500-calorie diet and daily injections of a growth hormone, HCG. HCG is human chorionic gonadotrophin, a placental hormone usually present only in pregnancy. The starvation diet, like a demanding fetus, stimulates the hormone to unlock the body's fat reserves.

Some scientists speculate that the obese may have a deficiency in HGH, human growth hormone, and that some fatties truly do eat like birds. Rats given HGH can gorge on rich foods yet remain lean.

For many years physical exercise has been debunked as a method of controlling weight. Now it appears that a reversal is in order. University of Edinburgh researchers found that briskly walking subjects released intermittent bursts of growth hormone. The growth hormone liberates stored fat. Interestingly enough, carbohydrate turns off the growth hormone. Walkers who ingested glucose while exercising did not release growth hormone.

Body wisdom is a curious kind of knowing. Children deficient in calcium have been known to eat chalk in the classroom. Children with diagnosed emotional dwarfism, a syndrome involving an apparent failure of the pituitary gland, steal fat from garbage cans and drink from toilets to satisfy their cravings.

Researchers at Rockefeller University loaded rats with water, then placed them in a maze. If the rats went to one arm of the T-maze they received an injection of antidiuretic hormone that interfered with water excretion. In the other arm, a saline injection would allow the excess water to be excreted. The rats learned to aim for the saline solution.

No phenomenon is stranger than the apparent primitive capacity of the brain to desire meat or feel distaste for it. The limbic brain seems to be the key.

An aversion to meat is seen in many individuals in altered states of consciousness, states in which the limbic brain seems to have gained ascendancy. Schizophrenics often refuse to eat meat because it seems suddenly distasteful. Psychedelic drugs sometimes engender a strong aversion to meat. Longtime meditators often say that they gave up meat because they had eventually lost their taste for it.

On the other hand, a null magnetic field, which apparently lowers the normal level of consciousness, causes cannibalism in mice. If the amygdala of a monkey is damaged, the animal tends to become carnivorous. And a Princeton research team recently announced evidence for a hypothalamic mechanism that can either activate killing in a rat or can suppress it. By injections that interfered with this system, they made killers out of rats that would not ordinarily kill mice.*

Malnutrition and specific vitamin or mineral deficiencies can devastate the brain's hierarchy, causing permanent retardation in a very young child, depression or psychosis in an adult. Neurologist Charles Sherrington's description of the body as "transformed groceries" is a graphic reminder of human dependence on nutrients.

Myron Winick of New York Hospital estimated that more than 300 million children are suffering malnutrition's effects on the brain. Winick and Pedro Rosso, a Santiago pediatrician, found that Chilean children who had been malnourished in their early years had measurably smaller-than-normal head circumferences, implying smaller brains and a lower number of brain cells.

"The vicious cycle begins in infancy and condemns a person to a lifetime of perhaps marginal function," Winick said. He pointed out that a dull adult is in no position to rescue his own children from a similar fate. Winick places indirect blame for

---

* The researchers injected crystalline carbachol, a cholinomimetic, into the lateral hypothalamus. The injection of various brain transmitters, drugs, and salts had no effect, and the carbachol was not effective elsewhere in the hypothalamus. "We infer that in the lateral hypothalamus, a cholinergic substance, probably acetylcholine, is a neurohumor in part of an innate system for killing," they said.

the worsening worldwide malnutrition on the industrialization which brings about a decline in the number of children who are breast-fed. Even when the mother herself is half-starved, the human body manufactures milk efficiently. Human milk is adequate to forestall malnutrition-caused retardation during the first year of life. In undeveloped countries, retardation's gross signs are not evident until after weaning.

One Winick-Rosso study reported that even after the semi-starved children were put on normal diets, over 90 percent remained limited in their capacity to adapt to the environment, and more than half were educable only with a special teaching system.

British pediatrician John Dobbing made a chilling point. Growth retardation does not alter the *timing* of the growth spurt in the brain. "There is no true retardation in the Oxford Dictionary sense of a delay in accomplishment. The trajectory is lower. The brain has a once-and-for-all opportunity. If its opportunity is lost, it can never be fully recovered."

The grave results of prenatal malnutrition were evident in a series of studies at UCLA. Stephen Zamenhof and his associates underfed pregnant rats, then measured the brain deficiencies in their progeny. Astonishingly, Zamenhof and his associates found that baby rats may reflect the poor prenatal diets of their *grandmothers*.

Very young human mothers bear a disproportionate number of underweight, retarded babies. Since teen-age girls are commonly undernourished, Zamenhof's experiments suggest that these human fetuses, like the gestating rats, were unable to mobilize enough nutrients from their mothers' supply.

Vitamin A plays a vital role in brain development. Too little can cause retardation, and so can too much. Indonesian children who were deficient in vitamin A as well as generally undernourished scored significantly lower on intelligence tests than those who had been malnourished but whose A-intake was adequate. On the other hand, an excess of vitamin A interferes with the differentiation of certain cells in the growing brain. Rats fed too much bear spastic, hyperactive offspring.

When female rats are fed a copper-deficient diet, their offspring are brain-damaged. They overreact to noise, convulse, and fall into catatonic postures.

Although adult brains are miraculously immune to permanent damage from starvation, specific nutritional shortages can seriously disrupt brain processes. Trace minerals or a lack thereof play a part in schizophrenia. Lack of magnesium can produce mental fatigue, irritability, even suicidal depression or maniacal behavior. Confusion and coma may also result.

Scientists in Switzerland and at Massachusetts Institute of Technology found that vitamin E-deficient rats lost quantities of the brain transmitter norepinephrine. In other studies rats fed diets low in vitamin E died at an early age; postmortems showed damage in the brain and spinal cord.

Vitamin D is vital for assimilation of calcium, and calcium is vital for nervous-system activity. There is some speculation that the lack of sunshine in northern countries may play a role in the high suicide rate, because there is an inadequate source of natural vitamin D.

The brain needs B_6, pyridoxine. Human infants on B_6-deficient formulas suffer convulsions. In experiments at the University of North Carolina, rats had seizures in exact proportion to the extent of their deficiency in pyridoxine. The greater the lack, the more frequent the convulsions.

Individuals may vary radically in their needs for specific vitamins and trace minerals. Ascorbic acid, vitamin C, is a case in point. Animals manufacture their own from glucose, but man presumably lost that ability through a genetic mutation.

Rats under stress synthesize vitamin C at a rate equivalent to fifteen or twenty grams daily in man. An agitated mouse manufactures it at a rate equal to one hundred grams in man. According to Irwin Stone, a New York biochemist, schizophrenics have been given thirty grams of vitamin C per day without satisfying enough of their heightened bodily demands to excrete any of the vitamin. That is roughly one thousand times greater than the federally recommended minimum daily requirement.

The properties of vitamin C are not understood but clearly powerful. Russian scientists administered a lethal mercury compound to sixty albino rats. Thirty of the rats were given ascorbic acid along with the poison. Postmortem examination showed profoundly greater damage in the brains of those that had not been given vitamin C.

Since glucose is the brain's only fuel, hypoglycemia, low blood sugar, serves as a vivid example of the mind-body continuum in disease. Some authorities have speculated that hypoglycemia is the most widespread functional disorder in the civilized world.

Although the overproduction of insulin in the body is sometimes caused by a tumor of the pancreas, most hypoglycemia is triggered by stress: grief, pregnancy, a severe injury, prolonged worry. The pancreas can also be overstimulated by a diet high in carbohydrates, all of which are converted quickly to sugar. Caffeine and alcohol indirectly affect the insulin response by stimulating the liver to release a stored sugar product.

The individual with hypoglycemia is on a wretched treadmill. Carbohydrates raise the blood sugar level, and the hair-trigger pancreas gushes insulin in such quantity that the sugar content plunges. As the sugar drops, the brain chemistry goes into a spin. At its extreme, the insulin response can produce shock, coma, even death. Animal experiments have shown that hypoglycemia produces bizarre brainwave patterns similar to epileptic seizures, even during a recovery period.

The disease goes hand in hand with hypocalcemia, a calcium deficiency. Calcium is critical in the transmission of the brain's hormonal activity and mediates activity throughout the nervous system. Little wonder, then, that hypoglycemia has been associated with sundry mental disorders.

THE MOST IMPORTANT SEX ORGAN

Sexuality, like illness, illustrates the dynamic nature of the interaction between brain and hormones, mind and body, nurture and nature. Intervention by either psychological factors or hormones can alter the balance of power.

The genes trigger the hormones that sexually differentiate the brain; the sexed hypothalamus affects the pituitary which measures the hormone levels. The hormone levels affect the brain, creating feelings of confidence and optimism—or anxiety and hostility. And the brain itself can alter the hormones.

Trying to determine to what extent side effects of the Pill were psychological, investigators conducted a study among younger women who had not yet used it as a contraceptive. After warning all of the participants to use another means of birth control as well, they gave one-third of the participants the Pill, with no comment as to typical side effects. Another third were given the Pill and briefed on common side effects.

The last third were given a placebo, an impotent sugar pill, but they were also briefed on the side effects of the Pill.

The warned women reported more side effects from the Pill than those who had not been briefed. But the women given the placebo also reported side effects, including cessation of menstruation! Clearly their anticipation had influenced the sex glands, which then suppressed ovulation.

Can we then conclude that the brain's expectations can override its regulatory mechanisms? It isn't that easy, alas, because there is also massive evidence that hormones affect mood, behavior, and mental efficiency in both sexes. Women show marked optimism and enhanced self-confidence, as measured by personality tests, at the time of ovulation. Estrogen and progesterone levels are high then. The same women are comparatively anxious or hostile when their hormone levels hit bottom during premenstrual and menstrual periods. One study estimated that 46 percent of the psychiatric hospitalizations and almost half the criminal acts took place then. Fifty-seven percent of attempted suicides by women took place during the menstrual period. And a woman's dreams are likely to be more lurid during the low period.

The alteration of hormonal levels may even bear on acute psychosis. Science has established that those women who become schizophrenic around the time they conceive are inclined to bear only live girl babies, probably because a factor in their blood plasma damages male (Y) chromosomes but not female (X) chromosomes. M. A. Taylor of New York Medical College studied the records of female schizophrenics. He noticed that those women whose full-blown schizophrenia appeared within a month after delivery had borne a preponderance of male children. He suggests that a hormone produced by the male fetus, circulating in the mother's blood, might have kept her schizophrenia in remission until after delivery.

Fluctuations of sex hormones may also affect males, some of whom have been noted to become schizophrenic at intervals of four and a half weeks. Men are subject to emotional ups and downs, and their cycles are not dissimilar to the menstrual rhythm. A Danish endocrinologist, Christian Hamburger, observed an almost monthly rhythm of 17-ketosteroids, sex hormones secreted by the adrenals.

Testosterone, a male sex hormone, fluctuates periodically throughout the day and is manufactured in spurts just before the onset of the rapid-eye-movement (REM) stages of sleep during the night. Whether or not dream content is erotic apparently is irrelevant.

Accustomed as we are to considering sex hormones in terms of ovaries and testicles, the brain's supremacy as a sexual "organ" comes as something of a surprise. Not only do the deep brain structures control the activity of the pituitary, but they contain regions where electrical stimulation produces a sensation very much like orgasm.

An example of the brain's critical role is the possibility that at least some women who fail to ovulate may unconsciously want to be sterile. Walter Herrmann, chairman of the obstet- rics-gynecology department at the University of Washington, pioneered the use of ovulation-inducing drugs in the United States. Herrmann later said that he had had some serious mis- givings about the wisdom of using the drugs.

As he saw it in retrospect, many of the infertile women may have shut off ovulation because of psychological conflicts. When friends and family pressure them to investigate the causes of their sterility, they may seek medical help. Herrmann observed that before the discovery of the drugs nothing could be done, and the infertile woman could "go home knowing that she had done her best."

Herrmann's later misgivings are based on the remarkably high percentage of difficult labors, intense postbirth depression, and marital problems that follow the births of babies whose mothers were treated with the drugs.

Mammalian brains are now believed to be basically female in their early stages, with maleness imposed in the womb by hor- mones released through the embryo's genetic code. It is as if the female brain were the basic model and the male brain a modification of it.

During the human infant's prenatal months, its brain differ- entiates. The hypothalamus becomes sensitive to the hormones appropriate to its sex. There is even evidence that certain men- tal attributes develop in a different half of the brain for males than for females. Mechanisms underlying artistic judgment and verbal ability may overlap in the female brain but are in oppo- site hemispheres for the male, according to one report. Six times as many boys as girls have congenital language problems. Males tend to be superior on maze tests, and they are less sen- sitive to electric shock stimulation during their first days of life. Girls show more interest in size and color than boys at age two, one researcher reported, and they build basically different kinds of structures with blocks.

Sexual differences in attention have been measured by Robert McCall of the Fels Research Institute. Judging from a pronounced slowing of the heart rate—a standard lab measurement of attention—infant girls habituated to a novelty more quickly than infant boys. The boys, strangely enough, habituated to a *green circle* more quickly than the girls.

The sexes seem to respond differently to the relationship between a stimulus pattern and its background. Boys are more likely to respond to an action-related stimulus, girls to a passive one.

The boys' aggressiveness is at least partly bolstered by the male hormone, testosterone. If immature female rats are masculinized by interfering scientists, they are likely to display the aggressive behavior of their male counterparts socially as well as sexually. The change is irreversible. If testosterone is administered during the critical first days after birth, replacement doses of estrogen at a later date cannot counteract it.

Pregnant rats subject to stress are likely to bear feminized males. The males later tend to assume the female position for copulation. Postnatal stress has no effect. The investigators conclude that stress causes a change in the normal ratio of the two male hormones to each other during the critical time sex differentiation occurs. Androgen is produced by the adrenals and gonads. Usually the potent androgen from the gonads is present in greater quantity than the androgen from the adrenals.

The implications for human homosexuality are interesting. Psychologists have long believed that male homosexuals typically have demanding, emotional mothers. Possibly such women were unusually susceptible to the effects of stress.

Researchers in Edinburgh and in Boston recently reported hormonal abnormalities in homosexuals. A number of impotent subjects also showed abnormally low levels of testosterone in their urine. A Los Angeles study reported that the normal ratio of the androgens to each other was reversed in homosexuals. Attacks of homosexuality affect some usually heterosexual individuals at intervals of four weeks. Perhaps the balance of the androgens is delicate enough to be tripped by slight fluctuations during the hormonal cycles.

Seymour Levine of the Institute of Psychiatry in London demonstrated that testosterone implantations could permanently change the sex of a rat's brain during the critical days after birth. (Unlike most mammals, rats are not sexually differentiated until a few days after they are born.) Noting that the experiment produced a profound and permanent change in the brain's sensitivity to sex hormones, he said, "Human sexuality may also depend in a fundamental sense on what the hormonal makeup of the individual happens to be during the development of the nervous system."

Too much prenatal androgen creates an ambiguous sexual appearance in the female child, with sometimes tragic results. Because the external genital structures have differentiated before birth into male as well as female sex organs, the individual may be reared as a male by mistake. By the time her true sexual identity is determined, the psychological problems may be beyond solving.

Males with the syndrome appear normal at birth, but later undergo a precocious puberty and a rapid physical growth that comes to a sudden halt, leaving them abnormally short. The syndrome can be treated with cortisone if it is diagnosed in time.

There is some preliminary evidence that high IQs may result from the syndrome.

Experts on intelligence have remarked that high-IQ males tend not to be strongly masculine, nor are high-IQ females extremely feminine. This can probably be explained without hormones, however. Personality tests tend to classify independence as a masculine attribute and sensitivity as feminine. Both these traits have been culturally assigned to some extent. The brightest individuals are likely to be both sensitive and independent, regardless of sex.

In *A Child's Mind,* Muriel Beadle cited a remark that attempting to separate genetics and experience is a little like trying to decide whether hydrogen or oxygen is more important to the properties of water. One might also liken the genetic code to an encyclopedic recipe book. The brain follows some of the recipes precisely, but others, because of environmental circumstances, are skipped altogether or concocted of whatever is in the house. Some young animals are preprogrammed to attach themselves after birth to someone or something. Ducks are imprinted to begin following whatever crosses their field of vision during a critical period shortly after birth. The genes do not specify that the something must be a mother duck, however, and the ducklings will waddle after a little red wagon if that is the stimulus that presents itself during the critical hours.

Infant monkeys fed by surrogate mothers—metal feeding stands covered with fabric—will become as emotionally attached to the dummy as if it were a female monkey, clinging to it when uncertain or frightened.

This subterfuge undermines yet another mechanism. Having no interaction with a real adult monkey, the young grow up sexually inadequate. Females so reared usually cannot conceive. The few that do are appalling mothers, rejecting their beseeching offspring, batting them away time and again.

Into the whirlpool of eddying, oscillating hormones of a human female toss a contraceptive pill. The vigilant brain, taking astonished note of the suddenly escalated progesterone and estrogen, behaves as if pregnancy had occurred. It measures, responds, shuts down ovulation, and attempts to adapt the body to the fictitious pregnancy.

That the adjustment is makeshift becomes apparent from a number of recent studies. Women who take the Pill in the non-sequential combination form show none of the emotional peaks and valleys of the normal cycle. Instead, because of the relatively high levels of hormones, they experience a steady state of moderate hostility and anxiety. The hormones seem to increase the activity of MAO, monoamine oxidase, an enzyme that sabotages the brain's neurotransmitters. Depression may ensue.

The sequential-type pill more nearly replicates the normal cycle; the relative levels of estrogen and progesterone simulate the natural proportions.

Masters and Johnson, the well-known sexologists, said that the Pill "appears to cause diminished libido or inability to achieve orgasm in some women after one-and-a-half to three years." A few women also report increased libido. This disparity may be psychological or may be due to the relative hormonal levels of the women before they began taking the Pill.

Paradoxically, women whose physical characteristics suggest high levels of the male hormone testosterone frequently have a greater sex drive than their voluptuous, estrogen-rich sisters.

Testosterone seems to increase the sexual urge in women as well as in men, and a woman with too little may have trouble achieving orgasm.

Sexual excitation, oddly enough, depends more on the brain than on the reproductive organs, as first evidenced by reports in the 1930s that female rats minus their uterus and vagina may still be in heat, and that anesthetizing a cat's penis does not inhibit his sexual aggression. A series of experiments, in which various brain structures were removed sequentially from animals, proved by a process of elimination that the site for sexual response is in the area of the hypothalamus.

Experimenters stimulated the vaginas of cats, with mixed results. Although the cat would adopt all the appearances of arousal, it would refuse to accept the male. It seemed that brain activation was necessary before the cat would follow through. Implanting estrogen directly in the hypothalamus was found to excite mating behavior even in cats whose ovaries had been removed.

Environmental triggers for sexual arousal may be very subtle indeed. Henry Wiener of Metropolitan Hospital in New York says that there is evidence that external chemical messengers—odors—may affect the subconscious mind. Tests have shown that women can detect the odor of testosterone acetate at much lower concentrations than men can, and that men are more sensitive to the odors of female hormone derivatives than women are. Olfactory stimuli too weak to penetrate conscious awareness apparently alter the electrical resistance of the skin, blood pressure, pulse rate, and respiration.

Human beings with dangerous, uncontrollable sexual compulsions can be relieved sometimes by experimental surgical lesions in the hypothalamus. Among those who have volunteered for surgery have been men troubled by the urge to seduce or attack children. After surgery their sexual interest apparently falls within the normal range.

Hypersexuality may reflect damage in another region of the hypothalamus, a postulated sexual satiation center. The inhibitory region probably lies in the border zone between the midbrain and the hypothalamus. As noted earlier, hypothalamic tumors may cause precocious puberty. When the child's inhibitory brain mechanism is destroyed, the reproductive machinery goes into action prematurely. One research journal reported that tumors are found in more than half the instances of sexual development in boys eight or younger.

Cyproterone acetate, marketed by a German pharmaceutical firm under the trade name Sinevir, seems to counteract hypersexuality. Thus far the drug has been used primarily in Germany and Britain. In Germany, the laws governing treatment of habitual sex criminals now include the drug as an alternative to castration.

Electronic stimulation of the brain (ESB) offers some hope for individuals with sexual problems. Robert Heath of Tulane has used ESB to condition a young homosexual who wanted to enjoy a heterosexual relationship. After weeks of treatment, the young man had intercourse with a girl while the EEG recorded his brainwaves for the research team in the next room.

Jose Delgado of Yale, a pioneer in ESB, noticed that mild sexual interest—flirtation, at any rate—could be neatly turned off and on by the positioning of electronic probes in the brain. The subjects were mostly epileptics undergoing the probing process so that the focal point of their seizures could be located. One reserved young woman suddenly became talkative, "openly expressed her fondness for the therapist (who was new to her), kissed his hands, and talked about her immense gratitude. . . ." A taciturn eleven-year-old boy spontaneously began verbalizing homosexual desires whenever the probe touched a certain point in his temporal lobe.

Delgado and his associates located three points in their brain-mapping studies where stimulation produced a sensation resembling orgasm. The patients expressed intense enjoyment, then suddenly were satisfied. Many more brain points are associated with a continuous euphoria.

Recent chemical discoveries may be more feasible than ESB in stimulating sexuality. Workers trying to determine which brain transmitter is responsible for sleep discovered that one of the chemicals they were using—PCPA (parachloralphenalamine)—had aphrodisiac qualities. Rabbits, for example, attempted to mate with cats. And adding the male hormone, testosterone, increased the effect. The combination caused even castrated rats to mount other rats. The sexual excitement, furthermore, was of long duration.

Gian L. Gessa and Allessandro and Paolo Tagliamonte of Italy are studying the possible therapeutic value of PCPA in treating human sexual disabilities.

Dosages of the substance as relatively high as those used in animal experiments would be toxic for man. However, a similar difficulty was circumvented in dopamine research (for the treatment of Parkinson's disease) by the development of L-dopa, a version of the chemical with a mirror-image molecular structure.

Impotent males are said to be learning to achieve erection at will through biofeedback training. A plethysmograph attached to the penis measures the changing blood volume. Through earphones the subject hears the voice of a female therapist who is monitoring the equipment in another room; she reports increases in blood volume and encourages him. The clinic using this therapy reports a success rate of "nearly a hundred per cent." That is, nearly all their patients eventually learn to produce an erection without the aid of biofeedback.

Although the mysteries of sexuality have not been resolved, research makes it increasingly clear that the brain is the primary erotic zone in man.

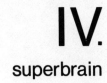

IV.
superbrain

"Too many are unawakened . . ."   —ANTOINE DE SAINT-EXUPÉRY

FIVE SENSES . . . OR TWENTY?

If the doors of perception were cleansed everything would appear to man as it is, infinite. For man has closed himself up till he sees all through narrow chinks of his cavern. —WILLIAM BLAKE

In *Mysterious Phenomena of the Human Psyche,* the Russian physiologist Leonid Vasiliev discussed the case of an apparently healthy man who reported a sudden remarkable sharpening of his visual senses. He could make out very small objects from astonishing distances. Within twenty-four hours he developed apoplexy and died. "An autopsy disclosed a brain blood clot of recent origin on the right side of the optic prominence," Vasiliev said, adding that other pathological states have long been associated with supernormal perception. As examples he mentioned the sharpened vision and hearing in hysterics and neurotics and the apparent connection between paranormal phenomena and brain injuries.

In 1962 an American team at the National Heart Institute furnished startling evidence of enhanced perception in Addison's disease, a condition in which the pituitary fails to produce enough adrenal cortical hormones. Drops of distilled water containing small amounts of salty, bitter, sweet, or sour substances were placed on the subjects' tongues. Those suffering from the pituitary disorder were 150 times more sensitive to taste stimulation than the normal subjects. They also heard sounds inaudible to normal subjects and their sense of smell was more acute. Treatment with cortisone eradicated the supersensitivity.

Intrigued by the high incidence of past brain injury among

gifted psychics,* Gertrude Schmeidler of New York University tested hospital patients suffering from concussion and a control group of nonconcussion patients. Those with the head injuries made higher scores on ESP tests. Some schizophrenics also demonstrate enhanced psi as well as keen sensory perception.

These phenomena strongly support Henri Bergson's theory that the brain is a reducing mechanism, designed to enable the organism to pay selective attention to stimuli for the purpose of appropriate action. According to this premise, if the brain did not act as a filter one would be assaulted by so many sights and sounds that he would be unable to function.† Several recent experiments support this view. It appears from EEG records and subjective reports that the brain responds continuously to incoming stimuli of which the individual is consciously unaware. The more primitive processing system seems to have the capability of determining which data are meaningful and altering the threshold accordingly.

William James also held that ordinary consciousness filters out the "larger reality." Recounting his intensified and enlarged perceptual field under the influence of psychedelics, Aldous Huxley expanded on Bergson's point and compared the brain to a reducing valve that allows only a trickle of reality through its apparatus. In altered states the filtration process is interrupted and a more intense experience of reality is reported.

In Bergson's view, artists and other creative types had only a transparent veil between themselves and the larger consciousness rather than the relatively opaque barrier limiting most human beings to reduced vision.

Raynor Johnson, a physics professor at the University of Melbourne and an eloquent writer on psi, compared the senses to narrow windows. "We are each rather like a prisoner in a

---

* Among them: Peter Hurkos, whose abilities were first evident when he regained consciousness after a 30-foot fall and a prolonged coma; Nelya Mikhailova, the Russian apparently able to move objects at a distance, who suffered a serious head injury during the Siege of Leningrad when she was fourteen; Rosa Kuleshova, known for her ability to "read" and perceive color through her skin, who became epileptic after a brain infection during her teens.

† Perhaps the most incredible example of the brain's inhibiting function is the praying mantis, who can't copulate unless the female first bites off his head to disinhibit him.

round tower permitted to look out through five slits in the wall at the landscape outside. It is presumptuous to suppose that we can perceive the whole of the landscape through these slits—although I think there is good evidence that the prisoner can sometimes have a glimpse out the top!"

The senses are theoretically capable of much greater acuity than is usually measured. R. L. Gregory, director of the perception laboratory at Cambridge University, pointed out that although the receptors in the eye's retina are so sensitive that they can be stimulated by a single quantum—the smallest unit of measurement of light—five to eight quanta are required before one experiences a flash of light. When the lens is surgically removed, human beings can see farther into the ultraviolet range.

One scientist found that the pulsed microwaves his subjects discerned as sound were experienced as higher in frequency than any audio mix he could create in the laboratory for matching purposes. The radio waves bypassed the mechanical transmission system of the ear's ossicles. The researcher, Allen Frey, speculated that perhaps the ossicle system cannot respond to as high a frequency as the rest of the auditory system, just as the lens diminishes the sensitivity of the retina.

Blind human beings develop something of a sonar system that enables them to discriminate between objects of various sizes on the basis of their different echoes. Stanford researchers demonstrated that four blind subjects could detect objects with remarkable accuracy. This ability is most highly developed in other species: Bats, porpoises, whales, swifts, and some other birds use echolocation. Pit vipers placed in total darkness can locate an object the size of a mouse within half a second at a distance of 40 centimeters. The elaborate eyes of bees and flies can receive more than 200 separate impressions per second, ten times the maximum seen by human beings. One species of bat hears best at 140,000 cycles, several octaves above normal human auditory perception. Although human beings are not usually conscious of tones above 20,000 cycles, various tests have shown that they can perceive the higher frequencies subliminally.

Raynor Johnson pointed out that if we had eyes sensitive to X rays rather than visible light, we would have an altogether different impression of the material world. A razor edge would look like a saw, "and much that we describe as opaque would be transparent, or porous." All appearance is relative. An individual with eyes sensitive only to ultraviolet or infrared rays would not see a painted canvas as we do, but he might sense its presence through smell or touch—yet is our world picture more valid than his? Color and solidity are irrelevant to the realm of whirling electrons, although they are a product of it. We perceive light in a very narrow band of vibration. Johnson quotes the scholar and pioneer psychic researcher, Frederic Myers, who asserted in the nineteenth century that investigators must look to the ultraviolet end of the spectrum for answers to some of the puzzling phenomena of mind. "The limits of our spectrum do not inhere in the sun that shines, but in the eye that marks his shining."

Ernst Mach, the German physicist for whom supersonic speeds have been named, said, "The expression 'sense illusion' proves that we are not yet fully conscious that *the senses represent things neither wrongly nor correctly. . . . Under different circumstances they produce different sensations and perceptions."* That statement is a key to understanding the marriage of brain research and theoretical physics. Through myriad transactions in the brain, we perceive; our senses select from the stimuli, cerebral structures interpret the data, but there is no ultimate model of reality out there against which our perceptions can be measured as true or false.

How the brain sees is not understood. Ordinary vision is still a mystery, despite brilliant advances. As Loren Eiseley said of contemporary science, "Huge shadows leaped triumphantly after every blinding illumination." Several years ago two Harvard researchers, David Hubel and Torsten Weisel, astonished their colleagues by demonstrating that some visual cells respond only to light of certain brightness, others only to lines at a certain angle, and so forth, and that the mosaic of their activity becomes the visual image experienced by the brain.

"In retrospect you can say, 'Of course, it makes perfect sense,' " Hubel told us. "We teach medical and biology students what is known about the various parts of the brain that *are* understood, and they sit back, not terribly excited, as if, 'Of course—how else *would* you expect the brain to work?' They don't realize that before you found that it works that way, you'd never have guessed it in a million years. That's often the way with science." Although it is biologically valuable for the visual cells to be sensitive to contours, lines of certain orientation, and so forth, "That possibility didn't enter into anybody's wildest guess."

As Hubel, Weisel, and their co-workers continue their painstaking exploration, moving from fourth- and fifth-order cells further back into the brain's visual center, they move into increasingly complex cellular integration. Hubel said, "We know nothing about what the next five steps—or ten, or thirty—are going to involve. We know, in fact, absolutely nothing about what comes next. Any guess that one can make is just a guess, and the chances aren't good that any individual will turn out to be correct."

The ideal brain researcher would be not only a physiologist but also a mathematician. Recently workers at Massachusetts General and the University of Massachusetts reported that the brain converts incoming visual stimuli into a Fourier transform, a mathematical device much used in modern physics.* If the brain uses a Fourier transform, there must be a timing mechanism in the brain. They say, "Evidence suggests that an excitability cycle in the alpha frequency band may provide this mechanism." They refer to an earlier hypothesis that alpha activity may exist in individual cells. The transform would not be dependent on "a grossly recordable alpha rhythm." The activity could be too subtle for EEG representation. Even so, if this theory were proved it might help explain the apparent memory enhancement of the recordable alpha rhythm.

Gregory said, "The senses do not give us a picture of the world directly; rather they provide evidence for checking hypotheses about what lies before us. Indeed, we may say that a perceived object *is* a hypothesis. . . ."

One researcher suggested that the sense of smell depends on the mathematics of "a complex holistic transform." Yet another investigator, Arnold Trehub, described the brain as "a parallel coherent detector." Trehub said that his research at the Veter-

---

* By this device, the complex cells would convert information received by the simple cells into the basic sets necessary for pattern recognition and memory.

ans Administration Hospital in Northampton, Massachusetts, supports the premise that the brain performs complex mathematics in building up its world picture. It apparently computes on the basis of limited information, Trehub said, and is "the most efficient stochastic * signal detection scheme known."

Research at Loyola in Chicago underscores the breathtaking efficiency of the perceptual system. Ordinarily the brain adapts as one looks at a grating; that is, the contrast between bars and background diminishes. When a subject views a grating partially blocked from view, adaptation occurs not only to the visible portions but also to that part of the grating not seen. The psychologist Naomi Weinstein said, "This may indicate the existence of a neural mechanism which conveys the information 'in back of.' "

The phenomena are numberless. If you stare at a moving spiral for a minute or two, then look away, you will see reverse movement. If the spiral had been turning outward, for instance, you will now see objects shrink. A group at McGill University discovered an even odder quirk of the brain. If the subjects stared at a moving spiral for fifteen minutes, they would see movement in the *stationary* spiral the next day. The motion occurred only when the stationary stimulus fell upon that part of the retina stimulated earlier by the spinning spiral.

"The brain," said R. L. Gregory, "is more complicated than a star and more mysterious." There are problems enough to employ visual-system researchers from now until infinity. One beautiful adaptation of the brain is size constancy. Gregory defines this phenomenon as "the tendency for the perceptual system to compensate for changes in the retinal image with viewing distance. It is a remarkable and fascinating process which, in certain conditions, we can see operating in ourselves."

One simple demonstration he described: Look at your two hands, one placed at arm's length, the other at half the distance. "They will look almost the same size, and yet the image of the further hand will be only half the linear size of the nearer. If the nearer hand is brought to overlap the further, then they *will* look quite different in size."

The geometric scaling—true perspective—is not what the

* Aiming for a mark by estimating.

brain sees, although experiments in the 1930s showed that highly critical individuals and trained artists are likelier than the average subject to see in true perspective. The disparity between the brain's picture and actual perspective was discussed by Giotto and Leonardo da Vinci. Gregory pointed out that Giotto designed the Campanile at Florence with slightly divergent towers to compensate for the eye's "inadequacy to correct for perspective." The Piazza San Marco, he said, is not a true rectangle but diverges toward the cathedral so that it appears to be rectangular when viewed from across the piazza. The Parthenon incorporates similar compensation for the visual effect.

Photographs often seem disappointing because they conflict with our constancy scaling. A tall building often appears in photographs to be falling backward. Figures seem smaller and more distant than when actually seen. Gregory believes that most artists use a modified perspective rather than the geometric perspective of photographs.

Occasionally the device functions erratically, and then the individual becomes disoriented for brief periods. Temporal-lobe epilepsy can cause objects suddenly to appear farther away or closer in space than they are. For unknown reasons this phenomenon happens in children in whom no dysfunction has been diagnosed. Strobe lights can jar the constancy scaling process —the scene jumps back and forth like a bad avant-garde movie. Some individuals have actually learned to alter the size of perceived objects at will. In the early 1900s Harvey Carr, psychologist at the Pratt Institute, published his studies of individuals who could voluntarily control the distance location of their visual field. They could cause objects to approach or recede. One, a New York businessman of forty, had first noticed the phenomenon while convalescing from typhoid fever. On a bright day he could move the entire visual field as near as two feet from his face or back to the horizon.

Another subject, a girl seventeen, had noticed a depth-displacement periodically since the age of nine. While describing the phenomenon to friends she found that she could induce it at will in dim artificial light within two minutes. Another individual told Carr that his visual displacement had first occurred after "a severe nervous attack." Intense illumination made displacement easier and he learned to induce it at will.

A universal displacement phenomenon has been observed by a group of contemporary researchers. When one is *about to look at an object,* the object moves in the field of vision fifty to one hundred milliseconds before the eyes have begun to move toward the object. It is displaced in the direction that the eyes will take in the future.

Eidetic imagery, like involuntary displacement, is more often seen in children than adults. The term describes the ability popularly known as photographic memory. But eidetic imagery is more than memory; the eidetiker sees a clear representation in his visual field, in color and often in three dimensions, of an object perceived days, months, even years before. He can hold the object in place and view it from several directions; it is not a retinal afterimage. If it is a page, he can read from it; if a tabby cat, as in one experiment, he can count the number of stripes on its tail.

Current testing methods have proved once and for all that eidetic imagery truly exists and is not just the product of a vivid imagination. Charles Stromeyer of the Bell Telephone Laboratories has studied a number of eidetikers. In one test, the subject scans a computer-generated, 10,000-dot pattern with one eye. He then looks at a second 10,000-dot picture. If he can generate an eidetic image of the first and superimpose it on the borders of the second picture, he will see a letter or figure. It would be impossible to fake the stereoscopic results or for them to be attributable to afterimages.

One of the most amazing eidetikers who ever lived was a young man known only as S, described by the neurophysiologist A. R. Luria in *The Mind of a Mnemonist: A Little Book About a Vast Memory.* S was pathetically unable to forget. As an adult, he spent much of his time working on techniques to help him unclutter his mind. For most of us the brain's selective memory enables us to retain in consciousness only somewhat relevant memories. Poor S experienced a constant flow of vivid memory that all but paralyzed him. His problem was intensified by a phenomenon sometimes seen in children, artists, and in the altered states—cross talk of the senses. This synesthesia intensified S's memory: certain words, for instance, would produce a color or tactile sensation every time he heard them, and this vivid sensory experience rendered those words or names more memorable.

A tone pitched at fifty cycles per second, played at a loudness of one hundred decibels, caused S to see a brown stripe against a dark background. The stripe had "red, tongue-like edges." Simultaneously he experienced a taste like sweet-and-sour borsch. A different tone and loudness produced the image of a wide stripe, reddish-orange in the center. Increasing the loudness transformed the image to a velvet cord with fibers jutting out on all sides.

S said that he could not escape from seeing colors, lines, blurs, or splashes upon hearing sounds. On meeting someone he would be so absorbed in the color of the individual's voice that he might not hear what was being said. On one occasion one of the brain researchers unthinkingly asked him if he'd have any trouble finding his way back to a certain location. S said, "Come now! How could I possibly forget? After all, here's this fence. It has such a salty taste and feels so rough; furthermore, it has such a sharp, piercing sound. . . ." *

Is synesthesia abnormal or supernormal? Does it have some curious validity? According to his biographers, Jean Sibelius perceived tones as colors. Musicians with absolute pitch have sometimes described the various keys as having characteristic colors.

Raynor Johnson commented on the frequency of synesthesia in mystical experiences. "If the brain is an organ of limitation, it is not surprising that apparently independent sensations on the physical level should be disclosed as related on higher levels of mind. A still higher apprehension would doubtless disclose

---

* S also showed remarkable control over internal processes and could raise the temperature of his right hand two degrees while lowering that of his left one and a half degrees—by visualizing the change. While sitting in a dentist's chair, he controlled pain by imagining that it was a thread he could cut. He could also imagine that someone else was sitting in the chair and that he himself was elsewhere. In fact, he reported several out-of-body experiences. By imagining various illuminations he could control his pupil size. He reported to the skeptical investigators that he could sometimes heal by visualizing, and that he could "make things happen"; if he clearly imagined a store clerk giving him too much change, the clerk would actually do so.

the unity which precipitates itself into sensory variety on the lower levels." He quoted one such account:

> I did not seem to be inside myself though I was still looking normally at the flower border. Everything had become a thousand times more brilliant. Everything had become transparent. But what was so amazing was the fact that I was not only seeing the colors—I was hearing the colors! Every color was an indescribably exquisite musical sound, the whole making a harmony that no instruments could produce. I do not know how long this illumination lasted, perhaps not more than a second or two, but as I came back to earth, so to speak, I knew that I had been in Reality.

E. R. Jaensch of the University of Marburg, Germany, who devoted a lifetime to the study of visual phenomena, believed that eidetic imagery and synesthesia were natural human abilities educated out of most individuals. He and his associates found eidetic imagery in 80 to 90 percent of the children attending special German schools in which there was an emphasis on sensory activities.

In Jaensch's view, the imagery was generally prevalent wherever there were no antagonistic processes in the environment. In other words, most human beings could preserve the phenomenon if they were not subject to a sterile, passive educational process. As early as the 1930s Jaensch maintained that the then-current findings about perceptual structures "show the range within which human nature is plastic to be far wider than even the most optimistic were willing to admit."

Eidetic imagery and synesthesia are found more often in highly creative adults than in the average subject. Jaensch spoke of the shift from passive to active educational experience as an unshackling: "liberation, the awakening of higher activity."

A sailor once remarked that, when he was at sea, he saw the color green only rarely, and after returning to land after a long absence he usually experienced the color as brilliant and thrilling; he couldn't seem to get enough of it. Within a day or two, however, it would lose its impact. We have all noticed similar instances of freshened perception. After a long separation, the familiar is experienced as more intensely beautiful, seamy, or whatever, than we had noticed on a daily basis. We become somehow anesthetized to our surroundings, a phenomenon that can be adaptive—or maladaptive, when we look at the world without seeing it. Erwin Schrödinger spoke of "the danger that custom will blunt our astonishment."

If the senses overadapt and give the impression of being fatigued, the process seems to be psychologically reversible. Perhaps, as Blake said, we need to cleanse the doors of perception so that we can experience the pristine, sensual world of children, artists, and mystics. In hypnotic subjects the senses can be selectively raised to supernormal levels. Sensory-awareness techniques, such as those used by Charlotte Selver, seem to result in long-term lowering of the perceptual threshold. Intense color perception sometimes persists after meditation, dreams, and psychedelic states. Negative ionization has a similar effect.

In *An Experiment in Mindfulness,* E. H. Shattuck, a retired admiral, narrated an incident that took place several months after he had begun to meditate in earnest:

> . . . I had just put my glass of wine down in a patch of sunlight that fell on the table. The sensation that accompanied it was so remarkable that it remains fresh in my memory. . . . The deep red of the wine came to me in a flash that was quite startling in its beauty. It completely engulfed me and invaded all my senses.
>
> It was a moment of pure breathtaking, absorbing ecstasy. It was terribly exciting and deeply satisfying. The color that saturated my being was very much a living power and I was emptying my heart in gratitude and at the same time was tense with fear that it might leave me.

Writing eloquently of the individual's role in perception, he maintained that one should take sensual enjoyment in the artistry created by his own mind. "A rose is only a rose because man sees it as such; without him it would only be a pattern of energy vortices."

Acknowledging that the visual processes are not understood, Raynor Johnson said, "But we *do* see . . . cathedrals and primroses, works of art and works of steel—what a world the mind has constructed from the electrical storms in a few cubic centimeters of grey matter which it has interpreted!"

The visual system has a phenomenal capacity to process data into memory. Investigators from the Bell Telephone Laboratories and New York University found that subjects can scan between 75 and 125 letters per second. Another study suggested that not only is visual scanning rapid, but the ability to remember what has been seen is almost limitless. Subjects were shown 2560 photographic slides at the rate of one every ten seconds. One hour after each subject had seen the last of the slides, he was shown 280 pairs of pictures. One member of each pair was a picture from the series he had seen, and the other picture was similar but had not been shown. The subjects chose correctly 85 to 95 percent of the time. Those who had seen the pictures in two days did as well on the testing as those who had seen them over four days. In one version of the experiment, subjects were shown mirror images of the originals. Still, the high scores were not affected.

The investigators found that image fixation seems to take a quarter of a second. If another image is imposed after an interval briefer than a quarter of a second, the first image is erased. The subjects say that they "didn't have time to see" the picture. The same rate of fixation applies almost universally to reading. The slow reader fixes his eyes on each word for a quarter of a second. During that same fraction of a second, the fast reader fixes on blocks of type.

Eye movements are essential to perception. This recalls the experiments in which a miniature projector was attached to the surface of the eye so that its image moved with the retina. The image soon disappeared. Gregory said that one function of the incessant eye movements is to "sweep the image over the receptors so that they do not adapt and so cease to signal to the brain the presence of the image in the eye."

But there is an odd exception to the disappearance phenomenon. If we stare at a sheet of white paper so that one region in its center is of the same brightness as another region, the eye is receiving constant identical stimuli, even though it moves. Yet the middle of the paper does not disappear. Apparently the brain—seeing borders and outlines—extrapolates that something must be between the boundaries. This possibility is supported by the reports that the brain has an amazing ability to speculate correctly on the basis of partial data.

Such guessing plays a vital role in normal hearing. Sounds that have been omitted but belong in context are heard by the brain. Also, when a word is repeated over and over to an adult subject, he begins to hear transformations. "Dish" might be perceived after a while as "wish" and then as "push" and finally as something as far removed as "put." Interestingly, young children and the very elderly do not hear distortions of the stimulus word. These phenomena are apparently normal and part of the brain's tendency to make sense of incomplete data.

There is even research to explain the cocktail-party phenomenon: the mysterious ability of the brain to understand what is being said by a single voice in a chorus of loud voices. University of Wisconsin workers reported that the brain apparently transforms loud sounds having an appropriate spectral composition in order to create missing faint sounds. The so-called auditory induction phenomenon apparently serves the purpose of enabling one to hear subtle stimuli in a noisy environment. It cancels the effect of masking.

The brain's guessmanship is the basis for much of our humor. It is evident on its most primitive level in such old doggerel as:

> ABCD cows?
> LMNO cows.
> SMR 2.

Et cetera. Visually it makes no sense. Spoken aloud, the letters and number are perceived, in context, as somewhat distorted words. Something in the brain is continually matching what it perceives with what it already knows, making comparisons and searching for meaning. Because its calculations take place with lightning speed, we are unaware of them except when we catch ourselves in error, as when, for example, a mumbled "Would you pass the butter?" becomes "Could you ask your brother?", if both would make sense under the circumstances.

This search for meaning is evident in the amusing mistakes all children make in hearing unfamiliar terms and phrases—for example, the revision of the Lord's prayer: "Give us this day our jelly bread." A similar orderly, if absurd, misperception was the high-school student's conviction that his biology teacher had told the class to read Darwin's *Oranges and Peaches*. The parlor game Gossip is based on the human tendency to try to render meaning from incompletely heard phrases; a message passed by whisper from one player to the next is so distorted along the way that the final version bears little resemblance to the original.

Sight gags are a visual counterpart of puns. Optical illusions, too, are at least partly caused by the brain's comparisons and expectations. R. L. Gregory noted that cultural differences affect susceptibility to optical illusions.

Babies and young children extrapolate from known quantities to new data at a remarkably early age. Objects in Impressionistic paintings and highly stylized animal drawings and figurines are correctly identified. Tiny children are surprisingly able to categorize a Chihuahua, a St. Bernard, and a poodle within whatever subtle parameters their brains have tagged dogness.

The stunning plasticity of the senses underscores that man, as Theodosius Dobzhansky, Nobel prizewinner for biology, said, is not a state but a process. Rats blinded at birth develop an abnormally large auditory region in the brain. Monkeys and kittens whose visual cortices have been removed may develop relatively normal vision after a time.

On the other hand, they have difficulty in making sense of what they see. Animals deprived of patterned light during a critical period of development also become behaviorally blind. The visual connections atrophy if they are not stimulated during certain sensitive periods.

A human being blinded by cataracts as an adult will regain relatively normal visual perception if the cataracts are surgically removed, even after ten or twenty years. But congenitally blind human beings who receive sight years later are often unable to recognize faces or objects without touching them. They may be able to discriminate between letters, especially if they learned the shapes by touch while blind, but they rarely learn to recognize an entire word. They must sound it out letter by letter.

Some damage caused by disuse and deprivation is apparently reversible, some irreversible. The effects vary with the individual. Austin Riesen of the University of California at Riverside, a pioneer investigator of the effects of early deprivation, told of one kitten that had been deprived of patterned light during the critical period. It should have been behaviorally blind due to irreversible cellular atrophy. After one of the researchers took it home for a pet, it developed visual acuity even keener than that of the typical nondeprived laboratory cat. "If I hadn't seen it myself," Riesen said, "I wouldn't have believed it."

Even nerve deafness might not mean an end to hearing. Radio-electronic hearing aids transmit sound directly to the brain. The low-frequency radio waves apparently stimulate dormant nerve cells. Tests at the University of Southern California school of medicine showed that thirty-six of seventy-eight experimental subjects showed significant gains in their hearing, averaging an 18-percent improvement over their usual measured ability to hear speech. The improvement lasted for three to five months.

The device used by the USC researchers was manufactured by Intelectron Corporation of New York. A smaller, more portable device, the Neurophone, has been patented. Its inventor, Patrick Flanagan of Glendale, California, said that it "couples complex modulated radio signals into the body by means of small insulated electrodes. Nerve-deaf individuals we've tested it on require from six to eight weeks' training before they begin to hear through the new sensory stimulus."

Meanwhile, the Chinese claim to have treated nerve-deaf children so successfully with acupuncture that they now hear without mechanical devices of any kind. Frank Z. Warren of New York University reported that a patient suffering from nerve deafness claimed to be helped by treatments she received from a neighborhood acupuncturist. Tests at NYU verified that her hearing seemed to improve measurably after the treatments.

Some human beings experience a hearing sensation related to light. Long before the current research interest in this kind of synesthesia, there were reports by individuals who heard fireballs and aurora borealis, the northern lights. Because the sound occurred with the appearance and over the trajectory of the fireballs even when the observer was some distance away, it is unlikely that it was caused by acoustic energy, which travels slowly.

The fireball sound is variously described as a hissing, sputtering, swishing noise, soft sh-sh, or occasionally a buzz. The sounds reported in connection with aurora borealis are similar. Ordinarily microwaves must be converted by radio before they are audible to the human ear. Researcher Allen Frey determined that pulsed microwaves create an auditory sensation in many subjects (including one individual who was clinically deaf). The sound—buzz, clicking, hiss, knocking—seemed to be coming from behind their heads, regardless of their turning. Blocking their ears only enabled them to perceive the microwave sound *more clearly!* (This was probably only relative, because the background noise was less distracting.) Frey found that the auditory sensations persisted even if he shielded portions of the skull, as long as the temporal region was exposed. If he shielded the temples, no sound was audible to his subjects.

Acknowledging that the auditory and visual systems have been classically distinguished by their responses to different types of energy—acoustic and electromagnetic—Frey commented that the human auditory system can demonstrably respond to electromagnetic energy in at least a portion of the radio frequency spectrum and that the human brain is only one order of magnitude less sensitive than a table radio.

One of the strangest examples of such sensitivity was the Santa Barbara, California, housewife who was apparently suffering pain and enduring great noise from the free electromagnetic energy in her home, caused by power lines and various appliances. The case was thoroughly investigated by an electronics engineer, Clarence Wieske, who reported it in a technical publication, *Biomedical Science Instrumentation. Newsweek* also ran an article on the report, which Wieske later said brought in a flood of mail from all over the country from individuals plagued by a similar sensitivity.

Through an unknown process, alternating current fields were apparently audible to the Santa Barbara woman, although so far as is known they had never been converted to sound waves. The wiring in her house, even the electricity transmitted via the water pipes, created an intolerable noise level. Unknown to her, the investigators connected a generator to the water pipe and to another ground, both a hundred feet from the house. She insisted she heard a dog barking. When the energy field was converted to audible sound waves, the tape recording did indeed sound like a low "Woof!" of a dog.

Since she also claimed to be hearing "extremely high-pitched Morse code," Wieske obtained a long-wave marine receiver and found that she was apparently hearing radio waves from long-wave, low-frequency stations. On one occasion during the months of the investigation an electrical storm knocked out the power in most of Santa Barbara. She had been lying on the sofa, resting, when suddenly everything became quiet. She heard almost none of the racket she had been living with day and night. Until she saw that the electric clock had stopped she was unaware of the power failure.

The utility companies and Wieske masked all the fields in her house with grounded metal shields, which helped for some time. Within two years or so, however, the nearby residential population increased so much that once again the utility noise level was intolerable. She developed shingles, a disease affecting the nerve endings, on the left side of her head—the side on which she was most sensitive to the noise. She said more than once that if it had not been for the noise, she would never have discovered the cause of her physical pain and discomfort, which were worse than the noise. At one point she developed an ear infection and temporarily lost most of her normal hearing, but the noise didn't diminish. She now lives in a relatively isolated house and has reported to Wieske that the noise level is tolerable.

Wieske related that in his conversations with nurses who worked in mental institutions he heard of a number of instances in which patients complained chronically of terrible noise inaudible to the staff. Stuffing their ears with cotton didn't help, but certain rooms seemed to them to be quieter than others.

Several laboratories are working on methods of enabling the blind to see through electronic stimulation of the brain's visual regions. Thus far only flashes of light have been seen, but patterns might eventually be programmed.

For some time it has been known that light patterns can be induced even in darkness by electricity applied to the brain or by a bar magnet, usually placed at the temples and pulsing at approximately the alpha rhythm (ten cycles per second). These patterns, usually known as phosphenes, can be tuned in at certain frequencies. Chemicals like LSD and mescaline alter and intensify them.

The geometric shapes are similar in both magnetic and electrical phosphenes. Changing the frequency of the electrical stimulus changes what is seen. Like the pattern hallucinations reported by some sensory isolation subjects, the phosphenes are commonly described as spirals, latticework, and vortices. The pattern found at a specific bandwidth in an individual can be induced again at that bandwidth months later; it can be tuned in.

Observing that chemicals could superimpose complex scenes over the simple patterns induced by electricity, Munich researchers suggested that a smaller brain region is probably involved in the electrical phosphenes than in psychedelic visions. "If this is true, the appearance of living or manmade objects can be expected to occur not only as a result of chemical stimulation," they said, "but also during meditation or fasting or sensory deprivation, where larger parts of the brain, e. g. the temporal cortex, are affected."

In their study, as the drug psilocybin took effect on the subject, electrically induced ornamental phosphenes were replaced by "thousands of blue asparagus," "a Japanese landscape," "dark blue bells and the view of a city like Moscow with many bulbous towers," "a ceiling of bananas with many small windows."

The electricity sustained these visions, and they would often disappear when the current was switched off. In some experiments the subject reported that the colors in a psychedelic vision would brighten as the current was turned on.

Another phenomenon, dermo-optic perception (DOP), offers hope to the blind. First discussed in the scientific literature in 1785, extraocular vision involving the skin was the subject of a 1924 book, *Vision Extra-Retienne,* by Jules Romains. During the 1960s researchers in the United States and USSR explored the curious ability of some people to detect color, light, and occasionally even pattern through the skin.

After dozens of Russia's top-level scientists had ascertained the genuineness of the ability in one subject, Rosa Kuleshova, researchers undertook to locate other individuals who could "see" without their eyes. A number of them turned up, mostly children and young people. Then the investigators began training volunteers to perceive colors through their fingertips. From that point, the state undertook to develop the perception in blind children. Reportedly some measure of fingertip vision could be trained *in all blind children* in whom the visual cortex was intact. The optic nerve does not seem to be necessary for this perception, but damage to the brain's visual center precludes it.

There are several theories about fingertip vision. P. G. Sniakin, one of the Russian experimenters, suggested that a certain range of electromagnetic energy affects the chemicals in the skin, creating molecular changes detected by sensitive individuals. Allen Frey suggested a simpler hypothesis and that the energy directly influences free nerve endings and causes shifts perceptible to the brain. Frey said that it is apparently even possible to influence neurons, including those deep in the brain, without the need for fiber optics.

Eyeless sight is usually not experienced as normal vision but rather as a tactile sensation or a sensation of light. Even when the skin is several inches from the test stimulus, the trained subject feels what he usually describes as stickiness, roughness, smoothness, coolness, heat, all characteristic of different colors. This response is somehow refined into genuine visual sensation in some subjects who, over a period of time, begin to describe subtle shades of color and detail of pictures, and who can read printed material via the new sense.

Most subjects "see" more accurately in bright light than dim, but two or three Russians, including Kuleshova, are said to have performed in total darkness. Red light seems to help the subjects detect redness in an object, yellow light intensifies the sensations of yellow. The Russians speculate that blind individuals might benefit from an environment in which certain key points such as doorknobs and oven controls were painted in a certain color and illuminated by light of the same color.

Much of the published scientific literature on dermo-optics is listed in *Bibliographies on Parapsychology* (*Psycho-energetics and Related Subjects*), published in March 1972 by the U.S. Chamber of Commerce.* Prepared by Russian scientists, the bibliographies give extensive technical references. The research is also described in less technical language in Ostrander

---

* JPRS 55557, National Technical Information Service, Springfield, Virginia 22151, $3.

and Schroeder's *Psychic Discoveries Behind the Iron Curtain.*

What sense does the brain use in learning control of the autonomic nervous system? The biofeedback lights and tones must be correlated with another kind of perception; the subject has to identify an inner state to reproduce it. For instance, one can't hear, see, smell, or taste a brainwave, nor is it felt in the usual kinesthetic sense. When a rat learns to control the rate at which his kidney filters urine, what senses is he employing? By what process do human beings, animals, birds, and insects detect magnetic fields?

In *The Human Brain* John Pfeiffer pointed out that the brain is constantly measuring the sugar level in the blood and monitoring hormone and enzyme activity. "Reports about the state of things inside the body come from built-in sense organs which give rise to sensations of muscular tension, hunger, thirst, nausea. The number of senses is not known exactly. It is certainly more than five and probably somewhere around twenty." Some of the unnamed senses involve brain transactions so remote from observation we can scarcely frame theories about them.

Until the recent scientific enthusiasm for biofeedback, the altered states, and psi phenomena, the five traditional senses were officially considered man's complete repertoire—and even they seemed quite limited. Many psychologists dismissed such anomalies as eidetic imagery as fraud. Conventional scientists assumed that schizophrenics only *seemed* abnormally sensitive to bright lights and loud noises.

The times, they are a-changin', as Bob Dylan put it. Increasing numbers of scientists have themselves experienced a shift in sensory perception by way of psychedelic drugs or meditative states. Because some unconventional mode of knowing must play a part in control of autonomic functions, the biofeedback revolution has also forced the issue.

And, after a hundred years of being dammed up on the fringes of respectable science, the psi phenomena have swollen, cracked the massive concrete of convention, and swept through. There is no turning the evidence back now. The physicist Raynor Johnson said in 1953 that psi must be regarded as "a fact established by as great a weight of observation and experiment as that which supports the basic facts in other sciences."

Johnson commented that at that time the average scientist was either apathetic or was openly hostile toward the experimental data in psi research—attitudes he attributed to a nonrational tendency to dismiss anything that is quite strange. "If we succeed in resisting this psychological tendency even for a moment," he said, "we can see quite clearly that there is no reason why our [traditional] senses should reveal the length and breadth of all existence." Nor is there any reason that nature should terminate at a point where our five traditional senses cease to register it.

When Carlos Castaneda, the author of *The Teachings of Don Juan, A Separate Reality,* and *Journey to Ixtlan,* appeared at the California Institute of Technology to talk about his most recent conversations with Don Juan, so many science students showed up that the lecture had to be moved outdoors.

Castaneda spoke of the intangibility of the stimuli that solicit our perception. Our interpretations of these stimuli, he said, can range widely once we break free of the shackles of our cultural adaptation. Much of what we see and hear is an agreement within our European heritage, based on our mutual experiences. Castaneda maintains that Don Juan and his fellow "men of knowledge" have learned to perceive a separate reality.

The Cal Tech students and their counterparts at other schools all over the world may prove to be the first entire generation of scientists to transcend the old physical-sense-based mold on a large scale. Ironically, the avant-garde physical scientists are more radical in their attitude toward mind phenomena than are traditional psychologists. Physicists, especially, are overrepresented among those pondering the wild phenomena of man's consciousness—perhaps for the reason Johnson tossed out for consideration twenty years ago, when he said that the critical-minded scientist is in a state of bewilderment. Sometimes he views the plain man's world of colors, tastes, and sounds as purely subjective—a world of appearance only—because he knows that it is interpreted from protons and electrons. Then again, where are the objective bricks of reality?

So we have the picture of sober physicists going into yogic meditation states in their search for an intuitive grasp of the whole curious business. Einstein himself once said that his first intimation of the theory of relativity was an ineffable physical sensation rather than an idea. He felt it before he understood it intellectually.

Sometimes in astronomy, a heavenly body has been virtually invisible until a single observer detects its presence and points it out to his colleagues, who then see it with increasing clarity. Perhaps a myriad of unknown senses are only awaiting our consciousness. Maybe we're like the congenitally sightless human beings whose vision has been restored but who are behaviorally blind, reverting to touch rather than using the alien data from their new sense.

After discussing the evidence for a multitude of senses from a physicist's viewpoint, Raynor Johnson said, "If such paranormal phenomena as telepathy, clairvoyance, and precognition are established, it is not too much to say that the bounds of Man's universe are widened without known limit, and he himself is a star of the first magnitude."

18

REVOLUTION IN THE CRADLE

We are only now on the threshold of knowing the range of educability of man—the perfectibility of man. We have never addressed ourselves to this problem before. —JEROME BRUNER, HARVARD

My hunch is, we've never really tapped the potential of human beings. —J. MCVICKER HUNT, UNIVERSITY OF ILLINOIS

In a postscript to *Wind, Sand, and Stars,* Antoine de Saint-Exupéry told of traveling in the 1930s on a train filled with Polish refugees leaving France. Between a work-worn peasant couple there lay a beautiful sleeping child. Saint-Exupéry recalled bending over the child and exclaiming to himself that here was the face of a musician. "This is a life of beautiful promise. Little princes in legends are not different from this. Protected, sheltered, cultivated, what could not this child become?"

After all, he thought, when a new rose is born in a garden, all the gardeners rejoice over the mutation. They isolate the rose, tend it, foster it.

> But there is no gardener for men. This little Mozart will be shaped like the rest by the common stamping machine. This little Mozart will love shoddy music in the stench of night dives. . . .
>
> Those who carry the wound do not feel it. It is the human race and not the individual that is wounded here, is outraged here. What torments me tonight is the gardener's point of view. . . . It is the sight, a little bit in all these men, of Mozart murdered.

Those who would take exception to this *cri de coeur* may protest that Mozart was a genetic accident. Now the ancient nurture/nature, hereditary/environment controversy may be in its death throes. Brain research and mountains of empirical evidence have proved beyond a reasonable doubt that both innate and experiential potential have been greatly underestimated. The intact human infant is neither a programmed computer nor a blank slate. As the biologist E. W. Sinnott expressed it, "What a gene determines is not a specific trait but a specific reaction to an environment." Every organism possesses a vastly greater developmental repertoire of such reactions than it is ever called upon to display. Every species has a greater repertoire than it may ever have displayed in its evolutionary history, Sinnott said. One example would be the recently observed ability of a species of grasshopper to convert a herbicide into a repellent it can use against its enemies.

What we usually think of as musical talent or athletic talent are not single abilities but complexes of various innate potentials. The musician may seem to have a naturally "good ear," or he may acquire perceptual subtlety by early exposure to tones. His sensorimotor processes are trained one way by cello lessons, differently for playing the trombone. Athletic potential may include superior coordination, stamina, quick reflexes. These qualities would be trained differently for different sports.

Some of the so-called genetic traits can be acquired. For years it has been believed that absolute (perfect) pitch, the ability to identify tones, is a rare, inherited characteristic. However, it is apparently common among the Vietnamese, whose language employs pitch to differentiate between words that are otherwise identical: a single word may mean six different things, depending on its pitch. And no one has yet found a tone-deaf Vietnamese.

Experience changes the brain. The implications of this discovery are as profound, as revolutionary, as $E = mc^2$. Tradition has espoused a fatalistic, fixed-capacity view of the individual. If the brain can change, all the rules must be rewritten.

Animal research has been essential in establishing objective evidence of brain changes, for obvious reasons. One would not likely stimulate human beings for the ultimate purpose of dissecting their brains.

The first animal study was reported in the late eighteenth century by Michele Malacarne, an Italian anatomist. Malacarne reported that postmortems showed more folds in the cerebellum of a trained animal than an untrained one.

There was no further interest in brain correlates of learning for almost a hundred years, until a French physician attempted to prove, by measuring head circumference, that training enlarged the brain. When other investigators were unable to verify such gross changes, the search was dropped.

It was resumed at the University of California at Berkeley in the 1950s by Mark Rosenweig, Edward Bennett, Marian Diamond, and David Krech. By that time refined techniques enabled the investigators to detect subtle changes in brain chemistry and to examine tissue minutely. They found indications that problem-solving experience had altered the level of a brain enzyme vital to transmission. To their surprise, they also found changes in the weight of the brain samples.

Most of their subsequent research involved the separation of rat litters into different environments to see whether brain changes would result. Typically, a group of three male rats would be placed in the standard laboratory colony cage. A second group from the same litter would live in an enriched environment; each day an assortment of playthings was placed in their cage. Each rat in the third group was placed in an impoverished environment, a cage in which he lived alone.

At the end of each experimental period, the rats were sacrificed, their brains dissected and analyzed. The Berkeley researchers first announced in 1964 the startling findings: Rats from the enriched environment had heavier, thicker cortices and greater total activity of two important brain enzymes.

Later they also found that the stimulated rats' brains contained more glial cells. Possibly vital to semiconductor properties of the nervous system, the glial cells also nourish and insulate the nerve cells.

Although the experienced rats had the same number of nerve cells as their deprived littermates, the enriched environment had apparently produced larger cell bodies. Also the ratio of RNA to DNA had changed.

The changes are not just an acceleration of normal maturation. In fact, one Berkeley investigator, Walter Riege, found that even fully mature rats respond to enrichment. They show as great an increase in brain weight as that seen in rats stimulated at a younger age, but the change requires a longer stimulation period. In infant rats as little as eight days of stimulation can cause measurable thickening of the cortex.

In 1959 other experimenters reported that rats reared in a stimulating setting were demonstrably superior to normally reared laboratory rats in their discrimination of three-dimensional objects. Another study reported that ten minutes' daily petting of Siamese kittens caused their color points to darken more rapidly than those of their siblings. (Siamese kittens are uniformly light-colored at birth; their characteristic dark points appear as they mature.) The petted kittens were more active, more attentive, and discriminated more accurately in a test situation. Nor was it merely affection that made the difference. In later studies, light and sound stimulation caused the same coloration phenomenon as the petting.

One research team shocked infant rats, expecting that they would later show greater emotionality and poor discrimination in a learning situation. To their astonishment, the stressed animals were superior to the unstressed controls by almost every measurement. Rats reared in a quiet, sheltered environment developed into jittery, emotional animals unable to cope with normal surroundings.

Critical periods are much talked about in studies of the effects of early experience. Some potentialities can develop only if the environment provides key input at a particular point in the organism's life. Other potentials, such as some aspects of the visual system and the sucking response, are virtually complete at birth but will degenerate if not used. Still other potentials can be developed before or after the critical period but at a much greater cost—and sometimes less fully.

The stress studies point up the specificness of some critical periods. If a rat pup is stimulated in the first five to ten days of life, he becomes a novelty seeker, eager to play with new objects, but his cognitive performance is not affected much. He behaves emotionally like a more mature rat, however.

Problem-solving and perceptual abilities are markedly improved if the rat is stimulated at about fourteen days, after his eyes are open. Manipulation limited to this period, however, will be less effective in improving emotional behavior than manipulation during the five-to-ten-day period.

Victor Denenberg and M. X. Zarrow at the University of Connecticut handled one group of rats during the first twenty days of life. Early handling affected later avoidance learning, discrimination learning, exploratory behavior, sexual precocity, maternal behavior, aggression, body weight, resistance to leukemia virus, rate of ascorbic acid depletion, and the ability to survive severe stress.

Why should such an array of stimuli—petting, shocking, light, sound, Tinkertoys—produce such similar changes? Denenberg proposed that stimulation in infancy may cause the adrenal cortex to release corticosterone. This hormone may "act on the brain, presumably on the hypothalamus, to modify the neural organization and make an animal less emotional." The pituitary and adrenal hormones, in their feedback relationship, are the master hormones, vital in learning as well as in the reaction to stress. Their activities affect the body's metabolism, excitability, immune reactions, and level of brain arousal.

The rat-stress studies have instigated considerable debate. Their possible relevance to man is certainly suggestive. Two researchers who recently undertook a cross-cultural study found that the mean superiority in height is two inches in those societies where infants are ritually cut, or their skin burned, to form a pattern, their lips or ears pierced, and so forth. The critical period for stress was the first two years.

If there were sufficient evidence that stress in infancy is ultimately beneficial, would we be willing to shock or otherwise stress human babies? Fortunately, other stimuli result in virtually the same changes in animals as the early stress. Colors, lights, sounds, gentle skin contact—all are powerful stimuli.

The development of the brain can be retarded by a variety of environmental factors. Premature weaning of rats has a deleterious effect on their later learning, according to Russian research. It also produces measurable effects on the RNA content of brain cells. Similar emotional and cognitive deficits have been seen in animals reared by an artificial mother-surrogate. The effects can be prevented if they are given the company of other young of their species. Isolation in infancy produces skittish animals that learn poorly.

What happens on a molecular level when the brain is stimulated by the environment? W. Ragan Callaway of the University of Toronto has suggested that the environment evokes enzyme production by the demands it makes on the cells' metabolic resources. The metabolic process becomes more efficient. He emphasized that the mechanisms involved are the same, "whether it is a muscle cell responding to exercise, a skin cell responding to injury, or a brain cell involved in the learning process."

The amount of transmitter fluid produced at the synapse of a brain cell may depend to some extent on its previous history. There is evidence that inactivity may decrease the amount, activity increase it.

Callaway pointed out that the evidence for brain changes due to experience abolishes two long-held assumptions: one, that genetic material is almost completely preprogrammed to perform all the necessary tasks, and two, that the structure of the central nervous system, once formed, is essentially stable. Earlier investigators made those assumptions on the basis of "the then infant science of genetics," Callaway said. "It is much more difficult to understand its current vogue, inasmuch as scientific evidence makes it completely untenable."

Although the intellectual changes vary with the species, the nature of the stimulus, and the timing, they undeniably are responses to experience. Man, with his prolonged infancy and childhood and his extraordinary plasticity, is even likelier to be affected by early stimulation than are rats or cats.

The average child reared according to tribal custom in Uganda walks at ten months, and many walk as early as seven months. The Uganda infant is closely attended by his mother, who takes him with her everywhere and is keenly attentive to his needs. If he attempts to sit or stand, she helps him. If he tries to talk, she encourages him. Between the fifth and seventh months, his language, adaptivity, and personal-social relations are at the level of European children two or three months older. But if a Uganda child is reared by native parents who have adopted European child-care methods, the precocity is not evident beyond the first month.

According to the Gesell-Thompson scale, the average child walks at a little over fourteen months. The various Gesell norms, for many decades the bible of American pediatricians and child psychologists, were derived from Arnold Gesell's careful observation of developmental milestones in thousands of children. But many psychologists now believe that, because these children lived in a specific culture with its own specific child-rearing practices, the norms are of limited validity in a discussion of human potential.

Recently a Boston team discovered a phenomenon that undermines whatever credibility such norms may still have. For some time it has been known that newborn babies have a curious innate tendency to attempt to walk. Since their musculature will not support their weight during the early weeks, they are rarely encouraged to exercise the reflex or the related foot-placing reflex. Normally these innate responses disappear at about eight weeks.

The researchers separated week-old infants into four groups. Six were not examined at all until the end of the experiment. Six others had no special exercise but were examined at intervals, so that it could be judged whether examination alone might have some effect. Another six received passive exercise. As they lay on their backs, their parents pumped their legs and arms.

The remaining six infants were given four three-minute sessions of active exercise of the walking reflex each day. They were held under their arms so that their bare feet could touch a flat surface; that stimulated them to "take steps."

Over the eight-week experimental period, what had been a reflex became a learned activity for the latter group. The babies were soon averaging thirty responses per minute. The three control groups were a sharp contrast. They averaged only eight per minute when tested at the end of the eight weeks. Their responses were poorly executed compared to those of the active-exercise infants. They became increasingly clumsy, especially by the eighth and final week. "Often the toes curled over," the researchers said. "The feet bent to the side, and extension of the legs failed to occur."

At the end of the eight weeks, all of the parents were informed of the research objectives and told how they could encourage their infants' motor development during the following months. There was no more supervision or training, but the investigators later recorded the date of each child's first independent steps.

Four of the active-exercise babies walked at nine months-plus. Only one of the other eighteen walked that young. The mean for the actives was more than two months younger than for the other babies.

This study suggests that nature has provided a response that, if exercised, facilitates walking. The researchers remarked that nature's characteristic efficiency and adaptability would be violated if these walking responses were programmed in the newborn only to fade with disuse. They speculated that since the brain's nerve fibers become more rapidly myelinated * with use, retention of this response may ease further development.

"If so," they said, "our widespread belief in the invariance of the motor sequence probably reflects more about our child-rearing practices than about the infant's capabilities." They suggested that a major benefit of encouraging early mobility would be the child's earlier sense of competence.

> Walking movements produce spatial, visual, and kinesthetic-tactile changes in his world, and these accompanying sensory changes may serve as the inherent reward that reinforces walking. Delaying the infant's opportunity . . . may result in some fading of his propensity for effectiveness. . . . The subtle forces in society that erode the self-rewarding activities underlying the infant's curiosity may begin their work during the first weeks of life.

The argument against a fixed capacity, although only recently supported by laboratory evidence, is by no means new. In the eighteenth century Karl Witte, an Austrian clergyman, argued that education overemphasized natural aptitude. He vowed that if ever he had a son he would educate him to be a superior man. He kept his promise. His child seemed slow as a baby, only average as a four-year-old. But by age six he was clearly precocious and at nine entered the University of Leipzig. At fourteen he earned his Ph.D. and at sixteen his doctor of laws degree.

The story of Karl Witte is discussed in greater detail in Siegfried and Therese Engelmann's *Give Your Child a Superior Mind*. The Englemanns note that a copy of Witte's cumbersome account of Karl's education was circulated within a group of Harvard and Tufts people during the early 1900s. A. A. Berle,

---

* The development of the myelin sheath around nerve cells is essential if they are to function.

a Tufts professor, was among those who followed Witte's advice. Of Berle's four remarkable children, a daughter entered Radcliffe at fifteen; a son, Harvard at thirteen. Berle said, "If this result had been secured with one child, the usual plea of 'unusual child' might possibly be raised. But it is unthinkable that there should be four 'prodigies' in one family!"

About that same time, Winifred Sackville Stoner wrote *Natural Education,* an account of how she taught her daughter to read at eighteen months and to speak several languages while still a toddler. Henry Olerich so believed in innate human potential that he decided to prove his theories on Viola, an eight-month-old orphan of apparently average development and in somewhat poor health. By age three Viola was a wunderkind, described as "the most advanced juvenile scholar on record."

During that era, Maria Montessori, Italy's first woman physician, was asked to take charge of the preschool children in a large public housing project in Rome. The scholastic achievements of Montessori's tiny urchins soon drew visitors to the Casa dei Bambini from all over the world. Quite by accident the *dottoressa* had discovered that the children could learn to read effortlessly at three and four. Shortly thereafter she realized that they were capable of understanding and using such terms as trapezoid and parallelogram, and that they seemed to be filled with insatiable curiosity. So long as the environment offered a rich variety of sensory stimulation, objects to explore and manipulate, there appeared to be no limit to the ability of the children to assimilate.

Montessori became obsessed with the growing conviction that this was true normalcy and that the usual haphazard environmental influences produced children who were less than normal—that is, not developing to their full potential.

As a worldwide Montessori movement got under way, there was considerable interest in the United States at first, but various factors militated against it, delaying American acceptance for nearly fifty years. Another radical approach had already gained a foothold; those dissatisfied with traditional methods had espoused John Dewey's progressive-education movement.

Another obstacle to American adoption of the Montessori views on latent intellectual potential was the giftedness research. Educators had put all their intelligence-theory eggs into one basket, Lewis Terman's monumental study of several thousand California children of genius IQ. Terman, whose research project was undertaken in the 1920s, was a linear theoretical descendant of Sir Francis Galton, author of *Hereditary Genius* (1869). Galton had observed that in various English families certain abilities seemed to flourish. Musicians, for example, were likely to be related to musicians. There were great literary clans and artistic clans. The great oarsmen tended to have sons who were fine oarsmen, wrestlers begat wrestlers.

There were at least two possible interpretations of Galton's accumulated data: (1) Great artistic, athletic, musical, and other specific talent is genetic in origin, or (2) artists, athletes, musicians, and so forth, tend to expose their children to their own specialties at a tender age, giving them a running start on developing any potential they might have.

Although he remarked that man is so educable an animal that it is difficult to tell where innate ability leaves off and training begins, Galton settled on the first possibility: innate ability. Similarly, when Terman observed that more than half his high-IQ subjects had learned to read before starting school, he and his followers assumed that the gifted children picked up that skill because they were so bright. They dismissed the possibility that some children might have scored in the gifted category on the Stanford-Binet test because they had learned to read so young.*

The Terman study, covering several decades, established the modern version of the fixed-capacity theory. Because the children of bright people tended to be bright, intelligence must be genetically determined. Yet there were disconcerting flaws in this theory. Adopted children of bright people also tend to be bright. Most tellingly, a disproportionate number of intellectually gifted persons are eldest children or only children. As the Englemanns remarked, the genes have no way of knowing whether they are combining to form a first child or a tenth child.

---

* The child whose language experience has been enriched will almost inevitably score high on IQ tests. There is a built-in bias favoring the verbal skills. Although the tests are notoriously imperfect, they are the only game in town at present, and are more useful than no indicator at all.

Despite the mounting evidence against it, the fixed-capacity school is dying a hard death. Many psychologists are still influenced by the views of Arnold Gesell, who maintained in 1929 that "there is no convincing evidence that the fundamental acceleration of development can be readily induced by either pernicious or enlightened methods of stimulation."

Forty-two years later, Louise Bates Ames, a psychologist with the Gesell Institute, warned parents against "Sesame Street," crib toys designed to stimulate perception, and early reading or typing.

"I urge any of you whose children are still preschoolers to relax," she said. "Let their minds alone. . . . Keep in mind that your children learned to walk and talk pretty much by themselves. . . . The results of early learning are seldom lasting."

After asserting that one can't really accelerate growth, Ames expressed fear that the readers might "raise a child who will be brighter than nature intended."

Gesell once likened the human child to "a precise and beautiful machine," containing the "mechanisms for growth" and "the machinery of behavior." Current research does not support a mechanistic concept. Readiness for various activities seems not to appear on a predetermined timetable, but in a sequence whose timing can be accelerated or retarded by the environment. For example, in Burton White's study at Harvard, infants who were mildly stimulated by crib toys developed top-level reaching in 60 percent of the time required by the unstimulated control group.

There is also astounding evidence that the human brain is innately endowed with such concepts as solidity and conservation. T. G. R. Bowers of the University of Edinburgh designed a number of experiments to investigate the role of what might be called preprogrammed genetic information. In one experiment he created a stereoscopic illusion of solidity. Infants between sixteen and twenty-four weeks old wore polarizing glasses to see an "object" created by two light projectors and a rear-projection screen. None of the infants showed any surprise on touching a real object, but whenever they failed to make contact with the illusory object, they became visibly upset.

Bowers also demonstrated that two-week-old babies were frightened by an illusory object approaching on a collision course. They pulled their heads back, attempted to block their faces with their hands. Their distress was so intense that the experiment had to be halted. Bowers said, "The precocity . . . is quite surprising from the traditional point of view. Indeed, it seems to me that these findings are fatal to traditional theories of human development."

An infant could hardly have learned the defensive reaction in his first two weeks of life. And if a newborn howls when he touches an illusory object and obviously expected solidity, Bowers inferred that at least one aspect of the eye-and-hand interaction is built into the nervous system.

He then wondered if a more complex concept, namely permanence, might also be built in. He then demonstrated that when an infant saw an object disappear briefly behind a screen, he apparently expected it to be there if the screen were moved away. More remarkably, if the object were moving on a trajectory and then disappeared behind the screen, even eight-week-old infants anticipated its reappearance on the other side. Their heads followed the trajectory.

There is also increasing evidence that the nervous system of the newborn human being is quite mature in its responses to changes in the environment. For many years it was believed that infants have no galvanic skin response to sensory stimulation. Then one investigator demonstrated its presence in babies from three to eleven months old. More recently a team at the University of Hawaii recorded this reflex in infants only hours old. Another study showed that newborns could discriminate between odors. A Leningrad researcher demonstrated that babies as young as two hours were able to orient to the direction of sounds. Other scientists have shown conclusively that infant human beings and newborn animals are awed or fearful when they perceive depth.

The brain was apparently genetically programmed to search for pattern from the beginning of life. Robert Fantz of Western Reserve University showed black-and-white patterns and plain colors to thirty-five infants under two weeks of age. The babies preferred pattern to color and showed definite preference in patterns. When eighteen five-day-old infants were given the

choice of looking at a schematically drawn face, bull's-eye, section of newsprint, or circles of various colors, eleven looked
longest at the face, five at the bull's-eye, and only two at the
newsprint. None stared at the plain colors. Later experiments
showed that most babies under twenty-four hours old preferred
the face pattern.

By not later than three months of age, babies learn to recognize complex configurations and prefer complex to simple patterns. "It would seem highly significant that the infant of three
months or so is able to learn complex patterns easily," said
W. Ragan Callaway, "because this is precisely what many children with reading problems cannot do."

Callaway pointed out that form perception in man regresses
if it is not exercised, citing as a gross example the lasting inability of human beings to recognize objects and faces when
their vision is restored after years of congenital blindness. The
reason for this is evident from the research on kittens and
chimpanzees reared in darkness. In the brain's visual cortex, the
cells have degenerated.

Many reading problems could be avoided, Callaway suggested, if children were exposed to letters and words much earlier than six years so that they could profit from the sensitive
period for form perception, which apparently begins at birth
and begins to diminish around four years of age.

It has been said that if children learned to speak by the same
methods that they learn to read, there might now be as many
nonspeakers as there are illiterates. Many researchers compare
language acquisition to form perception; both speech and reading seem to require similar skills of integration. Fortunately,
most children are exposed to spoken language. In fact, the ability of even somewhat dull children to acquire their native language has convinced many linguists that the human brain contains an innate language acquisition device. This capability, first
proposed by Noam Chomsky of MIT, theoretically enables
children to learn languages exactly as they hear them pronounced. They learn idioms, irregular verbs, and the complex
structure of grammar at an age when, by other measurements,
they are cognitively immature.

The transformational linguists believe that the task of learning a language would be overwhelming if it were not for the

presence of a genetic mechanism.* Eric Lenneberg of MIT speaks of "a biological matrix which forces speech to be of one and no other basic type."

Language seems to be important to overall perception. We seem to perceive objects more clearly when we have a name for them. In a Russian experiment, toddlers between one and two and a half required only one-third as many trials to "find the candy under the red hat" if they were first told the name for the color red. In another Russian study, the children were unable to match butterflies on other than a color basis until they were given the name for the wing patterns: spots, stripes, nets, etc. They then paired them rapidly—as if, for the first time, they could see them.

Scientists in the USSR are keenly interested in the phenomena of early learning. Kornei Chukovsky observed, "It is frightening to think what an enormous number of grammatical forms are poured over the poor head of the young child. And he, as if it were nothing at all, adjusts to this chaos, constantly sorting out into rubrics the disorderly elements of the words he hears, without noticing as he does this his gigantic effort. If an adult had to master so many grammatical rules within so short a time, his head would surely burst. . . ."

Yet this faculty diminishes with age. If a language is introduced to a human being after age eleven or twelve, the odds are against his learning to speak it without an accent. A three-year-old exposed to a foreign language will usually become conversant more rapidly than his six-year-old brother, who will learn much more easily than his older siblings or his parents.

A number of early-learning researchers have also observed that three-year-olds learned to read with less apparent difficulty than the average six-year-old. Controlled experiments have shown that four-year-olds who watched "Sesame Street" learned the material at least as well as the five-year-olds. Three-year-olds absorbed almost as much. Experimental programs in Denver and in Great Britain demonstrated that four-year-olds learned to read as easily as five- and six-year-olds. Researchers

---

* There is even a theory that the infant's vocal apparatus begins to vibrate spontaneously in response to the sounds he hears.

in St. Louis, who rewarded middle-class preschoolers for the number of words each learned to read, found that the two-year-olds learned about as well as the five-year-olds.*

First- and second-graders who read poorly have often been considered not ready. Because more boys than girls show reading disabilities at that age, a number of educators have speculated that boys should not be taught reading before the age of seven or eight.

Lewis Lipsitt of Brown University has remarked that a generation of psychologists have been eager and able to diagnose retardation but uninterested in the environmental factors that contribute to superior development. "If a four- or five-year-old child could not perform matching-to-sample tasks, or could not pick out the one object different from the rest, he was simply 'not ready to read.' He presumably suffered from some condition that limited his potential. No one ever suggested that the necessary conditions for acquiring the behavior had not been made available to the child."

W. Ragan Callaway suggested that learning to read at an earlier age, during the period of language acquisition, may offer special advantages. Possibly the mental activity involved in reading is transduced into permanent structural changes in the central nervous system, contributing to the general intellectual superiority early readers demonstrate as adults. Theoretically, then, it would not be reading, per se, that wholly accounts for superior intelligence so much as the brain changes caused by the early reading.

Mastering the complexities of reading calls for integration, observation, speculation, coordination, spatial orientation, visual discrimination, and sound discrimination. On the basis of his experiments at the University of Toronto, Paul Kolers commented that the skilled reader is engaged in a much more complex brain process than the piecemeal perception of individual letters and words. The reader is generating coherent messages.

---

* At the end of the year, all but one of the children tested at the so-called genius level. The scores on the Stanford-Binet individual tests had increased by as much as 36 points. The experimenters reported no average because three of the children had "topped out"—made something in excess of the maximum score possible on the test used.

"The process whereby the clues are selected and the messages are fashioned is one of the more challenging questions in the investigation of the way people process information."

Kolers quoted an earlier investigator of reading, E. G. Huey, who said:

> . . . to completely analyze what we do when we read would almost be the acme of a psychologist's achievements, for it would be to describe very many of the most intricate workings of the human mind, as well as to unravel the tangled story of the most remarkable specific performance that civilization has learned in all its history.

Citing several scholarly studies of the lives of geniuses, most of whom were taught to read long before school age, W. Ragan Callaway discarded the explanation that they learned to read because of their extreme intelligence. "Not only has this idea proved sterile, but, according to Piaget, there is no *a priori* reason to believe that anyone will learn anything regardless of mental age, if the requisite mental structures have not been developed by appropriate experience."

The extremely high incidence of early reading among our eminent intellectuals, he said, increases the likelihood that it has been an important factor in their adult achievement.

Although most parents in Terman's study said that they had merely let the children go at their own pace, more than half admitted furnishing paid private tutoring, an average of 6.5 hours per week including music, language, and art lessons. Nearly half the children read before starting school, and although many purportedly taught themselves, a later investigation of so-called spontaneous early readers drew from all parents the admission that the children had been given assistance of some kind, formal or informal.

Biographer William Fowler said, "In no instance (where documentation exists) have I found any individual of high ability who did *not* experience intensive early stimulation as a central component of his development." Victor and Mildred Goertzel studied the biographies of four hundred famous individuals while preparing their study, *Cradles of Eminence*. They reported that in more than nine out of ten homes one or both parents had expressed a love for learning. In a few cases the critical stimulation came from another relative or, rarely, a teacher. In a strikingly high percentage of the homes, a parent tutored the child on a one-to-one basis.

A scientist turned educator, W. Ragan Callaway was on the faculty of UCLA's school of education when his monograph on the effects of early stimulation was published. Some of the world's most prominent scientists expressed interest in his synthesis of contemporary research, and several expressed the fervent hope that educators would take notice.

Until very recently, most colleges of education seem to have existed apart from scientific research, as if learning had little to do with the physical brain. Who has been to blame? Harvard's Jerome Bruner, a leading figure in early-learning research, criticized himself and his colleagues for "allowing an educational-psychology ghetto to grow up and then mocking it."

To get education back into the mainstream of research, he proposed that schools of education might well be abolished and education made the responsibility of the entire university. "If we can give degrees in theoretical physics and experimental physics and applied physics, then we can surely give a degree in *pedagogical* physics. Let physicists train physics teachers and mathematicians train math teachers. . . . It won't be easy because many professional educators would think twice about losing their autonomy. But losing autonomy and gaining effectiveness may be what the new social invention is about."

A number of geneticists, brain researchers, and psychologists attacked educator Arthur Jensen of the University of California when he contended that blacks are genetically less favored in intelligence than other races. Callaway primarily objected to what he considered Jensen's consistent disregard of laboratory findings. "It is surprising to find a current, scholarly paper from so brilliant and erudite an educator anchored in a thoroughly antiquated biology."

The psychologists assailed Jensen's reliance on IQ tests as a scientific barometer of intelligence. Although the concept of measuring an intelligence quotient is unrealistic, psychologists still employ it because it is fairly reliably predictive of academic success and failure and because no one has yet designed a truly culture-free test.* Usually, however, it is considered a crude measurement indeed.

Benjamin Bloom of the University of Chicago estimated in a 1964 review of the relevant literature that the long-term effect of living in a deprived environment versus an abundant one is about twenty IQ points. Another researcher has estimated thirty points.

But the effects can be reversed. Rick Heber's project at the University of Wisconsin with children of subnormal mothers showed a 46-point gain of his experimental group over the controls. That is the difference between near-moronic and gifted intelligence.

Less intensive programs than Heber's have also produced remarkable changes in disadvantaged children. Four-year-olds gained an average of 23.5 points after one year in the Amote Pre-School in Long Beach, California. At Syracuse University's Children's Center, babies from poverty homes scored an average IQ of 120 (superior intelligence) after eighteen months in a special program. In the pressure-cooker program run by Seigfried Engelmann and Carl Bereiter at the University of Illinois, four-year-olds from a nearby public housing project learned so much in a year that their scores at age five were comparable to those of gifted middle-class children. In project Seed in Berkeley and Sacramento, volunteers are teaching college-level math to fifth- and sixth-grade ghetto children. Their idea is to offer the children an opportunity to succeed in a discipline where there is little cultural bias.

In a now-famous experiment, Harvard psychologist Robert Rosenthal and Lenore Jacobson, principal of a South San Francisco elementary school, told the teachers that certain students had been shown by a Harvard-designed test to be "about to bloom." Actually, they had been chosen at random. 47 percent

---

* The closest approach so far is a variation on the EEG called a "neural-efficiency analyzer," which records and analyzes the brain's processing of incoming stimuli. The speed with which the brain reacts seems to correlate fairly well with the scores on more conventional tests. Thus far John Ertl of the University of Ottawa, who developed the machine, has found no difference in racial or ethnic groups. He said, "Intelligence is not the score on an I. Q. test and it's not what our equipment measures."

of these children gained twenty or more total IQ points over the course of the school year. The average gain for the experimental children was more than twice that of the children not designated potential bloomers.

The phenomenon, now widely known as the Pygmalion effect, has since been verified by more than two hundred similar experiments. Lenore Jacobson said recently that the furore over the failures of disadvantaged children "has operated as a smoke screen for a much larger problem: We don't expect enough of *any* of the children in our schools."

Exciting as they are, the experimental programs are all, in one sense, remedial. Dramatic IQ advances, whether in ghetto children or in middle-class children, only point up the failure of an earlier environment to provide optimal learning opportunities. And there, Burton White said, "The mother is right on the hook, just where Freud put her."

Since 1965 White's Harvard Pre-School Project has been studying the intellectual development of young children. After long and careful observation of preschoolers and kindergartners, they designated major categories A and C. The three-year-old A child was more competent, logical, and socially mature than a six-year-old C child. In their investigation of what makes an A child markedly superior, the Harvard team began studying preschoolers of young and younger ages. They ultimately concluded that somewhere between ten months and eighteen months a child learned the skills and insights of an A child, or he probably never would.

The mothers were the key, and White has estimated that 90 percent fail to provide adequate stimulation for their preschoolers past the first nine months. Surprisingly, the mothers of babies who achieved remarkable competence were busier than the others and gave the baby only a little more than an hour of undivided attention during the course of a typical day. They were rarely meticulous housekeepers, and many held down part-time jobs. But they seemed to grasp intuitively the need to explore and understand. They answered questions, listened to the baby's attempts at speech, and helped him try his hand at new skills, like self-feeding. They elaborated briefly from time to time and stimulated curiosity. They participated in spontaneous play: a pretend game, a private joke, an extemporaneous walk in the neighborhood. They showed respect for the child's intelligence.

C mothers, on the other hand, were often well-intentioned, but they didn't stimulate their children. They didn't exploit learning opportunities. They failed to talk to their tiny children or they talked at them. Whatever curiosity their children displayed began to diminish because it was seldom rewarding. Some C mothers were restrictive, some permissive. Apparently it takes more than freedom to promote intellectual competence.

"If you do a lousy job of nourishing the child's basic intellectual curiosity," said Benjamin Bloom, "you have essentially wiped him out. This doesn't mean it is impossible to reverse the ill effects—nobody really knows. But very likely you have wiped him out."

Dickon Repucci of Yale believes that two-year-olds already have the tendency "to consider available information and to form a plan to guide behavior." He and other experimenters have suggested that the dimension influencing whether a grade-school child is reflective or impulsive might have been detected during his preschool years.

Most parents treat children differently according to their birth order. A study at the University of Oregon revealed that mothers interacting with five-year-olds tended to give more complex explanations when addressing firstborn children. They also seemed more anxious for the firstborn to succeed. For whatever reasons, firstborn children are disproportionately high on the IQ ladder and in achievement. Discussing this phenomenon, Matthew Besdine, a New York psychoanalyst, noted that there are a disproportionate number of firstborns in the *Encyclopædia Britannica* and *Who's Who*. Of sixty-four eminent scientists studied by Anne Roe, forty-one were firstborn or eldest surviving children.

As might be inferred, children in large families tend to have lower IQ scores, and there's a sharp downward trend in families of more than five children. Twins have lower average IQs by four to seven points than children of single birth. "To spread the mothering too thin," Besdine said, "is to retard all aspects of child development, while to increase the mothering is to stimulate and advance all aspects of growth."

Some scientists claim to have found a correlation between breast-feeding and a child's intelligence. Because the personal characteristics of the American women who wholeheartedly breast-feed tend to overlap the qualities of the superior mothers as defined by Burton White's group, the feeding might not be of primary importance. However, there are some intriguing findings.

Niles Newton of Northwestern University School of Medicine pointed out that in 1929, when American women often breast-fed for more than a year, investigators found that babies fed human milk walked almost two months earlier than bottle babies; another study reported that by the third or fourth day after birth, breast babies "showed stronger reactions to being aroused from sleep . . ." Still another researcher found significantly more body activity in breast-fed babies by the sixth day of life.

The latest biochemical research might have the partial answer. An amino acid, cystine, may be essential to the developing brain physiology of an immature human being. "Human milk is rich in cystine," Newton said. "Cow's milk is not."

Another clue might be found in the studies showing that babies learn by their effect on the environment. The Infant Laboratories at the Educational Testing Service in Princeton, New Jersey, reported that babies whose mothers responded promptly to crying and vocalizing showed more rapid learning in a test situation. A baby who realizes that his mother responds to his crying has learned to act on the environment. If there is a delay while his busy mother prepares or heats his formula, he may not draw the all-important conclusion that he has made a difference. So far as he can tell, he is impotent.

John Bowlby of the Tavistock Institute of Human Relations in London has suggested that the human infant is born with a species-specific repertoire of responses, including clinging, sucking, following with the eyes, crying, and smiling. Bowlby believes that this is how the human race has ensured its continued existence. It is up to the mother to integrate such responses into the next stage, attachment behavior, and this probably takes place during a sensitive period.*

* There may even be a maternal sensitive period, according to one study. Fourteen mothers were given their infants shortly after birth and for an extra five hours during the first three days after delivery. A control group of mothers had the brief early contact with their infants typi-

To parents who wonder if they are equipped to stimulate a child's brain, Burton White said, "You don't need to be terribly bright to do a good job. You don't need to be wealthy, you don't need a happy marriage, and you don't need to spend the whole day doing it." Donald Peters of Pennsylvania State remarked that it is important for the mother to be sensitive to the infant's reactions. If touch seems to trigger a great response, emphasize the tactile. If the child is intrigued by sounds, an alert mother might talk to him a great deal or sing to him. She would exploit the modality he seems to prefer.

Too often formal education fails to challenge the young brain or thwarts its natural momentum with monotony and rigidity. John M. Branan of Valdosta Stage College in Georgia asked 150 students to write up in detail the most distressing experiences in their lives, confrontations that hindered their development. More than half reported conflicts with teachers. In another experiment, adults visiting at a school open house were asked to record spontaneously their most vivid memories of school. All of the reports were of unhappy experiences.

The attempts to retool American education involve two major changes:

1. Early education, to exploit the postulated critical periods of brain development.

2. A more individualized approach to learning, offering greater freedom, more self-direction, and environments designed to foster (or preserve) creativity.

"Our traditional education approach was founded on a colossal error," John Tunney told his fellow U.S. senators. "The vast majority of children under five, at the age when the greatest change in intelligence can be brought about most easily, were not in school and were not receiving good enough training at home."

Public education for three-year-olds is common in other countries, including Japan, Israel, and the USSR. Urie Bronfen-

---

cal of most hospitals in the United States. A month later the experimental group of mothers were judged to be more reluctant to leave the baby with another person, soothed it more when it cried, indulged in more eye-to-eye contact and fondling.

brenner of Cornell reported that between his second and third birthday the Soviet preschooler is expected to learn to wash his hands before meals, dress himself, take care of his own possessions, and learn civilized table behavior. The two-and-a-half-year-old can help the nursery-school assistant place chairs and bring in the plates.

Between the ages of two and three, the typical child will have acquired a 1200-word vocabulary that includes nearly all parts of speech. By his third birthday, his pronunciation is basically correct. He can retell a fairy tale, walk a plank, go up and down a stepladder easily, and wait for signals ("One, two, three, run!").

But was he ready to learn all that? Compare the Soviet educators' expectations to Arnold Gesell's warning that the two-year-old is "sometimes too easily considered to be ripe for promotion to nursery school" and that he tends to be disruptive and destructive.

> More concessions ought to be made to his developmental immaturity. He is still an infant-child. There is a residual stagger in his walk. His running is amateurishly headlong. He cannot slow down or turn sharp corners. . . . He delights in the grosser forms of muscular activity—romping and rough and tumble play. He tends to express his emotions massively. . . . He has a robust sense of *mine*, but a very weak sense of *thine*. He can hoard but he cannot share.

Even infants in Soviet nurseries receive informal instruction —in speech, creeping, and standing. The babies are urged to experiment with sounds. They are tempted to reach and crawl. In one Russian study, adults quietly petted and conversed with institutionalized orphans (ages three to five months) for seven minutes, every other day. These babies were later significantly more active, more vocal, and better developed physically than those who had not received that minimal extra attention.

Since the publication of *Psychic Discoveries Behind the Iron Curtain*, competition-minded Westerners have expressed the fear that the United States is falling behind in psychic research as we once fell behind in space exploration. Perhaps it would be more appropriate to wonder about our lagging acknowledgment of the vast human potential for learning.

"We seek not wisdom but oracles," said Dwight Allen, dean of the school of education at the University of Massachusetts. "Thorndike, Hull, Dewey, Skinner, Bruner, Piaget—all have had the honor. At each swing we seem to assume that only one can have the right answer. . . ."

Although Jean Piaget has been this decade's hero, many early-learning theorists feel that his brilliant observations of young children are just that, observations. They believe that real potential is much greater than is evident in his schedules. Peter Bryant, an Oxford psychologist who studied 160 children for a year, concluded that young children could do almost as well as adults on certain Piaget-designed tasks, if they knew how to count. "Children as young as four have logical judgment," he said.

Middle-class American children have been shown to be two or three years ahead of Piaget's timetable on some tasks. W. H. Kooistra found that children whose IQs averaged 135 were two years ahead of Piaget's schedule in their ability to conserve volume, weight, and quantity. (An example of conservation would be the child's realization that pouring liquid into a container of a different shape doesn't change the amount.) Millie Almy of Columbia found that middle-class children were about a year ahead of lower-class children in their understanding of conservation.

"Piaget's genius," said Jerome Bruner, "is to study those aspects of mental functioning that show as little possible difference as you go from one school or class or culture or curriculum to another. So, for example, if I take his description of the typical formal operational thought processes, there is no way whatever to distinguish between an average 14-year-old boy and Einstein or John von Neumann."

Bruner believes that Piaget has not defined how the human being learns to use his operations and rules, how he scans a problem situation and finds possible ways to close a gap. Babies as young as six months are beginning to learn problem-solving strategies, Bruner said. "Furthermore, there is evidence that not only his estimates of age of occurrence are wrong, which is a relatively trivial fact, but also that the more specific details of the theory . . . may be questioned."

"The [recent] findings may well be the great breakthrough of our time," Fred Wilhelms observed in *The School Administrator*. Only a handful of educators realize the real significance of the discoveries about young children, he said. He called for "a forcing of vivid response . . . the awakening of precise perception, whether in the eyes or ears or fingertips. It includes endless attention to accurate, coherent, expressive language. It demands full play for creativity."

Newsweek reported on coming changes in education:

> As early education continues to grow, pouring ever better-prepared children into the primary grades, the public schools will inevitably come under fierce pressure for reform. . . . Nor have most kindergarten and first-grade programs yet adjusted to cope with the legions of *Sesame Street* graduates. . . .

TV Guide reported that school officials in Huntington, West Virginia, "were so startled by the erudition of the latest kindergarten crop that they launched a survey to find the causes." They learned that most of the children had watched "Sesame Street." A greater shock was imminent: Many preschoolers, building on "Sesame Street's" letter-and-number foundation, learned to read by watching "The Electric Company," its sister show for older children.

Maybe Maria Montessori's dream is emerging at last into reality. She had envisioned that one day the traditional primary program could be abandoned because already literate children would be ready to plunge into learning experiences more exciting than the rudiments of reading and counting. They would be the first generation of children whose innate potential has been fully developed—the truly normal children.

19

TRANCE LEARNING AND
MEMORY MOLECULES

In the late 1960s flurries in the press followed the astonishing announcements from several laboratories that some learning was apparently being transferred from one living creature to another. Planaria (flatworms) trained to contract at a light signal were fed to untrained planaria, which then seemed to know the response without being taught. Extracts from the brains of trained rats were injected into naïve rats, who then seemed to learn the appropriate behavior in record time.

For a while no one knew whether to laugh or cry. Either it was a hilarious mistake or a science-fiction nightmare. Would we homogenize scholars and serve them up, in lieu of education? Even the scientists engaged in the research poked fun at themselves. Much of their work was reported in a half-facetious journal, *Worm Runner's Digest*. Spoofs were included along with serious reports. Even to the believers the whole concept seemed almost too outrageous to be true.

In his 1970 book, *The Mind of Man,* Nigel Calder said of the memory-transfer researchers, "I am guessing that they are wrong; otherwise the shape and content of this book might have to be very different."

Indeed, stronger evidence for chemical transfer would have upset Calder's matter-of-fact report on the state of brain research. Since then, not only have hundreds of laboratories demonstrated chemical transfer of memory, but more recently

Georges Ungar of Baylor University College of Medicine, Wolfgang Parr of the University of Houston, and their associates have verified the existence of six specific behavior-producing peptides.

One such peptide has been isolated, purified, and synthesized. It was named scotophobin, from the Greek for "fear of the dark." Earlier experiments had shown that extracts from the brains of rats trained to avoid the dark produced dark-avoidance behavior in untrained rats. To accumulate enough material to locate the key substance, Ungar and his associates trained more than four thousand rats. More recently another research group reported that synthetic scotophobin affects dark-avoidance in goldfish as well.

The investigators have now partially isolated a substance extracted from the brains of rats habituated to a sound. They are also collecting material for the study of two substances extracted from goldfish; one group of fish was taught to avoid blue and prefer green, another group to do the opposite. This research will require the accumulation of *between ten and twenty thousand* donor fish. Researchers are also training fish in a motor skill, the ability to swim normally with a float attached that pulls the fish upward. Preliminary studies have shown that fish given an extract from trained fish acquire the skill without any training.

In 1973 the Baylor workers identified an eight-segment chain of six specific amino acids associated with trained rats' memory of the sound of a bell and their expected response. The identification of this peptide was acclaimed as a major breakthrough, comparable to the breaking of the genetic code some twenty years earlier.

What are the implications? Will it be possible someday to take a pill in lieu of learning to swim? Might we ingest foreign languages and higher mathematics as fractions from a trained brain?

Very little is known about learning. The brain processes involved might be viewed from a number of levels. The psychologist sometimes explores learning as a mental activity with only superficial reference to the physical brain. The anatomist may concern himself with certain brain structures vital to learning, such as the hippocampus. Or he may become absorbed in the study of cell structure.

A biophysicist or electroencephalographer might limit his research to the brain's electrical events. Some biochemists are devoting their careers to investigating the role of the various neurotransmitters in learning. Biochemists are among those who have wondered about the possibility of a molecular code that incorporates what the brain has learned.

In a wry parable called "The True Nature of the Book," Seymour Kety spelled out the problem. He asked the reader to imagine a country where the inhabitants had never seen a book. One day a million books appeared in their midst. The populace set up a scientific institute but insisted that each scientist examine these strange objects only with the tools of his own discipline.

The anatomists therefore reported that the specimen was a roughly rectangular block of material, covered ventrally and dorsally with two coarse, fibrous, encapsulated laminae approximately three millimeters thick . . . and so on. The chemists burned a book, computed the energy release. The analytical chemist checked out the composition, noting at one point that there were traces of elementary carbon in the pure compound —"probably impurities."

By centrifuging a specimen book, the biochemists eliminated the black contaminants altogether. The molecular biologists found that the book was fundamentally a twisted macromolecule. The physiologists studied the movement of the pages as the book was riffled. A cyberneticist was called in to help uncode tracings the biophysicists picked up with their electrodes.

A psychologist counted the number of letters in the words and came up with a frequency distribution of the words according to their length. Others classified the books. Finally a book was brought to a psychoanalyst in the hope that he would be able to read it.

That he does not do precisely, but instead asks the author to select portions and read them while he listens. Of course, the author is biased and reads what he wants to read, or if there is a 'good transference,' those passages which he thinks the analyst would like to hear. The analyst himself doesn't always hear with equal acuity but, depending on his school or on his preconceived notions, is deaf to greater or lesser portions of the data.

Admitting that his tale is only an "anecdotal, biased, and selected patchwork," Kety suggested that it serves as an approximation of the "rich and almost inexhaustible fund which reposes in the individual human brain. . . . There are no higher or lower, better or worse, disciplines except in respect to their relevance to particular problems."

Important insights in the various disciplines are unlikely to result in a glorious breakthrough, a dawn in which all the pieces suddenly fit, and science at last understands the mysteries of mind, learning, and memory. Some of the more remarkable findings can be shoved together in a vague, tantalizing fit, but the data are incomplete. The piecing together requires imagination and a large measure of speculation. It's like picturing the continents of the world united, as geologists suggest they once were. There are gaps, irregularities, and missing peninsulas. There is the irresistible need to postulate an Atlantis to fill up the holes.

Ungar and the other respected scientists engaged in chemical-transfer research are intrigued by the possibility that there is a molecular code in the nervous system. Phenomena observed earlier, particularly by Roger Sperry of California Institute of Technology, suggested the existence of neural signposts. Although Sperry's findings were first pronounced incredible by most of his colleagues, he proved repeatedly that regions of the brain recognize their appropriate pathways. Cutting the optic nerve of goldfish and newts, Sperry showed that the retina regenerated nerves to precisely the appropriate place. Somehow there had to be a system of passwords whereby the regenerating tissue found its way.

Traditional theory says that injured brain cells die and that the impaired region is left vacant. Recently a team headed by Gary Lynch and Carl Cotman, psychobiologists at the University of California at Irvine, reported that the brain possesses "an amazing and heretofore unsuspected capability for reorganization after brain damage." Lynch predicted that the findings would force a revision of the current theories about what the brain is capable of doing.

The research on rat brains showed that nerve cells near damaged cells move in to fill the vacancy, although not repairing the damage. Cotman said, "What we are excited about is that this research reveals a capacity of the brain that never before has been guessed at. The brain seems capable of doing tricks we were simply unaware of."

Their department chairman, James McGaugh, referred to the research results as "a phenomenal discovery with almost science-fiction implications for the treatment of brain disorders." Theoretically, if brain damage results in jumbled wiring rather than no connections at all, there is the possibility of rewiring. Shortly before Lynch and Cotman announced their findings, two Swedish scientists, Anders Bjorklund and Ulf Stenevi of the University of Lund, reported that they had successfully stimulated regenerative neuron growth in rat brains.

Intelligence on a cellular level has long fascinated thoughtful scientists. Kenneth Walker, a surgeon, observed that when he had surgically implanted the ureter in another part of the bladder, he was always appalled at the crudity of the appearance of the completed job.

> Yet when I examine it a year after, I am scarcely able to tell which is nature's joint and which is my own. Some intelligence in the patient's body has made good my failure, paring off redundant tissue here, adding new tissue there, until perfection has been attained.

Neal Miller, the biofeedback pioneer, marveled at the discoveries Hubel and Wiesel made about the brain of a newborn kitten whose eyes are not yet open:

> To their surprise they found that all of the specific types of responses seen in the adult cat's striate cortex are present in the newborn visually naive animal. What guides all of these millions of connections so that they are correctly formed during the growth of the fetus? . . . What a miraculous creation our brains are.

A neural code hypothesis evolved out of the discovery of the structure of the DNA molecule, "the secret of life." DNA carries the genetic code: The arrangement of substances along the spiral DNA molecule creates the equivalent of a four-letter alphabet from which three-letter words are formed, then transcribed via RNA into a specific amino acid. The twenty amino acids can also be combined as if they were letters of an alphabet. As Georges Ungar put it:

> These represent another alphabet that can form a practically infinite number of different proteins, each with a distinctive "meaning" representing different enzyme actions, structures characteristic of the species and even of the individual, and perhaps . . . records of specific neural information.

Ungar maintains that since learning requires the possibility of creating new connections, there must be a system of cells capable of linking the innate pathways. Such postulated cells have been called memory neurons by other scientists.

Because Karl Lashley proved that memory is distributed throughout the brain, Ungar said the circuit would have to be "replicated at a number of hierarchic levels." The electrical patterns of brain impulses may represent only quantitative elements of information.

Ungar believes his work supports the theory that specific molecules affect cellular interaction—that they are necessary for the consolidation of new junctions at the synapse, the gap between nerve cells. Information is theoretically recorded at the synapse and at the molecular level. The change at the synapse is like the signpost at the highway crossroads, guiding the nerve impulse.

When new information is acquired, the firing of neural circuits could maintain it temporarily by reverberation, but long-term storage would almost have to require that the synapses are permanently marked so that the nerve impulses recognize them. Ungar compares this recognition system to the color codes in complex electrical circuits. Because of this system, the neurons that belong to the same pathway can form synaptic junctions.

The principle could explain the organization of the neural pathways in the embryo, whereby at birth all such pathways are provided with molecular markers. "The question," Ungar said, "is whether this system of recognition molecules can also serve

as a basis for a molecular hypothesis of learning and memory."
He thinks that perhaps it can.

But he has pointed out that even if the hypothesis of a molecular code is confirmed in laboratory animals, the concept
will still have to be applied to man. Because language, both
spoken and written, is uniquely human, encoding of information in the human brain has to account for symbols as well as
raw sensory data.

Meanwhile, he said, "The most urgent need is to identify,
within the next few years, a large number of the behavior-inducing substances, to establish their role. . . ."

For a number of years Holger Hydén, a Swedish researcher,
has been analyzing incredibly subtle brain changes that follow
the learning process. He believes that proteins are likely to act
as executive molecules. When a memory is acquired, Hydén
said, "an external stimulus causes an internal transition in brain
cells from one state to another by a small energy expenditure."
This new state persists. When the item is recalled, or retrieved,
the stored information is matched with incoming data.

Hydén's work indicates that a rat that learns to reach for
food with its wrong paw, for instance, creates a unique protein
in the process. He believes that RNA is involved in the synthesis of this protein.

Karl Lashley searched for thirty years for the engram—the
site and substance of memory. He trained experimental animals
and then selectively damaged portions of the brain, assuming
that at some point he would scoop out the locus of what they
had learned. Removing parts of the brain did worsen the rats'
performance somewhat, but it seemed that, short of lethal brain
damage, it was impossible to eradicate what they had known.
At one point a nonplussed Lashley said wryly that his research
demonstrated that learning was just not possible.

His experiments were so thorough and so replicable that the
radical truth finally had to be accepted. Learning involved a
field of activity. There was a quantitative relationship between
the amount of tissue damage and the amount of memory loss.
But the engram was not to be found.

In the late 1960s, holography, an innovation in photography,
inspired a controversial new learning theory compatible with

Lashley's findings. Holography—which won a 1971 Nobel prize for its inventor, Dennis Gabor—records, as an interference pattern, the wave field of light scattered by an object. A coherent light, usually a laser beam, is split. Part is directed toward the photographic plate by a mirror and part shines directly on the object. The plate records the pattern of light waves that impinge on it. The interference caused by the reflected portion of light—the so-called reference beam—produces, by interference effects, a visible display of the lightwave patterns striking the plate.

Because there is no focusing lens, the plate does not receive a recognizable image. It appears a meaningless pattern of swirls. When the hologram is later placed in a beam of coherent light, the interaction of light and plate reconstruct the original image in three dimensions. The third dimension results from the recording of angle information.

The holographic theory of learning is attractive for several reasons. First, the brain is demonstrably capable of the intricate mathematics involved in transforming interference patterns into a coherent form. The hologram has another property even more exciting to brain theorists. Because the interference pattern of light from the object strikes the entire plate, any portion of the plate will reproduce the picture—not quite as clearly as that made by the entire plate, but it will be recognizable. The analogy to the diffusion of memory throughout the brain tissue is striking.

Brain scientists are quite sharply divided on the holographic theory. It is supported by recent evidence that the brain employs a Fourier transform in order to remember. On the other hand, many researchers are understandably leery of any technological model. The brain has proved, after all, not to be a switchboard, a computer, or any of the other mechanical devices to which it has been likened.

David Hubel commented that the holographic theory is very interesting and stands perhaps one chance in five of being correct. "But there are many other theories that wouldn't stand a chance in a thousand." Hubel's own experience has been that the way brain processes really work is often beyond the theorists' wildest imaginings. Sir John Eccles believes that the theory shows a "strange deviation from basic neurological thinking."

One of the foremost proponents of the theory, Karl Pribram of Stanford, emphasizes the storage capacity of a hologram. "Many different interference patterns can be superimposed on one hologram. Some ten billion bits of information have been stored holographically in one cubic centimeter!"

Pribram sees support for the hypothesis in recent findings of several other scientists, including the models for auditory and touch perception proposed by Georg von Békésy of the University of Hawaii. Pribram said that Von Békésy's models involve equations identical to those that describe the holographic process.

A line from Lincoln Barnett's *The Universe and Dr. Einstein* comes to mind: "Modern physicists who prefer to solve their problems without recourse to God (although this becomes more difficult all the time) emphasize that nature mysteriously operates on mathematical principles. . . ." Modern brain researchers find themselves in the same position.

Although the adult brain shows undeniably less plasticity than it had during its critical formative years, it is still astonishingly adaptable. Most of the breakthroughs in adult learning techniques have involved altering the state of consciousness. Ironically, trying too hard interferes with the learning process, perhaps because tension is usually correlated with beta rhythm production and is inimical to the relaxed but alert state marked by abundant alpha rhythms. If alpha rhythms play a part in the brain's lightning mathematical processing and recall, the mental prowess associated with some altered states is not so mysterious.

While mastery of a foreign language is usually considered difficult for a monolingual adult, trance techniques apparently drastically cut the learning time. At the now famous Suggestology Institute in Sofia, Bulgarians are employing a method called Suggestopedia to achieve fluency and large vocabularies in foreign languages and to learn technical subjects like physics.

The United Nations is introducing the technique into various parts of the world, and adaptations of it are successfully operating in the United States. The Suggestopedia approach was developed by Georgi Lozanov, the Bulgarian physician and psychotherapist. The method borrows heavily from both hypnosis and yoga. Students relax in reclining chairs, achieve something of a meditative state under the direction of the instructor, then supposedly listen to classical music. Against the musical background, the instructor begins intoning vocabulary grammar, idioms of the foreign language. The students have been instructed to listen to the music, not the lesson.

In this serene state, the mind seems to absorb information like the proverbial sponge. According to Lozanov's carefully documented *Suggestology and Suggestopedia,* the typical student learns in two or three months material that would ordinarily be covered in two years of college instruction. After a national commission investigated the claims made for the method and pronounced them legitimate, the Bulgarian Ministry of Education opened the center for Suggestopedia at the Institute of Suggestology and Parapsychology. Lozanov has twice accepted invitations to the United States to discuss his methods, and the UN has published a book about Suggestopedia.

This learning phenomenon is reminiscent of the uncanny memory of some hypotized subjects and the curious processing of data in sleep consciousness. Apparently, when the mind is not hampered by anxiety and busyness, its ability to assimilate and retrieve information is virtually limitless. Students in Suggestopedia classes have covered the material from fifteen French lessons in fifteen minutes. Biofeedback researchers have suggested that a twilight or hypnagogic state produced by brain-wave training or muscle-relaxation techniques might open new learning possibilities.

The brain's potential for adaptation is as spectacular as its powers of absorption. Karl Lashley told of "a student who, in the stress of a public recital, unknowingly transposed one-half tone upward an entire movement of a Beethoven sonata, a feat which she had never attempted before and could not duplicate afterward, even with some practice." Human beings can learn to breathe by action of the muscles of the larynx if their normal respiration is impaired. Rats with spinal or cerebellar injuries, whose motor control was grossly disturbed, could nonetheless get through a maze to the food reward. One would drag himself by his forepaws. Another would roll over completely in making each turn, yet managed not to roll into a cul-de-sac and made an errorless run.

The limbic brain, already implicated in the alteration of consciousness, plays an essential role in learning. It monitors the pituitary and adrenal hormones vital not only to learning but to *un*learning. If the hippocampus is damaged, animals are unable to inhibit old behavior in order to learn new material. Monkeys whose amygdalae are damaged can solve simple visual problems but can't generalize. They can't transfer their learning of one pattern to a similar but not identical pattern.

The hippocampus also stands out from the rest of the brain in its rapid turnover of protein. Protein activity is apparently involved in the coding and storage of new information. And while animals are learning a new task, electrical activity in the hippocampus changes dramatically and reverts to normal once the task is mastered.

Stimulation in certain limbic areas leads to an attention response, a riveting of consciousness and stilling of body movements. Such stimulation seems to bring about behavioral changes, too. Wild, enraged laboratory animals tend to lose abnormal fear, groom themselves more, and get along better with others in the colony after stimulation.

In human beings the hippocampus is apparently essential to long-term storage. Its loss following surgery can leave an individual with a memory of only fifteen minutes. Introducing zinc or potassium directly into the hippocampus sabotages learning. During learning the hippocampus shows a marked increase in RNA.

The chronological reruns of memory sometimes caused by probing during brain surgery can also be triggered by limbic stimulation. Apparently the stimulus spreads from the limbic brain to a site on the temporal lobe. There is also evidence that the limbic system integrates experience in the brain.

Critical involvement of the so-called emotional brain in the learning process underscores the importance of motivation, setting, expectation, and rewards. Apparently children are not alone in their need for a warm, cheerful learning environment. The adult brain too works more efficiently in a relaxed setting.

Nor do we outgrow our suggestibility to the expectations of others. The Pygmalion effect is seen in adult relationships as well as in the elementary classroom.

For example, psychiatric counselors were told that certain patients, according to tests, were ready to respond well to treatment. The patients did indeed respond well, although they had actually been chosen at random. In another experiment, vocational-training instructors were told that tests indicated that certain of the unemployable adults in their class had shown an aptitude for arc welding. Those special unemployables—whose names had been picked at random—did prove to be significantly better at arc welding than their classmates. On some subtle level, the expectation of success had been communicated.

Just as the expectation of failure is a self-fulfilling prophecy, so, apparently, is the anticipation of success. Anything that dissipates apprehension creates a better climate for learning.

And there is every reason for optimism. Look at Sarah. Sarah first learned to read at age five. Progress was slow but her teachers were patient. One by one, words and concepts were added to her 125-word reading vocabulary.

Then came a crucial point: Was Sarah capable of abstract thought?

Sarah's instructions were to find the brown block. *Brown [is the] color of chocolate,* she read. Although no one had taught her the color brown before, she now went to the table, sorted through an array of blocks, and selected the brown block.

Her teachers were overjoyed. Sarah had generalized. Teaching her had been "something like working with a retarded or autistic child." But after all, until then no one had ever taught a chimpanzee to read.

With his assistants, David Premack of the University of California at Santa Barbara has been teaching Sarah and another chimp to read over the course of several years. "Although I expected there would be a ceiling on what Sarah could learn, so far there's none in sight," Premack said.

The chimpanzees read a language expecially devised for them. Symbols are used. A blue triangle, for instance, means apple. Some symbols represent conditions, such as one meaning "if . . . then." (If Sarah takes the apple, then Mary will give Sarah candy. Mary was one of the lab assistants.)

"Sarah could have learned many more words than she has," Premack said. "We're mainly interested in teaching her concepts." Although the setup doesn't lend itself to innovation, Sarah has taken matters into her own hands from time to time. Ordinarily she is given only one piece of fruit. Once, when the board read, *Mary gives Sarah apple,* Sarah appended the symbols for banana and orange. On another occasion, when she was having difficulty answering a question, she substituted some symbols to change the problem and *then* answered it.

Sarah's achievements are sobering. The powers inherent in the mammalian brain render irrelevant such notions as a pill for French or calculus, extract of philosopher's brain for instant wisdom.

Michael Gazzaniga, a brain researcher at New York University, said of Premack's work with Sarah, "If a bright chimp has such potential but doesn't use it, what remarkable faculties might exist in man's brain that are not now in use?"

20

THE ANATOMY OF CREATIVITY

Every creative act involves . . . a new innocence of perception,
liberated from the cataract of accepted beliefs.
—ARTHUR KOESTLER, THE SLEEPWALKERS

At a symposium of educators, a keynote speaker remarked that it probably would not do to develop creativity in everyone. Who then would be willing to do society's menial work?

The speaker himself showed a lack of imagination, for if everyone in society were genuinely creative, the greatest part of drudgery could be eliminated. Take that classic example of meniality, garbage collecting. The invention of the in-sink disposer eliminated from millions of households the need to harbor eggshells and coffee grounds; untold man-hours have been saved for the sanitation department. More recently creative technology has come up with household trash compacters. The Japanese have invented a process to convert garbage into sealed, ordorless building blocks. In Germany, imaginative townspeople stacked their war rubble to create a man-made mountain.

Too often we think of creativity as a satisfying luxury—painting, for instance, or composing, or flower arranging. In reality creativity is at the very core of our lives. It invented the automobile and it will have to find a way to clean up our auto-polluted cities. Creativity is responsible for rapid transit, billboards, penicillin, movies, water beds, the hula hoop, the atomic bomb, and the Sistine Chapel.

There would have been no brain revolution if it were not for imaginative scientists. Most of the dramatic discoveries resulted from bold insights, not from the inevitable, painstaking assembly of existing data. Science itself, as Thomas Kuhn, the scientific historian, has pointed out, is a highly revolutionary enterprise.

According to one personality study, creative scientists are more like artists than like other scientists. Technique, tools, and hard work are the necessary handmaidens of the provocative idea—not the begetters. Breakthrough scientists are capable of asking silly questions: What if the autonomic nervous system could be controlled voluntarily? What if you could transfer learning from one organism to another? What would happen if you gave intense stimulation and training to the infants born to retarded women? Is it possible that babies are born knowing that heights are inherently dangerous? The answers are sometimes more preposterous than the questions.

The creative scientist is alert to accidents and anomalies, to the unexpected, unexplained findings in his own research or a colleague's work. Whereas the less imaginative scientist may dismiss a phenomenon that doesn't conform to the known facts, the breakthrough researcher often drops what he was doing to pursue the paradox. One example is James Olds's accidental discovery of the brain's pleasure centers. One rat in an experiment behaved as if it not only didn't mind being shocked but actually enjoyed it. It kept returning to the place where it had been shocked. Intrigued, Olds and his team examined the rat's brain and found that one of their implanted electrodes had missed its mark. After that they turned to investigating the strange effects of electronic stimulation of the pleasure centers.

"There are researchers who always seem to find significant things," said Froelich Rainey, director of the University of Pennsylvania Museum, "and there are others who don't." He suggested that some get caught up in a particular problem and their work becomes stereotyped, while their more flexible colleagues go on to more and more original discoveries. He placed part of the blame on "the strait jacket of academic training," the insistence that certain things must be true and others can't be.

He recalled that when he was in the Arctic, a biologist friend suggested that certain depressions in the ground might have been house sites. Rainey and a colleague, both trained archeologists familiar with the Arctic, pooh-poohed the possibility. They believed the depressions were frost cracks, but the biologist finally persuaded them to take a closer look, and they found important ruins. Rainey said, "It's always unique individuals who somehow look at the bumps instead of the depressions, and the depressions instead of the bumps. . . . They make the breakthroughs, I think."

Consensus is rare in psychology, but there is one area of general agreement: the characteristics of the creative thinker.

The creative person is playful. He entertains wild ideas and feels no need to pass immediate judgment on them. He is a one-man brainstorming session. He asks questions unceasingly. He is not satisfied with pat answers and has minimal respect for "established facts." Offered two alternatives, neither of which seems quite satisfying, he may devise a third. Even if he is a painter, poet, or composer, he does not think of his work as invention but rather as discovery. Drawing indiscriminately from chance observation and from outside his field, he is eclectic, always synthesizing and integrating.

His sensory perception is usually keen. He spends a lot of time in reverie and is inclined to be somewhat mystical. Often, he says, ideas come to him in dreams or idle fantasy. He enjoys surprises and challenges.

In the light of the great value placed upon creativity, a stranger to our planet might infer that it is rare indeed. Yet nearly all of the characteristics of the creative mind are present in young children! The child explores the environment, coins words, synthesizes phrases. He relishes surprises and copes with a challenge. He daydreams, discovers, asks questions unceasingly. His perceptions are fresh, strictly his own.

Frank Barron, a professor of psychology at the University of California at Santa Cruz, has spent his career studying and analyzing the creative personality. He vigorously disagrees with those psychoanalysts who see creativity as regression to childhood. He said:

Primary-process thinking is a *capability* that *may* be weakened in some individuals as they grow from childhood to adulthood. I emphasize *may* because we do not know that this is the case. Primary-process activity *may* also simply become muted. . . .

Creative power increases from childhood to adulthood in about the same way that general intelligence does. Creative individuals retain qualities of freshness, spontaneity, and joy, as well as a certain lack of cautious reality-testing—openness to the nonrational, if you will. They are in that sense childlike. But this is not regression; it is progression with courage. They bring their childhood along instead of leaving it behind.

Suddenly creativity is the popular goal. Ironically, a quality dissonant with our conventional educational process is greatly in demand in adults—and those who survive the system without losing their creative integrity are richly rewarded. The magic word in a book's title almost ensures sales: *Creative Stitchery, Creative Cookery, Creative Gardening*. . . . Big business sponsors creative management seminars. Encounter groups offer techniques for developing visual imagery. Specialists in education, having seen that intelligence does not necessarily equate with imagination, have devised tests of creativity and techniques for its enhancement.

Perhaps we are trying to develop something that was innately ours. Our marvelous, conjecturing brain was designed to make its choices on the basis of partial evidence. Our sensory processes are incredibly sensitive. We have the capability of imagining that our hands are hot or cold and making them so. The brain has an inherent ability to change gears, to switch to altered states of consciousness. An electronic probe in the temporal lobe can touch off a vivid re-creation of a past event, as intense as the artist's memory. In its visual processing, the brain detects anomalies, searches for pattern and particularly for symmetry.

George Leonard, author of *Education and Ecstasy,* expressed awe about the incalculable possibilities of neuronal interaction. "A brain composed of such neurons obviously can never be 'filled up.' Perhaps the more it knows, the more it can know and create. Perhaps, in fact, we can now propose an incredible hypothesis: *The ultimate creative capacity of the brain may be, for all practical purposes, infinite.*"

E. W. Sinnott ventures that the understanding of creativity will ultimately be found in an understanding of the nature of life itself. He thinks that life is the creative process by virtue of "its organizing, pattern-forming, questing quality, its most distinctive characteristic."

There is a strong likelihood that creativity does not need to be developed in man but simply liberated. Even the most conformist, cautious adult is creative every night, devising plot, assembling a cast of characters, and writing dialogue for bizarre, richly symbolic dreams. In a study of creativity and intelligence in young students, M. A. Wallach and N. Kogan found that children who had shown high intelligence and low creativity on earlier tests were capable of creative thinking when it was required of them—when there was no alternative. But they reverted to conformity whenever the test gave them that option. The investigators said:

> In both cases, the high intelligence, low creativity group is intolerant of unlikely, unconventional types of hypothesizing about the world. This particular group appears conspicuously loath to "stick its neck out," as it were, and try something that is far out, unconventional, and hence possibly "wrong."

The fear of being wrong seems to be a prime inhibitor of the creative process, and this phobia can be traced to the earliest influences. Emphasis on correctness, on right and wrong, black and white, true and false, deals a lethal blow to independence and imagination.

If creativity is a skill to be acquired, like water-skiing, perhaps a technology is necessary. If, on the other hand, it is an innate quality that has been muffled and shackled, perhaps we only need to give it its voice and freedom.

The directors of a psychiatric clinic remarked that treating phobias is relatively simple. The cure rate is nearly 100 percent, they said. Fear of flying, of animals, of sexual contact— all of these can be overcome because the patient learns to initiate behavior that is intrinsically rewarding. It is pleasanter to enjoy flying or sex than to fear it. But curbing a gratifying habit is hard. The prognosis is poor for the patient trying to stop smoking or overeating.

Being uncreative in the adult world is not rewarding. Creativity is rewarding. Yet in childhood, it is often the other way around. The child is not likely to be rewarded for his indepen-

dent discovery that glass breaks when thrown from a height
. . . or that water and dirt result—Eureka!—in mud. His ram-
bling narrative about his inner life may come at an inoppor-
tune time. If his parents are harried, they may ask him not to
interrupt so often, or they may overcorrect him or criticize him
for fantasizing.

Then there are the effects of school. Most of the famous
creative individuals discussed in Victor and Mildred Goertzel's
study strongly disliked their encounters with formal education.
In contrast, only 1 percent of the thousand children in Terman's famous study of giftedness expressed a dislike for school.

The Goertzels pointed out that Terman's subjects had been
recommended by their teachers. More recent studies indicate
that most teachers favor the high IQ-low creativity students
who are careful scholars and don't make waves. As adults Terman's subjects were solid citizens and high achievers, but he
himself remarked that there was a lack of outstanding accomplishment in the arts. No great musical composer or other creative artist appeared.

The Goertzels said, "If a potential Edison or Einstein or Pi-
casso or Churchill or Clements had been in school in California
in those days, he would surely not have been chosen to be
screened for inclusion in the Stanford study of genius." Indeed,
all of the above-named greats were trials to their teachers.

In his autobiography, Einstein recalled his relief at ending
his formal education:

> It is, in fact, nothing short of a miracle that the modern methods
> of instruction have not yet entirely strangled the holy curiosity
> of inquiry, for this delicate little plant, aside from stimulation,
> stands mostly in need of freedom; without this it goes to wreck
> and ruin without fail. It is a very grave mistake to think that the
> enjoyment of seeing and searching can be promoted by means of
> coercion and a sense of duty.

The very nature of intelligence tests sometimes militates
against the creative thinker. A very bright, creative child often
gives technically wrong answers for very intelligent reasons.
Sometimes he has introduced another dimension into the question. Or his definitions may reflect greater sophistication than
the test can account for.

"Where do ideas come from" may sound as juvenile as "Why can't you see the wind?" or "How high is up?" Yet research offers only theories at this point—no answers. Empirical evidence strongly implicates unconscious processes in the production of breakthrough ideas: scientific insights, invention, artistic inspiration. Having learned to draw on subliminal material, creative individuals typically report that their best ideas have come to them spontaneously, while they were not actively engaged in problem-solving.

Henri Poincaré was one of those exceptional individuals who are not only creative but are also intrigued by the creative process. Poincaré had observed that his own important insights resulted from unconscious work. Although hard conscious work always preceded the period of unconscious activity, conscious effort alone would not suffice. Many intelligent mathematicians seemed to Poincaré to lack intuition.

> They will learn by heart the details one after another; they can understand mathematics and sometimes make applications, but they cannot create. Others, finally, will possess in a less or greater degree the special intuition referred to, and then not only can they understand mathematics even if their memory is nothing extraordinary, but they may become creators.

Poincaré compared the conscious mind to an examiner for the second degree who would have to question only the candidates who had passed a previous examination. The unconscious does the screening if the conscious mind would but accept this bonus.

Because the contributions of intuition have been so thoroughly documented, many creativity theories assume that the subliminal mind is superior to the conscious mind. Poincaré offered an alternative hypothesis. He proposed that the unconscious actually performs all the calculations and makes all the combinations mathematically possible in search of a solution. With access to all of the data stored during a lifetime—everything observed, heard, or otherwise processed through the senses—this computing operation comes up with a wealth of possible answers. Poincaré further proposed that only the useful answers are admitted to consciousness.

All the combinations would be formed in consequence of the automatism of the subliminal self, but only the interesting ones would break into the domain of consciousness. And this is still very mysterious. What is the cause that, among the thousand products of our unconscious activity, some are called to pass the threshold, while others remain below. Is it simple chance which confers this privilege?

He believed not. He suggested that the privileged unconscious phenomena are those which, directly or indirectly, affect the emotional sensibility. *The useful combinations are precisely the most beautiful,* Poincaré said, meaning those most capable of charming the special sensibility, such as the mathematician's pleasure in harmony, symmetry, and geometrical elegance.

Poincaré offered his theory about the brain's permutations in 1924. If the sensory processes perform the complex calculations postulated by several recent theories, it is reasonable to conjecture that the brain is constantly problem-solving below the level of conscious awareness.

There is heartening evidence that most people could exploit that inner computer, as creative individuals do, if they could facilitate passage between the unconscious and conscious awareness. If we examine the childlike characteristics in the creative adult, we can see that the subjugation of the primary processes is neither necessary nor inevitable. That special sensibility Poincaré wrote about still may be viable even in individuals who consider themselves uncreative. Otherwise we would not react to a beautifully designed building, a song, or a well-crafted film.

Raynor Johnson suggests that the "buddhic" or intellectual self responds to the creation:

No man, however distinguished be the quality of his mind and however good his technique, can say, "I will now sit down and write a great poem or compose a great symphony or make an important discovery." There is a level deeper than Mind from which all inspirations and all creative insights arise. . . . When we respond to the greatness of these things, it is not because our minds have weighed their merit and pronounced them worthy to be appreciated, but because our own buddhi recognises immediately and intuitively the old authentic quality.

A mind capable of such recognition should be equally responsive to the elegant products of its own inmost processes if it were only able to re-establish communication with them. *The Imprisoned Splendour,* Johnson's brilliant treatise about mystical experience and physics, took its title from a poem in which Robert Browning portrayed truth as a clear inner perception, error the result of the search for external answers. Man is bound by a "carnal mesh."

> . . . and to *know*
> Rather consists in opening out a way
> Whence the imprisoned splendour may escape . . .

How does the creative individual keep the way open?

The most obvious answer is that he lets down the bars through the altered states of consciousness. It doesn't take Hercule Poirot to detect the association between creativity and the ASC phenomena: spontaneous imagery, rapid processing of ideas, enhanced sensory perception, exhilaration, the sudden falling into place of disparate data.

As the universal altered state, sleep offers the most accessible window to the unconscious. Elias Howe had come to an apparently insoluble problem in his development of a sewing machine. Then he had a dream in which symbolic spears suggested to him the idea of putting the eye at the bottom of the needle rather than the top. Working on the structure of the benzene molecule, August Kekule dreamed of snakes biting their own tails. This inspired his discovery of the benzene ring, a major insight in the annals of organic chemistry. An IBM inventor, Luther Woodrum, said that he often dreams about mathematics as a series of images, and he credits many of his most valuable ideas to dreams.

> In 1962 I was working on a program. . . . I'd spent a lot of time on the project but couldn't quite figure out how to optimize the program by relocating the instructions. One night, after supper, I took a nap. With the problem on my mind, I began dreaming about the program—with the mathematics of it seen as a group of images. To my surprise the instructions began relocating themselves.

Suppose that these or similar cue-laden dreams had come to less responsive individuals, as, according to Poincaré's theory and common sense, they well might. Does it not seem likely that they might have been forgotten, or dismissed as dreams about snakes or spears? The receptiveness of the creative person is an essential characteristic.

Roget, the author of the thesaurus, once tried inhaling nitrous oxide. He said, "My ideas succeeded one another with extreme rapidity, thoughts rushed like a torrent through my mind, as if their velocity had been suddenly *accelerated* by the bursting of a barrier which had before retained them in their natural and equable course."

In the eighteenth century Sir Humphrey Davy experimented with nitrous oxide. He described the exhilarating effects of what was then called laughing gas:

> I existed in a world of newly connected and newly modified ideas. I theorized, I imagined that I made discoveries. When I was awakened from this semi-delirious trance by Dr. Kingslake, who took the bag from my mouth . . . I exclaimed . . . "Nothing exists but thoughts!"

A versatile man indeed, Davy was not only one of the foremost chemists of his day but an accomplished poet as well. He used the gas for poetic inspiration and tried it out on Coleridge, Southey, and other of his literary friends.

The exploitation of drug ASCs by artists and would-be artists is nothing new, but these states are not a panacea. The pharmacologist Erwin DiCyan said, "The unfortunate myth has sprung up that psychedelic agents, known to accentuate creativeness, will make a poet of a sterile, emotionally flat, and shallow person. This is untrue. Poetry may spring forth with proper stimulation *if* there is an inner richness in which it spawns." DiCyan argued that creativity is not the mechanical screening of ideas but principally "the manner in which a curious mind transforms the wealth of material it has beachcombed, retrieved, and transcended into art."

For all practical purposes, the brain can only process and transmute that information it has on hand. If there is to be a creative product, the workshop must be stocked with rich, varied experience, a wide range of sensory data. Unfortunately, the need for raw material and for technique is often overlooked.

Many educators debate the relative merits of affective (emotional) learning versus cognitive (intellectual) learning, assuming that a choice must be made. A pediatrician and a psychiatrist, thinking along the same lines, advised the readers of *McCall's* not to worry about their children's sensitive periods in learning (whose existence they considered debatable anyway). "The stress on cognitive development ignores many other talents—those of the carpenter or poet, for instance."

But creative thinkers have warned that esthetic sensitivity cannot materialize in an intellectual vacuum. A poet needs words and a carpenter needs numbers. Igor Stravinsky described as a heresy the notion that art is something apart. He said, "In art as in everything else you can build only upon a firm resisting foundation. . . . So my liberty consists in moving inside the narrow bounds which I set for myself for each thing I undertake."

The view of creativity as a nonintellectual activity fails to take into account the dynamic, unitary, and coherent nature of the brain. Emotion and intellect, freedom and discipline, reason and intuition, the precise and the gossamer, primary and secondary processes, chaos and order—all of these apparent opposites can exist in creative harmony in the human brain.

In Wallach and Kogan's study of creativity and intellectual development in children, the subjects were divided into four groups. One group was high in intelligence but low in creativity. Another was high in creativity, low in intelligence. A third group was high in both, and a fourth was low in both. The high/high children showed the greatest attention span, concentration, and interest. They also tended to be somewhat disruptive, proposing novel possibilities to overcome their boredom with classroom routine. The investigators said, "These children can exercise within themselves both control and freedom, both adult-like and child-like kinds of behavior."

The researchers seriously questioned the 1961 study by Jacob Getzels and Phillip Jackson in which children who were highly creative but low in IQ scores were contrasted with a high-IQ, uncreative group. "If one wishes to establish generalizations about the nature of creativity and of intelligence as distinct characteristics, one cannot afford to ignore those children who are high in both and who are low in both," Kogan and

Wallach said. Creativity theorists have often cited the Getzels-Jackson study as evidence that imagination is superior to intelligence—another pointless comparison.

In his intensive study of fifty-six creative writers, Frank Barron reported that they were characterized by a high degree of intellectual capacity, and that they valued intellectual and cognitive matters. They were independent, productive, verbally fluent, and had strong esthetic reactions.

Their comparison to a group of institutionalized schizophrenics was interesting. About as many artists as psychotics reported odd sensations (ringing in the ears, peculiar odors, unaccountable numbness in parts of their bodies). Both groups preferred occasional solitude and expressed a proneness to impulsive outbursts. Kogan and Wallach said:

> These findings suggest an unusual state of psychic affairs in creative artists. They seem to be able to incorporate psychoticlike experiences and tendencies in a matrix of rationality, very high conceptual intelligence, honesty, and personal effectiveness.

Observation—acute sensory perception—plays a role in the creative personality. According to one study, there is a strong correlation between the sensory threshold of infants and their later imaginative tendencies. Those relatively insensitive when tested at a few months of age were later inclined to center their play around concrete objects, whereas low-threshold infants later tended to talk about imaginary playthings and imaginary companions. Although this suggests a genetic factor in sensory acuity, perception can be sharpened or dulled by experience. The sensibility of eye and ear become subtler with training, formal or informal.

Very recently, two writers independently published strikingly similar rebuttals to a traditional belief about creativity. Milton Knobler observed that children draw stick people and lollipop-shaped trees because no one has called their attention to specific trees and people.

> Did your teacher ever ask you, for example, to draw the big apple tree in the school yard? Not likely. What she probably said was, "Draw *a* tree." And so you drew one based on a vague, general impression. . . .

Knobler submitted that this is "nothing short of neglect—neglect in the vital area of developing a child's capacity for meaningful interaction with—and hence, meaningful interpretation of—his environment." He strenuously opposed the overwhelmingly popular view among educators that the child must be allowed to develop almost entirely on his own.

> The assumption here is that every child quite naturally develops the awareness and sensitivity necessary to interact meaningfully with his environment. That a structured program aimed at developing greater awareness represents an imposition of adult standards. That adult standards inhibit a child's creativity.
>
> The fact is, the typical 'child art' (the lollipop tree and its friends and relations) that is produced almost universally is itself the result of adult-imposed restraints. Because we adults insist on making such symbols sacrosanct, we deny our children an opportunity to observe and absorb the environment.

Knobler proposed to his fellow educators that "the child who is given the chance to run his hands over the bark of a tree, to investigate its structure, to compare its foliage with that of other trees and to listen to the music of the wind through its branches is not going to draw a lollipop. The lollipop simply would not satisfy his mental awareness of what a tree is—or can be."

Thomas Cottle of MIT took issue with the parents and teachers who lament the passing of creativity when a child's pictures or sculptures begin to show form and realism.

> . . . the act of artistic creativity requires techniques that allow one to control and shape expression. . . . The first drawings of early childhood are essentially an outpouring of impulses. In the next phase of a child's drawing, the representation of reality and an allegiance to detail become important. Still later, there can be a phase of what again appears to be pure spontaneity, but those who go through this phase will be able to speak about the meanings of their abstract renderings—as they were not in their kindergarten years. . . .

Some artists have unintentionally perpetuated the myth that technique is unimportant. A university music teacher complained that many accomplished pianists misled aspiring youngsters by telling them it is only necessary to "image" the way the music should sound. "They've forgotten that they had long ago acquired the technique that makes it possible for them to perform spontaneously now." The craft necessary to his calling sometimes becomes such a part of the individual that he is no longer aware of it. It is his second skin.

Many consciousness-altering methods are being explored for their potential in enhancing creativity. Sensory-awareness techniques seem to be effective. This approach has been compared to Zen. Psychosynthesis combines visualization with a meditative technique. Its proponents believe that it can stimulate intuition and creativity. They try to teach "what Fromm has called the forgotten language of images and symbols."

Hypnosis, meditation, and brainwave training have all proved valuable creativity generators. Virtually all imaginative people—whether artists, executives, or industrial designers— report that their best ideas consistently arise during trancelike periods, reverie, a hypnoidal state. W. B. Yeats said:

> The purpose of rhythm, it has always seemed to me, is to prolong the moment of contemplation, the moment when we are both asleep and awake, which is the one moment of creation, by hushing us with an alluring monotony . . . that state of perhaps real trance in which the mind, liberated from the pressure of the will, is unfolded in symbols.

That passage was quoted by the psychiatrist Wayne Barker, who believes that the brain's apparently spontaneous production of ideas—"fits"—is related to epileptic "fits." Some neurological series of events puts the pieces together, and the role of rhythm may be central in the creative process.

Current brain research strongly suggests that the altered states, with their abundant production of the regular alpha waves, may reflect an accelerated, uninterrupted processing of data. Since the alpha rhythm has been implicated as a possible timing device for the brain's mathematical transformation of stimuli into sensory data, perhaps psychology will investigate the data-processing uses of brainwave biofeedback and the related altered states. At the Menninger Foundation, where subjects are learning to increase alpha and theta brainwave production for the possible creative value, there are frequent reports of spontaneous imagery. The project researchers expressed the hope that such training "may make possible an enhancement of creativity in individuals whose potential is yet unrealized."

Spontaneous visual phenomena, even whole tableaus or playlets, are reported by creative artists and by individuals in other reverielike states. E. H. Shattuck said of a meditation period:

> Suddenly, without my noticing a change, instead of thoughts in words, pictures flashed into my mind. . . . I was walking along a dusty road when an old man came up to me, knelt down and offered me a bowl of soup. It was just a momentary flash, but startlingly vivid, and I was quite taken by surprise by this strange action. The whole thing was just as inconsequent as a dream, but I knew I was awake and it appeared convincingly solid and real.

Compare this passage from a memoir of Thomas Wolfe:

> I would be sitting, for example, on the terrace of a cafe . . . and suddenly I would remember the iron railing that goes along the boardwalk at Atlantic City. I could see it instantly just the way it was, the heavy iron pipe; its raw, galvanized look; the way the joints were fitted together. It was all so vivid and concrete that I could feel my hand upon it and know the exact dimensions, its size and weight and shape.

The most creative individuals are in an altered state much of the time. Their daily consciousness is apparently a free port, constantly admitting the rich cargo from the unconscious.

Sylvia Ashton-Warner has written a superb account of her experiences teaching the Maori children in New Zealand. She developed what she calls "organic teaching" to enable the children to build "the bridge from the inner world outward." She agreed with Erich Fromm's contention that destructiveness is creativity gone wrong. "Yet all this can be expelled through the creative vent," she said. "The more violent the boy, the more I see that he creates. . . . I put clay in his hands, or chalk. He can create bombs if he likes or draw my house in flames, but it is the creative vent that is widening all the time and the destructive one atrophying."

Rather than subject the children to what she considered insipid readers ("Come, John, come. See the boats."), she allowed them to choose their own first reading words. A typical vocabulary might include: Daddy, Mummy, ghost, bomb, kiss, brothers, butcher knife, jail, love, dance, cry, fight, hat, bulldog, touch, wild piggy. From such words the children constructed their own stories and shared them with each other.

Many American teachers of the disadvantaged have turned to similar methods of teaching reading and, simultaneously, creative writing—allowing children to narrate stories on tape cassettes, then typing up copies for the entire class.

Sometimes the stories are shown by an overhead slide projector.

John La Monte a teacher in Glendale, California, had his fifth-graders take turns making "constellations." The stars consisted of chalk marks they made on the blackboard while wearing paper bags over their heads. Then, like the mythmakers of old, each child decided what the constellation looked like to him—and composed a story about it. It was the diamond necklace an angry queen threw at a wildcat; a crown drawn by a boy for his dying mother; a palette discarded by an unsuccessful painter; a kite lost during a scuffle between two boys.

Often creativity-in-education buffs have emphasized positive feelings exclusively. Sylvia Ashton-Warner noted that Janet and John of the primary readers are not only two-dimensional representatives of upper-class England, but they are also sorrowless. And of the readers published in the United States, she said, "Has the American child no fears? Does it never rain or blow in America? Why is it always fine in primer books?"

Wallach and Kogan suggested that perhaps studies seeming to show neurotic tendencies in imaginative subjects were instead reflecting the creative person's greater awareness of emotions and his honesty in reporting them. In their own study, the children high in creativity and intelligence reported more anxiety about the test-taking situation than their high IQ, uncreative classmates. The authors suggested that the high/high children were more sensitive to their inmost feelings or freer about confessing them.

Tension is certainly a component of the creative process, but it should be compared to a pleasurable excitement, such as sexual arousal, rather than crippling anxiety. It has been said that the brightest students probably work best at the brink of frustration. Stanley Rosner and Lawrence Abt, in their excellent anthology, *The Creative Experience,* remarked on the emotional tension expressed by the gifted individuals they had interviewed:

> This sense of excitement, which some refer to as sensual or even sexual, is experienced by both artists and scientists. A sense of urgency is also present, stimulated by a fear that unless the idea is worked on immediately it will be lost. . . . [Molecular chemist Paul] Saltman sums it up well: "Those days when everything is hitting and you're seeing new relationships and each experiment works—this is a wonderful, wild whole life."

The individuals interviewed in the anthology spoke frequently of the importance of unconscious processes at work arranging the material they have attacked. They emphasized the importance of an open mind.

Wilder Penfield, the neurosurgeon who discovered the memory phenomena of temporal-lobe stimulation, was asked by the interviewers if any single figure in his life had played a significant role in his formulation of hypotheses in brain research. Penfield said, "Oh, yes—Sir Charles Sherrington." Sherrington won the Nobel prize for his discoveries in neurology.

"He was the least prejudiced man I've ever known," Penfield said. ". . . Sherrington's mind was so open that he expected each of us working under him to teach him something, and he was constantly asking us questions with the hope that we would give him something." Sherrington remained alert and enthusiastic about new ideas until his death at ninety-four.

He was probably of the breed of whom W. Grey Walter wrote, "In those few effective outstanding personalities whose brain functions we have been privileged to study, versatility of both function and brain activity seems the only common factor." Walter said that for most people, an analysis of thirty seconds' EEG was enough to provide a representative sample. "In that time, left to itself, the brain goes through its modest repertory of motions. But in the efficient genius brain . . . several minutes of analysis are needed before the picture begins to repeat itself, even in the most tranquil conditions. . . . It is surely time that we studied also the conditions which favour the development of the versatile genius."

Perhaps the intricacies of the creative brain, hinted at in the

EEG, grow out of the multiplicity of levels on which such minds operate. Sir John Eccles suggested that every neurophysiologist should be familiar with the following passage by the Italian poet Leopardi:

> To a sensitive and imaginative man, who would live, as I have been living for a long time, continuously feeling and imagining, the world and all objects are in a certain way double. He will see with his eyes a tower, a field; he will hear with his ears the ringing of a bell; and at the same time in his imagination he will see another tower, another field, will hear another sound. . . . Sad is that life (and life is usually so) which sees, hears, and feels nothing but those simple objects that our eyes and ears and other senses are able to perceive.

It would be reasonable to infer that creative individuals would tend to be more mystical than the average person. Research bears this out. Frank Barron reported that of the writers he studied, more than half of the male writers and two-thirds of the female writers reported vivid sensory experiences of persons or objects not really there. One reported a flickering blue light (commonly seen by purported psychics) around his radio and speaker and also had seen apparitions. Half the writers of both sexes reported that they had had intense experiences of mystical communion. (In connection with Sylvia Ashton-Warner's insistence that negative emotions are an important part of creativity, it should also be noted that more than half the writers had also experienced overwhelming emptiness, desolation, and loneliness.) Twenty percent reported that they believed they had had prophetic dreams. Many of the subjects reported detailed experiences they attributed to extrasensory perception.

There are famous examples of apparent ESP in creative people. In the nineteenth century, Jules Verne described the first lunar rocket launch. His account of the moon shot originating in Florida resembled the actual 1970 Apollo 11 trip in remarkable detail. In 1898, fourteen years before the sinking of the *Titanic,* a sailor named Morgan Robertson wrote *The Titan.* In Robertson's book, produced after what he described as a long trance, the ship resembled the *Titanic* not only in name but in size, number of passengers, and number of lifeboats. Like the *Titanic,* the *Titan* was making its maiden voyage in April when it struck an iceberg and sank.

One of the most famous examples of prophetic art is Tennyson's 1892 poem, *Locksley Hall,* in which he "dipt into the future" to envision commercial aviation, aerial warfare, world war, armistice, and the founding of a world federation. Parapsychologists might find it fruitful to consider the possible connection between his prophetic visions and his technique for altering consciousness, the monotonous, Hindu-like repetition of his own name. In his creative trances, Tennyson saw "vast images" that were "broken and withdrawn." He said that something touched him, "like glimpses of forgotten dreams," events that had happened he knew not where.

Henry Miller, the novelist, told an interviewer that if he were to be asked for his last word, he would reply, "Mystery." Everything seems more and more mysterious to him, he said.

> I think that scientists would say the same thing. The more and more they get into their particular realm, the more and more mystified they are. Knowledge is like cutting into a limitless cake. Cut a chunk, it's bigger. Cut another, the cake is still bigger. . . . So what is the most important thing in life? It is the spiritual, after all.

Albert Einstein maintained that the sensation of the mystical is the sower of all true science. "He to whom this emotion is a stranger, who can no longer wonder and stand rapt in awe, is as good as dead."

To explore, someone has said, is to tolerate uncertainty. The intense promise of the unknown, so tempting to the human child, gives the creative brain its lifelong drive. It is open to all of experience, yet sensitive to its rich, inner resources: recall, problem-solving, imagery, insight, intuition. "Heaven," said Tennyson, "opens inward."

V.

consciousness
and the supraconscious

We have found a strange footprint on the shores of the unknown. We have devised theories, one after another, to account for its origin. At last we have succeeded in reconstructing the creature that made the footprint. And lo! It is our own. —SIR ARTHUR EDDINGTON

21

MIND AND EVOLUTION

We should not pretend that consciousness is not a mystery.

—SIR JOHN ECCLES

Sooner or later, the brain sciences bump up against a Gibraltar of a problem—a riddle no nearer solution today than it was a thousand years ago. No one knows what consciousness is, what mind is. Nor is there reason to expect any blinding illumination from researchers next year or next decade.

Even contemplating this awesome problem has its bewildering aspects. There is man, intently studying the human brain, seeking the germinal clue, the heart of his self-awareness. Surely this is the cosmic *koan*.

Science breaks down very early in the mind problem, as soon as it attempts to define will. One decides to lift his hand. He lifts it. What could be simpler? But what moved the nerves and muscles? If a thought caused the movement, then we are invoking mind over matter. Mind, in this case, caused matter to move. Psychokinesis begins at home.

Roger Sperry has suggested that consciousness is an emergent phenomenon of the brain and simultaneously plays a causal role in determining neural activity. Answering his critics, Sperry agreed that he had not concretely defined the exact organizational features of the neural process responsible for conscious effects.

Anyone who does so will, of course, no longer have a hypothesis but the proven answer. Most of us who work in the area have become reconciled to seeking a solution to the problem of consciousness only through a series of successive approximations rather than by any single breakthrough that is complete and definitive.

He believes that his approach offers a compromise between materialism and mentalism, "proposing a mutual mind-matter interaction in the upper realms of a single, continuous hierarchy."

There is growing evidence that certain brain states correlate with consciousness phenomena, and that, conversely, consciousness phenomena affect brain activity. For example, brainwave biofeedback techniques—learned control of brainwave patterns—can create a changed psychological state. On the other hand, meditation techniques, whose goal is a shift in consciousness, alter the brainwave activity. Sorting mental events from physiological becomes tantamount to isolating the waters of the Atlantic from the Pacific. And there is a very real possibility that such manmade labels as mind and matter are as irrelevant and arbitrary as the naming of oceans.

"Does the cell, freely moving in the pond or in our body, seek its food?" asked Sherrington in 1940. "Is there some modicum of mind in it? That's a natural question to ask. It is not decisively answerable. It has seemed to some patient observers that the free single cell, for instance, paramecium, can be trained to some extent. . . .

"Not that there would seem any inherent unlikelihood in mind attaching in some degree to an individual consisting of one single cell."

Research in subsequent years has proved to the satisfaction of many scientists that the paramecium, a protozoan, can indeed learn. That is, researchers taught paramecia to cling to a platinum wire in hope of finding food. James McConnell, whose planarian (flatworm) studies at the University of Michigan opened a new field of research, said, "We would probably be well advised to accept the position that behavioral changes that *most* psychologists would consider to be learning have surely been demonstrated in protozoans." It even appeared that learning was transferred from mother cells to daughter cells.

What rudimentary knowing is involved in the body's formation of unique antibodies to fight off its invaders? How do damaged organs repair themselves? There is evidence that individual brain cells have alpha rhythms affected by daily and seasonal changes. How does the severed nerve of the frog's eye know its way back to the appropriate region of the brain?

If an embryonic tadpole brain is transplanted to another place, the skin over the new site will dip down to form the lens of an eye. If, on the other hand, the skin over the original embryonic brain is removed and other skin grafted on, the new skin will also form a lens. Noting this phenomenon, Raynor Johnson said:

> Someday all the actual *mechanism* of growth control may be demonstrated as chemical in character, but the crucial point is the existence of an intelligent plan. We cannot have a plan without a planner. Mind is the only thing known to us with purpose, memory, and intelligence, and we may infer that it is the source and sustainer of the plans.

Sherrington pointed out that although the cell is blind and has no senses as we know them, "it 'finds,' even to the 'fingertips,' the nerve-cell with which it should touch fingers. It is as if an immanent principle inspired each cell with the knowledge for the carrying out of a design."

The growing scientific respect for the exquisite intelligence underlying nature has resulted in reappraisal of Darwin's theory of natural selection. Survival of the fittest seems inadequate to explain the thrust of evolution. R. L. Gregory said:

> The problem of how eyes have developed has presented a major challenge to the Darwinian theory of evolution by natural selection. We can make many entirely useless experimental models when designing a new instrument, but this was impossible for natural selection, for each step must confer some advantage upon its owner, to be selected and transmitted through the generations. But what use is a half-made lens? What use is a lens giving an image if there is no nervous system to interpret the information? How could a visual nervous system come about before there was an eye to give it information?

Raynor Johnson questioned the applicability of the Darwinian theory to the evolution of, for example, birds. The development of a wing implies a whole group of related variations, he pointed out: scales into feathers, musculature, and shoulder-girdle modifications. Without them, wings would be useless and would have no survival value. All of these modifications would have had to arise as a coordinated group. Johnson maintains that the accidental simultaneous arrival of such groups is highly improbable. To him, such phenomena are suggestive of purpose and planning. He hopes that a basis of understanding might be found in the theory that there is a field of the organism, subject to "the pull of the future" as well as "the push of the past." To Johnson, the concept of field is irresistibly reminiscent of mind.

Many anthropologists now doubt that "chance mutation and natural selection are sufficient to explain evolution as a whole, or whether other processes, in the course of long time periods, render inheritable acquired properties."

Loren Eiseley has pointed out that four changes had to take place simultaneously in man's evolutionary history to achieve the brain that distinguishes him from the lower orders. "One is amazed and humble that man was achieved at all . . . yet all of this moved apparently with rapidity. It is a dizzying spectacle with which we have nothing to compare. . . . What touched it off is hidden. . . ."

In the current preoccupation with consciousness, the term evolution is used rather freely, often in reference to personal change. A highly evolved individual is supposed to have refined the stress out of his nervous system. He is unflappable, healthy, compassionate. Because he experiences the human comedy from a timeless rather than a temporal vantage point, he is rarely upset.

Are we evolving as a species? That seems to be the question of the hour. A surprising number of scientists are wondering aloud if man is on the verge of biological innovation and if he will save himself from Armageddon by evolving into a race possessed of a higher consciousness.

That possibility is not unthinkable. Speaking of the "next age of man," Eiseley described natural selection as real, but at the same time, "a shifting chimera, less a 'law' than making its own law from age to age. . . . The world, we know now, is open-ended, unpredictable." He cited a prominent linguist who places the emergence of true language at not more than 40,000 years ago.

Theodosius Dobzhansky called evolution a source of hope for man. "Man, this mysterious product of the world's evolution, may also be its protagonist, and eventually, its pilot. . . . The world is not fixed, finished, and unchangeable. Everything in it is a product of evolutionary flux and development."

Dobzhansky emphasized the need for evolution if man is to realize his potentialities. "The evolutionary process does not flow like a quiet river, always at the same speed. It may have periods of relative calm, and others of intense innovation." Man, he said, is the only form of life capable of directing its own evolution.

The notion that evolution need not be gradual was anticipated by Luther Burbank, who subjected plants to stress and what he called "perturbation" to change their heredity and produce a larger array of mutations. He said that it was not the duration of an environment that affected heredity but the amount of pressure exerted. "The more sensitive the plant or man, the more readily he takes the impressions his surroundings or situations give off. It is all a matter of vibrations—a matter of response to vibrations."

Growers are now stressing plants with nuclear radiation to change their heredity. If perturbation is a factor in rapid mutation, modern man should be undergoing considerable change. There are those who believe that stress is the epidemic of our age, and that its ravages will be survived by those who are fittest in the Darwinian sense.

The dynamic spearhead theory of evolution supports the premise that man is capable of rapid change. It holds that the spearhead, an advance unit of life, moved swiftly through the stages of evolution, and that the process may be ongoing. In a dynamic organism, theoretically, something unstabilizes heredity under stress to promote better adaptation.

The biophysicist J. R. Platt said in 1967 that man may now be in the time of the most rapid change in all of human evolution. "It is a kind of cultural shock front, like the shock fronts that occur in aerodynamics when the leading edge of an airplane wing moves faster than the speed of sound and generates the sharp pressure wave that causes the . . . sonic boom."

Man's next stage of evolution is envisioned as a transformation of consciousness, an expanding awareness of his own potential and his place in the universe. Shortly before his death in 1961, Carl Jung said that modern man was faced with the necessity of rediscovering the life of the spirit because "it is the only way in which we can break the spell that binds us to the cycle of biological events." Jung, Burbank, and Pierre Teilhard de Chardin predicted that the line between the physical and the psychic would disappear. Teilhard said, "Matter no longer exists. There is nothing but spirit."

Like Jung, Dobzhansky expressed the belief that man ignores the metaphysical side of his nature at his peril. He compared the repression of the nonrational core, the spiritual impulse, to the repression of sex. He remarked that very few can abstain permanently from metaphysics.

Jung saw the archetypal modern man as one who has freed himself from unconsciousness by drawing more and more of his psyche into consciousness. "Every step forward means an act of tearing himself loose from that all-embracing . . . unconsciousness which claims the bulk of mankind almost entirely." The modern man has "come to the very edge of the world, leaving behind him all that has been discarded and outgrown . . . acknowledging that he stands before a void out of which all things may grow."

Recounting the failure of man's brilliant technology to fulfill his urgent need for transcendence, Eiseley said, "A greater sacrifice is demanded—the act of a truly great magician, the man capable of transforming himself." Eiseley suggested that man himself may be slowly achieving powers over "a dimension capable of presenting him with a wisdom he has barely begun to discern."

The problem, as Lincoln Barnett has pointed out, is that there is no mystery in the physical world which does not point to a mystery beyond itself.

> Man is thus his own greatest mystery. He does not understand the vast veiled universe into which he has been cast for the reason that he does not understand himself. . . . Least of all does he understand his noblest and most mysterious faculty: the ability to transcend himself and perceive himself in the act of perception.

In a now-famous *Punch* cartoon, a scientist confides to his associate, "Don't laugh, Hartley—but every time I begin a new experiment, I wonder if this will be the one where I find religion." Those who have peered most intently through microscope or telescope seem to be awed by the infinitely great and the infinitely small.

Sir John Eccles, who has explored the physiological workings of the brain as intimately as anyone living, said:

> I believe that there is a fundamental mystery in my existence, transcending any biological account of the development of my body (including my brain) with its genetic inheritance and its evolutionary origin. . . . I woke up in life, as it were, to find myself existing as an embodied self with this body and brain—so I cannot believe that this wonderful divine gift of a conscious existence has no further future, no possibility of another existence under some other unimaginable conditions.

Eccles said that his own beliefs were well expressed by a colleague, W. H. Thorpe, who saw science as "a supremely religious activity." Thorpe maintained "the absolute necessity for belief in a spiritual world which is interpenetrating with and yet transcending what we see as the material world." The great physicist, Max Planck, saw science as a quest for spiritual enlightenment.

Another famous physicist, Sir James Jeans, said, "Mind no longer appears as an accidental intruder into the realm of matter; we are beginning to suspect that we ought rather to hail it as the creator and governor of the realm of matter. . . ."

Perhaps we are in the stressful, perturbed throes of a step in our evolution, the transformation of consciousness. Maybe the race is about to realize the centuries-old hope of a Tibetan monk, Kunto Zangpo, who blamed the endless stream of human suffering on the failure of most individuals to perceive their source in universal mind. "May all beings," he prayed, "recognize their own radiant awareness."

22

THE BRAIN AND PSI

We are undergoing a fast transformation. In the future mankind
will look back and say that the psychic age began in the 1970s.
— WILLIAM TILLER, LECTURE AT UCLA SYMPOSIUM ON HEALING

Luther Burbank, that giant of horticulture, was often called a
wizard, a magician, because his colleagues could find no reasonable explanation for his intuitive, highly successful approach
to plant breeding. Burbank denied that anything in his method
was unscientific. In 1926 he prophesied:

> I think it not unlikely that there will come later an age when sci-
> ence will concentrate on the wonders of the mind of man and on
> the subjects that we now consider mystical and psychic. We have
> five senses, but all around us we see evidence that there may be a
> sixth sense, or some additional power of getting impressions and
> knowledge. . . . Undoubtedly we have a great field to work in
> —a field now almost untouched. We may someday find psychol-
> ogy only the first of a great body of sciences concerning them-
> selves with what is now but hinted at in the present state of this
> department of knowledge.

Burbank also predicted that the time would come when there
would be no line left between force and matter. He believed
that scientists could not get the right perspective unless they
went beyond the traditional senses. "A universe of force alone
is probable, but requires great effort to make it conceivable because we must conceive it in the terms of our sense experience."

As Burbank anticipated, the assertion of modern physics that
the universe is not tangible at all, that solidity is *maya,* an illu-

sion, is unsettling to the nonphysicist. From a sober servant science became a tyrant, and now, a mystic. Quite suddenly a number of physicists have gone a short step further, into paraphysics.

Paraphysics embraces much of the scientific investigation once generally bracketed as parapsychology. It explores the mysterious relationship of mind and brain, primarily through the measurement of the secondary effects of unidentified energies.

Until quite recently, the majority of parapsychologists believed that psychic phenomena were attributable only to mind, and that correlates in the physical spectrum were unlikely. The emphasis was metaphysical, beyond the realm of matter. Normal science, naturally, could not concern itself with ethereal ponderables. Over the years a few lonely voices from both camps had insisted that mind and matter were two sides of the universal coin, that there was surely a link.

The thriving Soviet and Czech research on the phenomena hastened the shift in worldwide parapsychology. Changes in the physical environment and/or changes in the subjects' physiology are measured by increasingly sophisticated devices. The popular report, *Psychic Discoveries Behind the Iron Curtain,* provoked keen academic, governmental, and even commercial interest in the postulated unknown energies. Since the book's publication in 1970, intrigued scientists from the West have been making pilgrimages to the psi laboratories of Czechoslovakia, Bulgaria, and the USSR, just as their curious counterparts in medicine have trekked to China's acupuncture hospitals. And sometimes the twain meet; the psi research has cast new light on the ancient Chinese technique.

The book was pivotal in alerting the West to innovative, government-supported research on human potential. Many more physical scientists are entering a field once dominated by psychologists. Although our interdisciplinary approach is not yet as eclectic as that in the Soviet Union, the number of western physicists, electronics engineers, physicians, and biologists involved has probably quadrupled since 1970.

Many scientists had been performing experiments on their own time, sometimes in their official laboratories, often in garages, basements, or spare bedrooms. Others are new to psi research, having been intrigued by the phenomena for years but just now comfortable about openly admitting their fascination. What had long been an underground of interest is moving into public view. Many of the scientists have formed groups, formal and informal, for the pooling of data, methods, and theories. The National Institute of Mental Health has funded several ESP-related studies, including a two-year study of paranormal factors in dreams by the Maimonides Dream Laboratory. Serious scientific interest in psychic phenomena is at the highest pitch in history, and there is every indication of a groundswell.

William Tiller, chairman of the department of materials science at Stanford and an international authority on crystallization, said recently that worldwide research into psychoenergetic phenomena has been such that "mankind has now exceeded the 'critical mass' condition for a self-sustaining reaction, and we can anticipate a continued growth. . . ."

In 1971 Tiller was among a group of respected American scientists, physicians, and scholars who formed the Academy of Parapsychology and Medicine to draw their colleagues into research on unorthodox healing. A standing-room-only crowd of nearly three thousand attended their inaugural symposium at De Anza College in Cupertino, California. Several subsequent symposia on science and psychic phenomena have drawn capacity audiences at major universities.

Meanwhile, ESP classes for credit are being offered at a number of high schools, as well as at the University of Connecticut, Stanford University, New York University, UCLA, Berkeley, and the University of Colorado. In Santa Clara County, California, the bureau of mental health sponsored a class on psychic phenomena. Similar classes are being offered by a number of churches and synagogues.

Because of the need for a program of some kind, R. A. McConnell, a biophysicist at the University of Pittsburgh, wrote an *ESP Curriculum Guide* (Simon and Schuster, 1970). McConnell discussed the scientific study of psi, suggesting study programs for various age groups.

McConnell pointed out that several Nobel prizewinning scientists have encouraged parapsychology. Lord Rayleigh (John William Strutt), discoverer of argon, J. J. Thompson, discoverer of the electron, and Charles Richet, the French physiologist who first defined anaphylaxis, were officers in the British Society for Psychical Research. Richet described his lifelong pursuit of psi in *Traite de Metaphysique* (*Thirty Years of Psychical Research*). Other Nobel laureates keenly interested in the metaphysical were Alexis Carrel, Charles Sherrington, Max Planck, Albert Einstein, Pierre and Marie Curie, and Erwin Schrödinger. In a foreword to Upton Sinclair's *Mental Radio*, Einstein urged an investigation of clairvoyant phenomena.

Perhaps it is no longer necessary for parapsychology to name-drop, but the inclination is understandable. Anyone who ranges into the region of the nonrational, what Sidney Cohen called unsanity, finds comfort in the knowledge that he is in sane company. On confronting the inexplicable, there is a natural tendency for the most level-headed of men to turn to each other, like Abbott and Costello in a haunted house, and say, "Did you see what I just saw?"

Psychic research has been plagued by a number of problems not found in any other field. Its funding has often depended on gifts and popular support, and therefore it is not only underfunded but overrun with lay interpreters. If a neurophysiologist reports a newly observed phenomenon in the optic system, he need not worry that an avid public will blame the mystery on astrology, numerology, or UFOs. If he wishes to explore the new finding further, he is not criticized by fellow scientists who point out that no one has yet identified the nature of light, much less explained how the visual system perceives. Yet parapsychologists have been criticized for studying an observable effect on the grounds that they do not yet have a coherent general theory.

But there is increasing evidence that the benchmark has been passed. More and more scientists and science writers make passing references to such phenomena as telepathy and psychokinesis without adding the apologetic qualifying remarks that were once de rigeur. And the weight of the evidence for psychic phenomena has become so great that it is more difficult to explain away than to accept. As was pointed out by H. J. Eysenck, psychology chairman at the University of London, one would otherwise have to postulate a gigantic worldwide conspiracy involving dozens of universities and hundreds of scientists.

Resistance is understandable. Thomas Kuhn, the scientific historian, pointed out that a new paradigm, or framework within which to operate, seldom converts the community of older, established scientists. Their own productive life's work may seem threatened by a new insight. He quoted Max Planck's comment: "A new scientific truth does not triumph by convincing its opponents and making them see the light, but rather because its opponents eventually die, and a new generation grows up that is familiar with it."

And there has been a historic apology.

In 1955 *Science* published an article, "Science and the Supernatural," by George R. Price, a chemist. Price denounced J. B. Rhine's research at Duke University and the work of S. G. Soal in England. He did not question their statistical method, but said that, since the results were incompatible with modern science, and since some men lie, the alternatives were clear.

"The choice," he said, "is between believing in something 'truly revolutionary' and 'radically contradictory to contemporary thought' and believing in the occurrence of fraud and self-delusion. Which is more reasonable?" He also remarked that he would not accept the existence of ESP if there were "1,000 experiments with 10 million trials and by 100 separate investigators giving total odds of 10^{1000} to one."

January 28, 1972, seventeen years after that famous denunciation, *Science* published a letter from Price stating that he had recently had correspondence with Rhine which convinced him that he had been "highly unfair" in charging possible fraud. He suspected that he had been similarly unfair in what he said about S. G. Soal. Price later acknowledged that although he still refuses to accept ESP as a natural and scientifically explicable power of the brain, he believes that "God sometimes reveals to someone a little of what another is thinking, or of what is happening in a distant place, or of what will happen."

The great Russian scientist, Leonid Vasiliev, secretly pursued psi research for decades under the Stalin regime and did not reveal the scope of his monumental work until shortly before his death. Vasiliev's legacy is the industrious investigation of the paranormal now going on in the Soviet Union. He cited the admonition of the French mathematician, Pierre Laplace: "We are so far from knowing all the forces of nature and the various modes of their action that it is not worthy of a philosopher to deny phenomena only because they are inexplicable in the present state of our knowledge."

The American scientist whose theories have aroused the greatest current interest is Tiller. He has been responsible for attracting a number of physicists into the field. With ex-astronaut Edgar Mitchell, he has effected a warm relationship with the Soviet psychical researchers. He and the physicist Victor Adamenko conferred at length during Tiller's 1970 visit to the USSR.

Based on what is known in the field, and particularly on the Soviet findings, Tiller has listed the following apparent characteristics of psychoenergetic phenomena:

1. The energy fields seem to be completely different from those known via conventional science.

2. Experiments suggest that there is a level of substance whose characteristics are predominantly magnetic, with an organizing rather than a disorganizing tendency as temperature increases (in seeming violation of the second law of thermodynamics).

3. There seems to be a radiation pattern or hologram of energy that acts as a force envelope for the organization of substance at a physical level.

4. There is mounting evidence, from experiments on plants, animals, and human beings, that there is "an interconnectedness at some level of substance in the universe, between all things in the universe."

5. There are indications of energy manifestations that are stable in different space-time frames than we are familiar with. Space and time might be constructs of waves at these levels of substance.

Heady speculations indeed, but Tiller is a hard-nosed scientist. He recommends that American researchers begin by developing devices similar to those used in the Soviet Union, for the documenting of psi effects with as much objective data as possible. He and several other American researchers have set up laboratories similar to that of the Kirlian laboratory in the USSR, for the purpose of photographing the bioplasma.

In the light of the existing data, Tiller has suggested models from physics in the hope that even a crude thesis might at least serve as a springboard. He suggested that there is a matter-mind continuum, several interpenetrating levels of substance ranging from the coarsest and densest, the physical, through several strata of mind to one he has called spirit. He said:

> We have an inadequately developed sensory system for sensing the information coming to us from other spaces, and so we must recreate within ourselves the network to recognize this information. Because of our attention to physical space and the seeming realities therein, we have become polarized to it. We want to talk about oranges, but we have only the language to talk about apples. Because we are using a language not perfectly suitable, we must be patient with ourselves. We will probably muck things up a bit semantically.

John Lilly, on the other hand, suggests that the new insights might have to be expressed abstractly, in mathematics.

As one moves up the continuum, the levels of substance become finer, more coherent, Tiller believes. The importance of such coherence would be seen in the comparison of a ten-watt light bulb to a laser beam. In the ten-watt light bulb the energy is incoherent, the waves canceling each other. The waves in the laser beam are coherent energy, powerful enough to do a job or destroy. In the ultimate level of substance he postulates, all the waves are truly coherent and therefore immensely powerful.

He likened the theoretical levels of substance to various microscopes through which one can look at the universe. "We have looked through the physical microscope so steadily that our eyes have become more or less glued to the lens, so that we tend to think it's all there is. We must detach ourselves and look through another microscope."

At UCLA, Thelma Moss has replicated the Russian findings that some sort of energy is apparently released by healers and transferred to the subjects. Using field-radiation photography, a method similar to the Kirlian process, she and her associate, Kendall Johnson, were able to obtain photographs showing that the energy surrounding the patient's fingertips was weak before the experiment and flared brightly afterward. The healer's fingertip showed the reverse effect—flamboyant, then faint. In another experiment, a hole torn in a leaf appeared black on the film until the leaf had been treated by the healer. When it was next photographed, the leaf's glittering pattern showed no gap. (Such obvious factors as moisture are apparently not responsible for the effect. Sweat, for example, interferes with the process.)

Using a live Kirlian process, the Russians watched a healer's hand as he was attempting to affect a patient. The hand's acupuncture points flared, their luminosity increasing until they steadied into a disc in the palm of his hand about the size of a dime; at that point the patient said, "Now I really feel it." The Russian workers first reported several years ago that they had correlated the acupuncture points with the major flare points of the bioplasma effect. They say that differences in the electrical potential between one's acupuncture points are seen in pathology, and that, after healing, the patient's energies are apparently aligned and the healer's are not.

The Soviet researchers say that they have observed a no-energy zone near the operator in psychokinesis. When Nelya Mikhailova and Alla Vinogravada move objects without touching them, the energy near the object is detected in plant and insect electrical responses and in liquid crystals (particularly barium titanate), which become luminous. Film under the target object is imprinted by the energy.

Interestingly, Vinogravada is the young artist-wife of Victor Adamenko, the physicist who participated in the early investigation of Mikhailova's powers. She has said that she had an intuitive feeling that she too would be capable of psychokinesis. Using autogenic training methods for relaxation, she spontaneously began to demonstrate the ability. Whereas Mikhailova draws objects toward herself, Vinogravada repels them.

Mikhailova expends incredible physiological energy in her efforts. The American physician William McGarey, who accompanied Tiller and other Americans to Russia, reported that he measured her pulse; it went from 75 to an uncountable 150–200. She is sometimes temporarily blinded and reportedly loses as much as eight pounds in a thirty-minute session. Vinogravada, on the other hand, is relaxed. The energy pulsations recorded in the vicinity of the target object are reportedly synchronized with alpha brainwave rhythms, heart, and respiration.

The Russians pioneered in the careful measurement of physiological changes during paranormal events. In human subjects, brain activity typically shows arousal a few seconds before the human receiver displays awareness of telepathic transmission. In one grim experiment, they recorded the brainwave activity of a female rabbit in a university laboratory while her progeny were being killed, one at a time, in a submarine. The EEG showed a pronounced arousal simultaneous with the death of each baby rabbit.

On one occasion Soviet researchers pulsed strobe lights in one eye of the sender at one rate and in the other eye at a different rate. This caused a characteristic unstable, complex brainwave pattern, which also appeared in the receiver's EEG. The sender was able to prepare for the strobe effect, but the receiver became ill.

In this and a number of other aspects, so-called extrasensory perception displays a certain lawfulness strikingly like that noted in studies of subliminal perception. In both cases, emotion enhances the threshold at which information is admitted to consciousness, and the EEG shows activation before there is conscious awareness. In one subliminal-perception experiment, the subjects saw emotionally loaded words more readily than neutral words when they were projected on a translucent screen, faintly at first and then with increasing brightness. *Their EEG showed activation before they signaled awareness;* recognition was also preceded by an increase in heart rate and the incidence of theta rhythms in the brainwave pattern.

Norman Dixon of University College in London believes that these and other experiments form a strong basis for the belief that there are two perceptual systems in the mammalian brain, and that the two can operate independently. The brain can elaborate conscious experience such as dreams and hallucinations in the absence of external stimuli, and it can also receive, classify and respond to sensory information without such data penetrating consciousness.

Dixon cites a study in which investigators recorded directly from the exposed cortex of conscious patients. The brain clearly showed electrical responses to external stimuli of which the patients were unaware. Furthermore, the brainwave pattern appeared to be specific to the external stimulus. There seemed to be no contribution from the brain's reticular system, which is vital to conscious experience.

But when repeated stimulation finally resulted in conscious awareness, *there was simultaneous evidence on the EEG that the reticular system had been activated.* Dixon cites another study implicating the reticular system in expanding consciousness. Stimulation in that region of monkeys' brains resulted in a lower threshold for the recognition of briefly exposed stimuli.

He suggests that this duality of perception was necessary to man's survival. Consciousness, a limited-capacity system, needed to be used to maximal advantage. Limiting the inflow of data would be detrimental, but if the brain could maintain a variable restriction on what enters consciousness, the organism could have its cake and eat it, too. Dixon believes that the experimental data suggest that at some preconscious stage of the perceptual process the brain detects the meaning of the incoming information, then initiates an appropriate change in its level of sensitivity. Important, meaningful data are likelier than trivial information to achieve conscious representation.

The literal translation of subliminal is "below the threshold." Once again we encounter the concept of a gate, veil, or barrier between consciousness and the unconscious. The height of that threshold, the penetrability of that barrier, varies not only among people but also within the individual, depending on his mood or circumstances. The state of restful alertness associated with the alpha brainwave pattern seems to enhance subliminal perception. A similar state is usually employed for the purpose of experimental ESP. The relative lawfulness of ESP phenomena suggest that they are not the result of something totally apart from the brain and senses but are an *unknown* perceptual process. Individuals apparently vary in their capacity for admitting psi stimuli into consciousness.

In the Soviet experiment, the female rabbit's EEG activation simultaneous with the consecutive deaths of her progeny may or may not have indicated conscious awareness of what had happened. In his discourse on subliminal perception, Dixon pointed out that the EEG records of cats with severed brainstems showed that they were still able to discriminate between two patterns learned before the surgery. In theory, the operation had deprived them of what, in human beings, would be considered conscious experiences. Nonetheless, "a differential analysis of incoming sensory information continued to occur."

S. Figan in Czechoslovakia and Aristide Esser, Thomas Etter, and William Chamberlain of Rockland State Hospital in Orangeburg, New York, undertook separate experiments measuring changes in the volume of blood in the capillaries. This level is recorded on a device called a plethysmograph. A sudden increase in blood volume is usually indicative of strong emotion.

The investigators obtained evidence that individuals with close emotional or biological rapport share physiological reactions, even when only one of a pair has received the stimulus. In one of Figan's experiments, a newlywed man was shown the photograph of a former fiancée. His plethysmograph showed an instantaneous reaction—and so did that of his bride, who was isolated from him and unaware of what had happened.

Esser, director of the hospital's Psychiatric Research Foundation, found that identical twins isolated from each other displayed simultaneous plethysmographic changes even when the agent twin reacted to statements of only mild emotional impact. Esser and Douglas Dean found that a dog in isolation would show a strong physiological reaction when researchers threw ice water on his master in another room.

"The world is a rich interconnectedness," said Harold Cahn, a biologist and psychic researcher at Northern Arizona University. One team of scientists has suggested that organisms of the same species employ a communications system using modulated, coherent electromagnetic radiation. Most parapsychologists would probably agree with the hypothesis but might amend it to include an unknown energy.

Esser and Etter pointed out that such speculation is inherent in major scientific discovery. "Be it wild guessing or an intuitive grasping of a basic order or a willful juxtaposition of disparate facts—speculation must be for parapsychology today what it has been for the physical sciences." The scientific method, they said, gives the investigator progressively powerful means to dispatch wrong speculations.

"The history of science," they said, "teaches us that 'queer' facts point to a misunderstanding of the commonplace. The explanation for something as strange as precognition could not help but throw new light on the most ordinary behavior of mind and matter and create a new wealth of prospects for shaping our environment. By a new light, we do not mean *more* light, but light of a new *kind*. . . ."

Sister Justa Smith, a biochemist and head of the natural sciences concentration at Rosary Hill College in Buffalo, has conducted a number of healing experiments growing out of her earlier discovery that strong magnetic fields activate enzyme activity. She reported that Oskar Estebany, a retired Hungarian army colonel and reputed healer, accelerated the activity of damaged enzymes by holding the vial in his hands for a few minutes daily.

"Healing is qualitatively and quantitatively similar to the effects of magnetic fields," she said. She stated her belief that the human race is inching its way toward psychic faculties through evolution in the cerebrospinal system. Estebany's activities were also investigated by Bernard Grad of McGill University in Montreal. His ministrations markedly accelerated the growth of plants and the healing of wounds in mice.

In 1971 Robert Miller, an industrial research scientist, formerly professor of chemical engineering at Georgia Tech, conducted a remarkable experiment with Ambrose and Olga Worrall. The Worralls, who were well known for their reputed healing gifts, were in Baltimore. Miller was in Atlanta, where he had been recording the slow, steady growth of a rye grass seedling. The growth had stabilized at 0.00625 inch per hour.

As scheduled, at 9 P.M., the Worralls visualized the plant growing vigorously in a white light. Over the next ten-hour period the growth rate increased 840 percent. Although it decreased slightly over the subsequent 48-hour period, it did not fall back to the original rate. There was no known environmental variable to which the sudden spurt could be attributed.

At Rhine's Foundation for Research on the Nature of Man, the researchers anesthetize two mice, then ask subjects to try to influence one mouse to recover more quickly than the other. According to Rhine, the subjects have demonstrated that they can influence living matter. Helmut Schmidt, a physicist at

Duke University, has had encouraging results in experiments designed to enable animals to exercise psychokinesis. A cat, for example, apparently can influence the random mechanism that turns on a heat lamp in a cold building.

At the University of California at Davis, Charles Tart has been carrying on a continuing investigation of the brainwave patterns of individuals claiming to experience out-of-body states (OOBEs). Several teams of investigators are attempting to settle the controversy of whether or not enhanced alpha brainwave activity correlates with high ESP scoring runs. Various researchers have been studying the effects of drugs on paranormal perception. Small amounts of alcohol seem to have a beneficial effect, they say, but a stiff drink doesn't. Caffeine helps somewhat. The effects of dextroamphetamine are being explored.

Douglas Dean, a veteran parapsychology researcher, has written about what he calls executive ESP, the ability of successful company presidents to act intuitively. Dean found that the earnings of sixty companies correlated strikingly with the results of the presidents' computer-scored psi tests.

The startling evidence of some sort of primary perception in plants has caused a proliferation of projects around the United States. At least thirty universities and a number of private laboratories are reportedly replicating Cleve Backster's major experiment—in which sophisticated equipment recorded the reaction of plants to the "execution" of brine shrimp.

The theory that there is some rudimentary perception in plant life is not new; the idea interested Luther Burbank greatly and was extensively explored, with positive results, by Sir Chandra Bose, an Indian physiologist. Bose's works, published around the turn of the century, are much sought after by current investigators, who pore over his charts and theories. Charles Darwin speculated that plants might be susceptible to the effects of music and hired a bassoonist to play in his greenhouse.

Recently Backster, whose precise research instigated the revival of interest, accidentally discovered that laboratory plants reacted to the cracking of eggs. He then began investigating the sensitivity of the eggs themselves, and to his astonishment found that they also showed evidence of primary perception.

He said, "We've also been working with cell cultures and with amoeba, paramecia, fresh fruits and vegetables, mold cultures, and blood samples. We find they all appear to have the same capability as plants. . . . Our experiments imply that total memory may go down to a single-cell level, at least."

Even the line between organic and inorganic matter has become blurred. Language is inadequate to describe the dynamics of life. As Nobel-laureate physicist Max Born said, "We distinguish between living and dead matter: between moving bodies and bodies at rest. This is a primitive point of view. What seems dead, a stone or the proverbial doornail, say, is actually forever in motion. We have merely become accustomed to judge by outward appearances; by the deceptive impressions we get through our senses. We shall have to learn to describe things in new and better ways."

Judith Groch, in *You and Your Brain,* said of ESP:

> Merely because we cannot explain such phenomena and because the data stubbornly refuse to accommodate themselves to the framework of our knowledge, we do not have the right to discard such inconvenient information. . . . Although the psi phenomena are no more than a whisper, they hint that all may not be well with our concepts as they are today. It would certainly not be the first time in the history of science that stubborn problems and persistent contradictions have finally forced the revision or expansion of established beliefs.

Noting that Einstein, unable to reconcile inconsistencies within Newton's physics, unlocked "a theoretical door through which scientists then poured in pursuit of the knowledge which lay on the other side," Groch suggested that perhaps the brain still awaits its Einstein, and that eventually brain literature might include chapter titles "we could not even imagine today."

Einstein himself said, ". . . for us believing physicists, the distinction between past, present, and future is only an illusion, even if a stubborn one."

Of all the psychic phenomena, precognition is the most unsettling. Although modern physics has already questioned our concepts of causality, we find it difficult to abandon our commonsense view of time and space. This philosophical dilemma was expressed by Charles Richet's description of premonitions:

"I will not say that it is possible. I will only say that it is true."

The hard evidence for precognition is virtually unassailable. Three times in France and six times in the United States, scientists have proved, at odds averaging a thousand to one, that jirds (North African gerbils) and mice could predict in which half of a box an electric shock would be discharged, although the side receiving the shock was determined randomly, by the rate of radioactive decay. As early as the 1930s J. B. Rhine had amassed statistical evidence for precognition but delayed publication because he felt that his findings on telepathy and clairvoyance were jarring enough to the scientific community.

At the 1971 meeting of the American Association for the Advancement of Science, researchers from Maimonides Dream Laboratory reported on a careful series of experiments supporting the existence of precognition. The experiments were designed to eliminate all psychic phenomena except precognition. They wondered whether Malcolm Bessent, an Englishman with a history of spontaneous precognitive experiences, could dream about an event to be created on the following day. In order to eliminate the effects of telepathy or clairvoyance, no one knew what those events were to be. Their exact nature would be randomly determined after the dreams.

For eight consecutive nights in one experiment and for sixteen nights in a second run, Bessent's EEG was monitored as he slept in the laboratory, and he was periodically awakened for dream reports. The reports were held by the interviewer. In the morning two other experimenters each drew a random number and turned the numbers over to yet another individual, referred to as the recorder. One number determined the page in Hall and Van de Castle's *The Content Analysis of Dreams*. The second determined which item on that page would serve as the key word.

After establishing the key word, the recorder checked through a pool of several hundred art prints to find the one that best depicted the word. Next he created a multisensory environment inspired by the print. Bessent was then brought into the environment to experience this randomly determined situation. As scored by three outside judges, he had five direct hits out of the first eight nights and a similar score on the second run. That is, five of his eight reports foretold what would happen.

An example: For the target word corridor the recorder chose a Van Gogh painting, *Corridor of St. Paul Hospital*. The painting depicts a lone figure standing in the corridor of a mental institution constructed of light-colored concrete. For the environment, Bessent was led down a darkened corridor to the accompaniment of music suggesting madness. Someone was laughing maniacally in the background. Bessent was given a niacinamide tablet and a glass of water. His skin was daubed with acetone to give the impression of disinfectant.

The dream-report files were then checked. Twice during the night he had reported dreams about a large concrete building with an unhappy patient in it. Three of his dreams dealt with doctors or other medical personnel. He repeatedly said that a patient had escaped. Twice he dreamed about drinking, once from a cup and once from a glass.

The physicist J. E. Orme asserted that because of positive experimental findings, "spontaneous occurrences of apparent precognition cannot be entirely dismissed as the product of fantasy, superstition, and folklore. Nor should it be ignored because of the theoretical difficulties it raises in many fields."

No one pretends to have an answer to the precognition puzzle, but physicists have suggested possible approaches. Sir Adrian Dobbs suggested that there may be particles of energy he called psitrons, operating in another time dimension and having imaginary mass (in the mathematical sense). According to the relativity theory, psitrons could travel faster than light indefinitely. William Tiller postulated the existence of particles he called perceptrons to account for what we might think of as a radiation from the future. A number of scientists are already searching for the tachyon, a faster-than-light-particle whose existence was first suggested by Gerald Feinberg of Columbia University. Definite evidence of the elusive tachyon would play havoc with our conventional sense of time.

A number of scientists and philosophers have proposed that time is a human construct, an artificial system whereby we measure our experiences, and that our limited understanding requires this concept, much as the kindergartner needs a lined tablet to guide his first halting letters.

Orme, Louisa Rhine, J. W. Dunne, and others have suggested that the common but eerie *déjà vu* phenomenon might be accounted for by precognition. That is, the experience involves the fragmentary recollection of a long-ago precognitive dream.* We are now living for the first time an event that we once dreamed.

It may be that the precognitive dream was disregarded earlier because, being out of chronological context, it made no sense. Carl A. Meier of the Jung Institute said, "The material may be too strange, too alien, or too 'advanced' and will consequently either make a very strange but strong impression or be immediately forgotten . . . simply because the conscious system still lacks the necessary concepts to assimilate it properly."

The case for *déjà vu* as evidence of precognition is supported by its increased incidence in individuals experimenting with such altered states as meditation and psychedelic intoxication. The liberation of unconscious material common to those states might sharpen the recollection of old dream material.

In a more general sense, scientific theories that time is an artificial construct align with experiential reports from the altered states, reports that time and space are transcended, that causality is seen as an illusion. Although individuals cannot explain this conviction in terms of logic, they insist that it is very real. The sense of being beyond time has been reported frequently from psychedelic states, epileptic aura, meditation, mystical experience, early acute schizophrenia, hypnosis, and during electronic stimulation of certain regions of the limbic brain.

Edgar Mitchell has expressed that hope that he can contribute to a breakthrough in psychic research by bringing together scientists from various disciplines. Many in parapsychology

* These dreams would probably have been the product of slow-wave sleep, non-REM mentation, known to be realistic, plausible. Also, NREM sleep is more amnesic, harder to arouse from. Because it is relatively deep sleep and the mental activity unremarkable, we are unlikely to retain more than an ephemeral fraction in consciousness. It is interesting that whereas the brain cells fire randomly in REM sleep, during NREM mentation they fire simultaneously and in synchronized bursts. This activity might be compared to the curious rhythmicity of the other altered states, known to facilitate paranormal phenomena.

Jung classified precognitive dream phenomena as synchronicity because it seemed to him that the dreams occurred in close proximity to the actual event. But perhaps the dream is only recalled in those cases where the foreshadowed event occurs within a day or two. Those experienced years later might provoke only a sensation of *déjà vu*.

look to Mitchell as the man of the hour. As a member of the establishment, educated in the scientific method, and as a former astronaut, he is accorded respect by the public and by the scientific community.

Mitchell attributes his sense of urgency to his experience in space. Looking back at what Loren Eiseley has called "this planetary jewel," he was overwhelmed by the conviction that mankind will annihilate earth by apathy or by accident within a few generations if business goes on as usual.

He sees the evolution of a higher state of consciousness as the only hope for man, and deplores the tendency of scientists to dismiss psi and the phenomena of the altered states without investigating them experientially. "Many of the physical scientists feel threatened. They're like the learned men of Galileo's day, who refused to look through his telescope for fear that he might be right."

Mitchell said, "If the old-line parapsychologists were to be accepted, they had to use the techniques and methodology of physical science. They proved the phenomena using noise-level statistics, moving things away from chance by two or three percent. But we will never get beyond that point until we're willing to look at the experiential side. Many of these older researchers have not engaged in meditation themselves or otherwise attempted to enter an altered state."

Mitchell compared the experiential research to putting a magnet into a magnetic field; the field is changed. The investigator becomes the measuring rod.

Charles Tart urged his colleagues to undertake research of the phenomena of the altered states.

> My own impressions are that very large numbers of scientists are now personally exploring ASCs but few have begun to connect this personal exploration with their scientific activities.
>   . . . Will scientific method be extended to the development of state-specific sciences so as to improve our human situation? Or will the immense power of ASCs be left in the hands of many cults and sects?

In a recent essay on parapsychology and physics, Arthur Koestler remarked that the limitations of our biological equipment may condemn us to the role of Peeping Toms at the keyhole of eternity. "But at least let us take the stuffing out of the keyhole, which blocks even our limited view."

As man moves into new inner spaces, the danger is twofold. First, there will be psychiatric casualties. In many individuals, dabbling in psi may jar the central nervous system beyond its capacity. William Tiller, Elmer Green, and other scientists interested in parapsychology have stressed the importance of a stabilizing technique, such as meditation. Secondly, there is a genuine concern that we will become so preoccupied by the psi phenomena that we fail to progress beyond them. Most interested scientists do not see them as an end or a curiosity; to them the phenomena are a clue to the transcendental powers of the human brain.

23

TOMORROW

"To fly as fast as thought, to anywhere that is," he said, "you must begin by knowing that you have already arrived."
— RICHARD D. BACH, JONATHAN LIVINGSTON SEAGULL

There are those who see the future as an amalgam of fiction and behavioral psychology, *Brave New World* in a Skinner box. Keeper and kept, the human race will be socially aligned by conditioning, and life will be packaged like Fritos.

Prediction has become a popular sport. In *Future Shock,* Alvin Toffler envisioned subterranean cities, disposable wedding gowns, professional parents who will rear children by contract for their biological parents. Relying on the predictions of E. S. E. Hafez, a biologist at Washington State University, Toffler described tomorrow's woman venturing into the market to buy a tiny frozen embryo to be implanted by her doctor and borne by her as if she had conceived it. Toffler said:

> The embryo would, in effect, be sold with a guarantee that the resultant baby would be free of genetic defects. The purchaser would also be told in advance the color of the baby's eyes and hair, its sex, its probable size at maturity, and its probable I.Q.

Or fertilized human eggs could be carried in spaceships for the future colonization of planets, to be reared to term by a competent biologist.

Robert Rimmer, author of *The Harrad Experiment* and *Proposition 31,* foresees the corporate family, a mini-commune. Several couples will enter multiple marriage, rearing their children in common. B. F. Skinner postulates that we will soon be *Beyond Freedom and Dignity*. He has said that the duty of society is "to attempt actively to control human behavior in such a way as to achieve the effects we consider desirable before some other group becomes more proficient at controlling behavior and directing it into paths we consider undesirable."

In *The Biological Time Bomb,* Gordon Rattray Taylor imagined the day when we might talk to a brain created artificially in the laboratory, to learn whether it differs in any respect from our own. He also predicts that human beings will no longer have to tolerate moods. Pills will produce amiability or aggression, serenity or anxiety.

Toffler, Taylor, and R. C. W. Ettinger discuss the difficulties and promises facing society if immortality should become a reality within the near future. In *Man into Superman,* Ettinger warns his readers that if they are obtuse about the possibilities for the future, they may be among the last human beings to die, while the immortals dance on their graves.

Now that science has the capability of cloning—of producing genetic copies from the parent cell—various futurists are talking about the mass production of statesmen, brilliant scientists, and superb athletes. Some writers are prophesying the breeding of a superior race through genetic engineering. A pet prediction is that man will arrange for the development of a larger brain. Toffler quotes George Miller of Rockefeller University, a psychologist, who maintains that "there are severe limitations on the amount of information that we are able to receive, process, and remember." Scientists have predicted head transplants. The Russians have already demonstrated that a disembodied mammalian brain can remain alive very briefly.

Based on the projections of various scientists he interviewed, Gordon Rattray Taylor compiled a timetable of probable developments. In Phase One, by 1975, he predicts, there should be extensive transplantation of limbs and organs, memory erasure, and considerable power to postpone clinical death. Phase Two, by the year 2000, should see memory injection and memory editing, hibernation and prolonged coma, extensive mind modification and personality reconstruction, perfected artificial placenta and a true baby factory. After 2000 we can expect to see cloned people, synthesis of complex living organism, and indefinite postponement of death—according to Taylor's scientists. That golden age will be Phase Three.

If there seems to be something absurdly wrong with these predictions, it may be that most scientists are notoriously poor prophets. In *New Scientist,* George Gale remarked:

> I do not myself have much of an idea along what lines scientific activity will develop and I do not suppose that scientists have much idea, either. I note that the best prophecies in recent times have been made by a poet (Tennyson), a self-educated novelist (H. G. Wells), and a science-fiction writer (Arthur C. Clarke), and that some of the best-known prophecies of scientists have been fatuous.

Gale said that his worst fear for the future is that through excessive regard for the scientist's specialness, the public and press may create a tyranny of scientist-priests more powerful than that of any historic church.

Perhaps the predictions of many scientists have failed because they were based on potential technological capability without a realistic appreciation of the unplumbable mysteries of human nature. Multi-couple marriages, the farming-out of children, commercial marketing of babies, the cloning of offspring in one's own image, and similar innovations may be incompatible with aspects of man's innate makeup.

However warm the mutual affection of the communal family, it probably would not afford most people the depth and permanence of relationships within the traditional nuclear family. Furthermore, there is mounting evidence that human babies thrive best intellectually and emotionally with a primary caretaker. Some studies have even suggested that human infants require a single strong attachment in order to develop normally. When they are reared by a number of interchangeable caretakers, they seem to grow up deficient in the capacity to form attachments.

Carl Rogers, the influential psychologist who first introduced group therapy, has written extensively about alternatives to traditional marriage. Rogers said, "Basically, I think most people will continue to opt for one-to-one monogamous relationships with partners, not communes or group sex or homosexuality. People are like that."

The futurists have mentioned the theoretical implications of cloning people like Abraham Lincoln, Albert Einstein, or

Adolf Hitler. For the most part the speculation ignores the powerful role environment plays in the development of a human being. Genes alone do not produce a Lincoln.

The anticipation that cloning would become widespread assumes a powerful narcissism in human beings. In reality, only a fraction of married couples give their own first names to their children; why do we suppose that they would want to give them their faces? As for the supermarket dispensing of guaranteed embryos, it is clearly impossible, in the light of scientific evidence against fixed capacity, to guarantee "probable IQ." It may even be impossible to guarantee height, at least not in the sense of quality controlled mass production. According to recent reports from several researchers, height can be affected by emotional factors as well as nutrition and genes.

And worse yet, this prediction ignores man's innate enchantment with the unknown. Anticipating the uniqueness of an unborn child is one of life's major thrills for many human beings, perhaps most, and not likely to be exchanged for the store-bought embryo whose ingredients are listed like the contents of a TV dinner.

Wholesale organ transplants are not probable by 1975, as predicted. Heart transplants have now become uncommon because we have not yet overcome the rejection phenomenon. "Memory erasure" cannot be inferred from any contemporary research. The postulated editing and injection of memory presume a far greater understanding of the brain than even the most arrogant scientist now claims to have.

In reality, man is becoming increasingly conscious of both his immediate potential for change and his impressive racial endowment. At a time when we are confirming the subtle superiority of human milk over artificial feeding, it seems unlikely that we would throw our technology into the development of an artificial placenta for the nourishment of human fetuses.

When we are discovering just now the almost infinite capacity for dynamic change from within ourselves, would we rely exclusively on the reconstruction of personality from without?

If we can extrapolate from recent findings and current social trends, predictions of a cold-blooded, hypertechnological society are groundless. Assuming a modicum of good will and

good sense, we stand a chance of emerging from relative unconsciousness into the fuller awareness prophesied by such multidi-
mensional scientists and philosophers as William James, Carl
Jung, and Teilhard de Chardin. This, then, is the real implica-
tion of contemporary brain research.

The medical community will turn increasingly to biofeedback, acupuncture, and other healing tools now considered
unorthodox. Adults will learn to control the fight-or-flight syndrome of the sympathetic nervous system through biofeedback
or autogenic techniques. Children will learn such control on a
preventive basis, probably without the need for biofeedback devices. Meditation and similar relaxation techniques will become
part of western folk knowledge. Everyone will become familiar
through education with the psychological components of physical illness and the biochemical components of mental illness.
Psychic self-healing will become common, whether through
meditation, autogenic training, or relaxation-visualization techniques.

The Kirlian techniques now being used diagnostically in the
Soviet Union will be widely adopted in the West when the
equipment can be efficiently manufactured and there is adequate proof that high-frequency fields are no more hazardous
than X rays. As this process is further refined and investigated,
scientists will report increasing evidence that the unknown energy fields are vitally affected by mental processes.

The mentally ill will be treated in increasingly informal environments. The biochemical causes of schizophrenia, depressive
illness, and autism may be discovered, and perhaps will respond to preventive medication. But more and more psychiatrists may choose not to interfere with an acute schizophrenic
episode on the premise that it may be a survival tactic, a regenerative process of a mind under pressure.

Sexual disabilities and deviations will be treated biochemi-
cally, sometimes in combination with biofeedback. Recent findings of hormonal abnormalities in impotent individuals and
homosexuals may radicalize their treatment. Pubertal screening
might detect some abnormalities. Whether the physician or
family chooses to intervene for the sake of preventing homosexuality will depend on several factors. Despite their growing ac-

ceptance by society, many confirmed homosexuals consider themselves relatively unhappy, especially as they enter their forties and fifties.

Pain will be diminished by electronic means, by acupuncture, and by learned inner control. If the restrictions on psychedelic experimentation are loosened, LSD therapy will probably be used increasingly for terminally ill patients. New neurophysiological findings may furnish support for further exploration of LSD therapy for alcoholics, autistic children, and psychopathic personalities.

The genetic components of alcoholism will probably be identified within the next few years, along with the exact metabolic pathway in normal individuals and alcoholics. Perhaps biochemical analysis will pinpoint those adolescents who have the predisposition to become alcoholics so that they can find an alternative mind-altering drug or abstain altogether. Early EEG screening might detect incipient sociopaths by the absence of an expectancy wave. If intervention is early enough, perhaps they can be helped by therapy. But there is also the possibility that research will reveal that early emotional deprivation during a critical period plays a large part in the development of such abnormalities—in which case, strong preventive programs will have to be designed.

Psychosurgery and electronic stimulation of the brain will be used cautiously. Again, early diagnosis of such problems as the episodic violence syndrome and temporal-lobe epilepsy might make it possible to intervene with medicine or surgery at a period when the brain's plasticity can compensate for untoward side effects. Early recognition of severe disorders will benefit both society and the sufferer. There will be less tragic wastage of lives as we begin to understand the neurological, as well as environmental, causes of the so-called criminal mind.

There is little danger that man will be controlled by sinister drugs, subliminal brainwashing, brain surgery, or electronic stimulation. Seymour Kety pointed out, "Anyone influential enough to get an entire population to consent to having electrodes placed in its heads would already have achieved his goal without firing a single volt."

Although Jose Delgado remarked that electronic stimulation could possibly become a master control of human behavior by means of man-made plans and instruments, he also noted that even laboratory animals are influenced only to a degree. Norman Dixon doubted that a nation could be propagandized by subliminal messages. In one experiment, the subliminal instructions, "Eat roast beef," had the effect of making the subjects hungrier than the controls, but when allowed to order sandwiches they expressed no preference for beef. Dixon observed that one can hardly expect to change ideologies if he can't even affect food preferences.

It is unlikely that most parents will place their children in day nurseries on a full-time basis, as projected by some writers. For one thing, a shortened work week would reduce the number of hours such care would be essential. For those children placed in nurseries, a more enlightened approach is already evident in experimental programs around the country and well established in some other parts of the world. Rather than a team of impersonal caretakers, such nurseries are staffed with affectionate teachers and parent-substitutes who offer their young charges a continuing relationship and responsive adult give-and-take.

The awareness of the critical importance of this human interaction will lead to greater paternal participation in child-rearing. Many fathers are better suited than their wives to stimulate and care for their children. In one reported case, the father took over the care of a four-year-old during her mother's long-term illness. Under his tutelage, the child went from a diagnosis of borderline retardation to a superior IQ.

The primary trend in the brain revolution is a growing interest in expanding awareness, for creativity, health, learning, problem-solving, and for intrinsically rewarding ecstatic experiences. This culture-wide phenomenon has been misread by some of the futurists, Toffler among them. He dismisses it as a fad:

> The religious fervor and bizarre behavior of certain hippie cultists may arise not merely from drug abuse but from group experimentation with both sensory deprivation and bombardment. The chanting of monotonous mantras, the attempt to focus the individual's attention on interior bodily sensation to the exclu-

sion of outside stimuli, are efforts to induce the weird and sometimes hallucinatory effects of understimulation.

Dreaming, that expressway to the unconscious, will attract growing interest. The widening fascination with the dream technology of the Senoi tribe will almost certainly bear experimental fruit. Perhaps one day children all over the world will offer their dream reports at the breakfast table.

Psychic research will continue to integrate with various scientific disciplines. The energy-oriented Soviet approach will be the prevalent model for research.

The need for ombudsmen in science will become more urgent with every passing month. More and more data are being acquired by increasing numbers of specialties, to which fewer and fewer generalists are prepared to attach relevance. P. K. Anokhin pointed out to his fellow brain researchers that the accumulation of facts creates "a dangerous illusion of progress. . . ."

In America particularly, the education of scientists has been narrow, impoverished in the humanities. Yet a gradual shift is apparent, even now. There is every indication that a new generation of scientists will include many more researchers genuinely concerned with the philosophical and metaphysical implications of their work. Scientists are convening oftener to discuss the ethics of such developments as psychosurgery, electronic stimulation of the brain, and the possible abuses of genetic programming, transplants, and cloning. As someone observed, scientists can no longer drop their discoveries as foundlings on the doorstep of society. Their collective conscience is beginning to speak loudly and articulately.

The distinguished scientist René Dubos said that it is apparent today, as in the past, that "many scientists—among them some of the most brilliant and most effective—are eager to escape from the austere discipline of factual knowledge and to experience again the intoxication of philosophical thought."

Growing numbers of the younger professors and legions of students are exploring altered states of consciousness, whether out of curiosity or in the hope of enhancing insights. Whatever their motivation, the experiences will inevitably have their effect on attitudes and orientation.

Charles Bures, professor of philosophy at California Institute of Technology, said that the atmosphere at the school is changing. "There's a loosening. I can now teach courses and say things I couldn't have said even five years ago." Bures warns his students against the dangers of what he calls imbeddedness and tries to get them to look at different paradigms so they won't become too entrenched in their future research to examine the unexpected and the radical.

The education of psychologists may also change. Sigmund Koch, professor of psychology and philosophy at the University of Texas, has said that psychology cannot be a coherent science. Just as Jerome Bruner suggested that the responsibilities of education schools should be fragmented and integrated with other disciplines, Koch foresees the necessary disassembling of psychology.

"Anything so awesome as the total domain comprised by the functioning of all organisms can hardly be thought the subject matter of a coherent discipline," Koch said. "As the beginning of a therapeutic humility, we might re-christen psychology and speak instead of *the psychological studies.*" Koch believes that what is solid of psychology could best be pursued "in association with the germane scientific and humanistic disciplines." Biological psychology would be part of biology, psycholinguistics a part of linguistics, and so on.

The late Gordon Allport deplored what he called "arrogance in psychological theorizing." He insisted that it was better to be "tentative, eclectic, and humble. . . . 'Our knowledge is a drop and our ignorance is a sea.' " And a number of psychologists are saying that their specialty can never successfully imitate the methods of hard science.

Although demoted from its former pedestal as man's potential redeemer, technology will continue to play a vital role in the brain revolution. Computers are becoming more important than ever, and should be viewed as tools, not threats. W. Grey Walter recommended their increased use in brain research:

Such machines have been decried and ridiculed . . . fictionalized into superhuman idiocy and malevolence. As a child frightened by a teased puppy will say he met a bear, so we tend to project into these docile slaves of the laboratory our feelings of guilt, apprehension, inferiority, and insignificance. In fact, they are domestic servants, as truly the friend of man as are the dogs and horses. . . .

Recent developments have enabled computers to diagnose possible brain abnormalities in a fraction of the time it would take an encephalographer to interpret the tedious miles of EEG paper. Computers have made it possible for paralyzed monkeys to move artificial limbs (via implanted electrodes). Individualized computer programs are already ending wasteful, lockstep education in some elementary schools.

Technological sophistication will make possible the increasing use of genetic counseling and the early detection of embryonic defects. Carriers of Tay-Sachs disease can already learn whether a fetus is the victim of the devastating, fatal illness and can have the pregnancy terminated.

More specialized biofeedback equipment will open the way to investigate the clinical application of, for example, the control of histamine flow. There has been speculation that biofeedback could enable an individual to starve a malignant tumor of its blood supply, an application beyond current technology but within the realm of the possible.

But something more is needed to cope with society's practical problems. As the architect Ulrich Franzen observed:

> Technology is a useful tool, but the basic problem, I'm convinced, is a human one. It's perfectly apparent we don't need a new technology to put up decent housing. We just need the will to do it.
>
> If we as human beings say that a good portion of the people should be better off and should be more attractively accommodated, we can do it tomorrow morning. If we want to.

The desire to effect Utopian change has to come from within the individuals comprising society. It will not likely be the product of the smug, sophomoric Consciousness III postulated in Charles Reich's *The Greening of America*. It will more likely arise from the conviction that the bell tolls for us all. Teilhard de Chardin insisted that men will not evolve as isolated mutants but together. "The consummation of the World," he said, "the gates of the Future, the entrance into the Superhuman, they do not open either to a few privileged or to one chosen people among peoples! They will admit only an advance of all together. . . ."

Education, now in the early throes of revolution, will change radically. As the research findings about early experience are publicized more widely, the resistance to preschool cognitive learning will continue to weaken and will shortly collapse. The public schools are already expanding their programs to include younger children.

Those parents who feel inadequate to the challenge of intellectually stimulating their children will probably resort to books, just as in generations past they read Dr. Spock to find out how to toilet-train. The horror with which the old-line educators and child psychologists regard this cognitive interaction is disproportionate to the risks involved. Most of the books and psychologists recommending intellectual stimulation of the young child make it clear that he will only learn in a warm, supportive environment and that he must never be forced. The emphasis is always on the joyful aspects of learning.

The classroom is changing. Little by little, rows of desks are disappearing as teachers convert on their own to open education. The early excesses exemplified in the private free-school movement seem to have dissipated, and the healthy aspects have been preserved in the open classroom.

Education is at last coming into its own, both as folk art and fine art, a profoundly creative process dependent on both spontaneity and design. Like all successful art, open education is not formless, but its structure is unobtrusive. In *Education and Ecstasy,* George Leonard envisioned the changes:

> Life has one ultimate message, "Yes!" repeated in infinite number and variety. Human life, channeled for millennia by civilization, is only just beginning to express the diversity and range of which it is easily capable. . . . To affirm, to follow ecstasy in learning—in spite of injustice, suffering, confusion, and disappointment—is to move more easily toward an education, a society that would free the enormous potential of man.

Those futurists who conjecture that man will shortly engineer himself a larger brain show an appalling ignorance of the brain we already have. W. Grey Walter said, "We need not yearn for greater masses of gray matter. We already dispose of enough nerve units to enumerate in their permutations every particle of Eddington's universe."

Marcus Johnson, a biophysicist at Johns Hopkins, said of the brain, "It is a perfect instrument. It can take man wherever we might want it to take us."

Wherever we might want it to take us . . .

The popular prophets have underestimated how strange the truth can be. The human brain, that "perfect instrument," that "fabulous electronic dance," can be our open sesame to an infinitely richer life than we have believed possible. The fluent, liberating, creative, healing attributes of the altered states can be incorporated into consciousness.

We are just beginning to realize that we can truly open the doors of perception and creep out of the cavern.

bibliography and notes

About the bibliography:

The Brain Revolution has attempted to present the exciting developments in this subject in language that is clear, yet with sufficient documentation to satisfy those who wish to go to the scientific literature for supporting references and suggested reading.

As a compromise, in the informal bibliography that follows, references are categorized by topic under chapter headings. Popular periodicals such as *Science News, Psychology Today,* and *Scientific American* are designated by date. Technical references are shown by volume, issue number, and page numbers.

The extent of this bibliography made it impractical to name the thousands of authors of the journal references. This omission does not imply a lack of appreciation for the achievements of the individuals and teams of workers whose findings are cited in this book.

Chapter 2   FIRST CLUES: THE WHIRLPOOL

Man on the molecular level: *The Unexpected Universe* by Loren Eiseley (Harcourt, Brace, 1969); *The Human Brain* by John Pfeiffer (Harper, 1955); *Scientific American,* October 1970 (on the rebuilding of bones); *Man on His Nature* by Charles Sherrington (Macmillan, 1941).

Brain sensitivity to light: *Scientific American,* March 1972; *Body Time* by Gay Gaer Luce (Pantheon, 1971); see also references for Chapter 17. Innate rhythms: *Body Time* (see above); *Biological Rhythms and Human Performance,* edited by W. P. Colquhoun (Academic Press, 1971); *Time, Experience, and Behavior* by J. E. Orme (Iliffe, 1969).

Sensitivity to energy fields: "Very Low Frequency Electromagnetic Fields and Behavior" by Burton Milburn, doctoral dissertation, University of California at Los Angeles, 1971; *Virginia Journal of Science:* 21 (2) (re the Army's experiments with the dowsing effect); *Popular Electronics,* July 1971. See also *The Effect of Electromagnetic and Magnetic Fields on the Central Nervous System,* NASA TT f-564, translation from Russian, available from Clearing House for Federal Scientific and Technical Information, Springfield, Virginia; *A Review of the Biological Effects of Very Low Magnetic Fields,* NASA TN-D-5902 A-3415, National Aeronautics and Space Administration, Washington, D.C.; *Biological Effects of Magnetic Fields,* edited by M. F. Barnothy (Plenum Press, 1969); *Psychical Physics* by S. W. Tromp (Elsevier, 1949); *Electromagnetic Fields and Life* by A. S. Presman, translation from the Russian (Plenum, 1969); *Biological Prototypes and Synthetic Systems,* E. Bernard and M. R. Kare, editors (Plenum, 1962); *New York State Journal of Medicine* 2215–2219. Presman's speculation about entrainment by electromagnetic fields: *Biulleten Eksperimental'noi Biologii i Meditsiny* 53:41-45.

The effects of geomagnetic fields on psychiatric-hospital admissions and suicide rates: *Deutsche Medizinische Wochenschrift* 61 (3):95; *Nature* (London) 200:626-628; 205:1050-1053. Magnetic fields and reaction time: *Nature* 213:949-956.

Bioelectric field, disease and healing: *Science* 134:101-102; 175:1118-1121; *Proceedings of the First National Biomedical Society Symposium,* Los Angeles, 1963; *Proceedings of the XIV International Congress of Zoology* 3:179-184; *Proceedings of the XI International Congress of Radiology* 2:1753-1757. Liquid crystal characteristics of nervous system: *Genetic Psychology Monographs,* 1971 (2):177-235; *Biomedical Sciences Instrumentation,* Volume I, edited by R. D. Barnard (Plenum, 1963). Retinal cells as microscopic circuits: *American Journal of Medical Electronics* 1:112-121. Magnetic susceptibility of biological systems: *International Journal of Biometeorology* 12 (2):93-98. Magnetic field and cancer: *Nature* 177:577; 181:1785. Magnetic fields produced by alpha brainwaves: *Science* 161:784-786; 175:664-666. Near-infrared emission from mammalian cerebral cortex: Alexandria Defense Documentation Center, DDC 417125. Ionization and reaction time: *American Journal of Physical Medicine* 36:353-358. Ionization effect on brain chemicals: *Journal of General Physiology* 43:533-540.

Kirlian photography: *A. R. E. Journal,* March 1972; *Psychic Discoveries Behind the Iron Curtain* by Lynn Schroeder and Sheila Ostrander (Prentice-Hall, 1970); *Proceedings of First Western Hemisphere Conference on High Frequency Photography, Acupuncture, and the Human Aura* (Gordon and Breech, 1972); lectures by William Tiller, Stanford and UCLA, 1971, 1972; lectures by Thelma Moss, UCLA and Golden West College, 1972; *Bioenergetic Questions: Material of the Scientific*

Seminar in Alma-ata, edited by B. A. Dombrovsky, G. A. Sergeev, and B. M. Inyoushin, translated by George Schepak for the Southern California Society for Psychical Research, copyright 1972, available from the SCSPR, Room 314, 170 South Beverly Drive, Beverly Hills, California. This volume includes several papers by the Kirlians, who invented the process.

A number of relevant bibliographies are available. From the Brain Information Service, UCLA: *Biological Effects of Electromagnetic Fields (September 1970–August 1971); Biological Effects of Electromagnetic Fields (Below Visible Frequencies) Especially in the Central Nervous System (1964–1970); Irradiation Effects on the Central Nervous System,* bibliographies available for three periods: 1967–July 1969; August 1969–August 1970; September 1970–August 1971.

Detailed references are compiled in a major bibliography translated from the Russian and available from the Joint Publications Research Service, National Technical Information Service, U.S. Department of Commerce, Springfield, Virginia. Title: *Bibliography on Parapsychology (Psychoenergetics) and Related Subjects.*

Chapter 3 BIOFEEDBACK: MASTERMINDING THE BODY

The early research of Neal Miller et al. is summarized in *Science* 163:434-445. Other references concerning those studies: *Communications in Behavioral Biology* 1:209; 2:19; *Journal of Comparative Physiological Psychology* 65:9; *Science* 159:1485; *American Journal of Physiology* 215:684; *Scientific American,* October 1970.

General coverage of recent biofeedback experimentation: *Current Status of Physiological Psychology,* edited by D. Singh and C. T. Morgan (Brooks/Cole, 1972); *Biofeedback and Self-control: An Aldine Reader* and *Biofeedback and Self-control 1970,* both edited by Theodore X. Barber et al. and published by Aldine-Atherton.

Autogenic training: *Proceedings of Third International Congress of Psychiatrists,* Montreal, 1961 (McGill University Press, 1962); *Autogenic Therapy,* edited by Wolfgang Luthe (multilingual edition, Grune & Stratton, 1969); *Autogenic Training: A Psychophysiologic Approach in Psychotherapy* by Johannes Schultz and Wolfgang Luthe (Grune & Stratton, 1959); *Diseases of the Nervous System* 23:383.

Heart rate control: *Psychology Today,* October 1970; *Journal of Comparative Physiological Psychology* 68:338-342; 73:208-216; *Proceedings of the National Academy of Science, USA,* 1970, 65:293-299; *Psychosomatic Medicine* 32:417-424. Blood pressure: *Psychophysiology* 6:283-290; *Science* 163:588. Hand temperature (migraine therapy): *Menninger Perspectives* 1 (1) 22–27. Muscular relaxation: *Journal of Behavioral Therapy and Experimental Psychiatry* 1:205-211.

A broad general survey: *The New York Times Magazine,* September 2, 1971. Neurological mechanisms implicated in voluntary control of internal processes: *Subcortical Mechanisms of Behavior,* edited by Robert A. McCleary and Robert Y. Moore (Basic Books, 1969).

Chapter 4   STRESS AND HEALING

General adaptation syndrome: *The Stress of Life* by Hans Selye (McGraw-Hill, 1956). Columbia University stress experiment: *Science News,* November 21, 1970. Air controllers' diseases: study reported by Richard Grayson, president of American Academy of Air Traffic Control Medicine. Statement by René Dubos: *Psychology Today,* February 1971.

Somatic approaches to psychotherapy: *Psychology Today,* October 1970; *Mental Hygiene* 53:451-458; section by R. F. Hefferline in *Experimental Foundations of Clinical Psychology,* edited by A. J. Bachrach (Basic Books, 1962); *A Catalogue of the Ways People Grow* by Severin Peterson (Ballantine, 1971); *Bodies in Revolt* by Thomas Hanna (Holt, Rinehart & Winston 1970).

Meditation therapy for cancer patients: lectures by Carl Simonton, transcripts of symposia titled *Science and Psi,* Stanford and UCLA, October 1972, available from the Academy of Parapsychology and Medicine, 314A Second Street, Los Altos, California 94022.

Electrical abnormalities of cancer cells: paper presented by Clarence Cone, Twelfth Annual Science Writers' Seminar sponsored by American Cancer Society, San Antonio, 1970; *Journal of Theoretical Biology* 30:151-181; 183-194; *Oncology* 25:168-182; *Transactions of the New York Academy of Sciences,* Series II, 31 (4):404-427.

Kirlian photography: See references under Chapter 2 section.

Stress hormones: discussions by Diana Johnson of symposium held at Downstate Medical Center, Brooklyn, 1970, "The Influence of Hormones on the Nervous System," and a conference at UCLA, 1970, "Steroid Hormones and Brain Function," available from the Brain Information Service, UCLA.

Stress and cardiac function: *Psychophysiology* 8 (1):462-467; *Science* 173:1144-1146. Cancer and stress: see references under category titled "bioelectric field, disease, and healing" under Chapter 2 bibliography.

Note: Until recently scientists believed that the body's cells were separate units and that transmission occurred only along the surface membranes. In the 1960s researchers at Columbia University College of Physicians and Surgeons and at Harvard discovered that small inorganic ions were moving freely from one cell to another.

According to Werner Loewenstein of Columbia, "The exciting possibility presented itself that the . . . junction [between cells] is instrumental in conveying substances that control the growth and differentiation of cells." He and his associates conjectured that cancerous growth might be due to poor junctional communication from cell to cell. Experimenting electrically with tumors, they could detect no communication. With some exceptions, the membrane of cancerous cells was apparently *impermeable,* even where in contact with nervous cells. On the other hand, benign growth activity, such as liver regeneration, showed normal communication.

The attempts of Simonton's patients consciously to activate their immune systems to throw off the cancer might well tie in with the findings about (1) the electrical abnormalities of many malignant cells, and (2) R. O. Becker's speculation about a direct-current bioelectric energy field that controls growth, tissue repair, and tumors, an ancient web of communication directed by the central nervous system.

Chapter 5 INNER CONTROL OF PAIN

Peter Mezan's account: *Esquire,* January 1972; John Coleman's account: *The Quiet Mind* (Harper & Row, 1971). Phantom limb pain: *Psychology Today,* October 1970. Gate-control theory explained more technically in *Science* 150:971-979, and in *Brain and Behavior,* Volume 2, "Perception and Action," edited by K. H. Pribram (Penguin, 1969). Also, *Experimental Neurology* 25:416-428. Reverberatory circuit: *Pain Mechanisms* by W. K. Livingston (Macmillan, 1943). General theory about mechanisms: *Touch, Tickle and Pain,* Part Two, by Yngve Zotterman (Pergamon, 1971). Psychedelics and pain: *Psychedelics: The Uses and Implications of Hallucinogenic Drugs,* edited by Bernard Aaronson and Humphry Osmond (Doubleday, 1970); *Psychedelic Review,* no. 11, 1970–71.

Lamaze theory: *Childbirth With Confidence* by Pierre Vellay (Macmillan, 1965). Removal of hippocampus for pain alleviation: *Journal of Neurosurgery* 26:300-398.

Pain and alpha brainwaves: *The New York Times Magazine,* September 2, 1971; *Journal of Behavior Therapy and Experimental Psychiatry* 25:481-489. General pain phenomena: *Pain and Religion: A Psychophysiological Study* by Steven Brena (Thomas, 1972).

Acupuncture anesthesia: *Chinese Acupuncture* by Desmond K. Shieu (Oriental Society, 1972); *Acupuncture: The Ancient Chinese Art of Healing* by Felix Mann (W. Heinemann Medical Books, 1971); *Acupuncture Anesthesia* (Foreign Languages Press, 1972); *Acupuncture and You* by Louis Moss (Elek Books, 1964); *Journal of the American Medical Association* 218:1558-1563; *Transcript of the Acupuncture Symposium* (Stanford, June 17, 1972), published by the Academy of Parapsychology and Medicine, 314A Second Street, Los Altos, California 94022.

Chapter 6 ALTERED STATES AND THE LIMBIC BRAIN

The first two mystical experiences described are from Sir Alister Hardy's ongoing study of religious experiences as reported in *Science Digest,* September 1971; the next from *Watchers on the Hills* by Raynor

Johnson (Harper, 1959). The first psychedelic account: *Be Here Now* by Baba Ram Dass (Richard Alpert) (Lama Foundation, 1971); the subsequent psychedelic experiences from *Psychedelics: The Uses and Implications of Psychedelic Drugs* by Bernard Aaronson and Humphry Osmond (Doubleday, 1970). The first two prepsychotic experiences: *Altered States of Consciousness*, edited by Charles Tart (John Wiley, 1970). The third prepsychotic: from Raynor Johnson's *Watchers on the Hills*. Kundalini phenomena: *Mysterious Fires and Lights* by Vincent Gaddis (McKay, 1967); *Kundalini: Evolutionary Energy in Man* by Gopi Krishna (Berkeley/Shambala, 1967); Deikman's experimental meditation accounts: *Altered States of Consciousness*, see above.

Flicker phenomenon and epileptic aura: *The Living Brain* by W. Grey Walter (Norton, 1953). Sensory deprivation phenomena: *Sensory Deprivation: A Symposium*, edited by P. Solomon (Harvard University Press, 1965); *Psychology Today* (interview with John Lilly); *Beyond Time* by Michel Siffre (McGraw-Hill, 1964). Mystical and peak experience: *Ecstasy: A Study of Some Secular and Religious Experiences* by Marghanita Laski (Cresset, 1961); *Religious Values and Peak Experiences* by Abraham Maslow (Ohio State University Press, 1962).

Inseparability of functions of limbic system and reticular formation: *The Functioning Brain of Man*, Pfizer Laboratories; *The Mind: Biological Approaches to Its Functions*, edited by William Corning and Martin Balaban (John Wiley, 1968). Inclusion of hypothalamus in limbic system: James Olds in *Brain and Behavior*, Volume 4, "Adaptation," edited by K. H. Pribram (Penguin, 1969); *Subcortical Mechanisms of Behavior* by Robert A. McCleary and Robert Y. Moore (Basic Books, 1965). General: *Journal of Comparative and Physiological Psychology* 68 (3):437-441; *Science News*, July 27, 1968.

Effects of electronic stimulation of the brain: *Archives of Neurology* 21:157-169; lecture by James Olds, UCLA, 1971; *Physical Control of the Mind* by Jose M. R. Delgado (Harper & Row, 1969); *Biology of Mind* by W. R. Hess (University of Chicago Press, 1964). The role of the limbic system as mediator of cortical and subcortical activities: *Frontiers of the Brain*, edited by John French (Columbia University Press, 1962); *Autonomic-Somatic Integrations* by Ernest Gellhorn (University of Minnesota Press, 1967); *Subcortical Mechanisms of Behavior*, see above.

Déjà vu phenomenon and temporal-lobe lesions: *Journal of the American Medical Association* 216 (6):1025-1034; *Time, Experience, and Behavior* by J. R. Orme (Iliffe, 1969). Limbic system and hormones: *Neurosciences Research Program Bulletin* 9 (2):232; *Scientific American*, April 1966 and January 1971; *Science* 153:767-769; *Neuropsychologia* 7:235-244; *Neurological Foundations of Psychiatry* by T. Smythies (Academic Press, 1966); *Angiology* 20:325-333. Effects of minute variations in stimulation of limbic brain: *The Human Mind*, edited by J. Roslansky (North Holland, 1967); *Brain and Conscious Experience*, edited by John C. Eccles (Springer Verlag, 1965); *Subcortical Mechanisms of Behavior*, see above. For references concerning the role of the limbic brain in learning, see bibliography for Chapter 19. Other useful references to the limbic brain are included in a Brain Information Service (UCLA) bibliography, *Hippocampus and Behavior Bibliography (Excluding Sleep): Stimulation, Recording, Lesions (1967—August 1970).*

Altered states of consciousness, general: *Psychology Today,* February 1967; *New Scientist* (1972), pp. 696–697; *The Natural Mind* by Andrew Weil (Houghton Mifflin, 1972), excerpted in *Psychology Today,* October 1972; *Archives of General Psychiatry* 15:225-234; 25:481-489; *Journal of Nervous and Mental Diseases* 149:68-79; *Cosmic Consciousness* by R. M. Bucke (various editions); *The Varieties of Religious Experience* by William James (various editions); *Psychologia* 8:145-150; *Journal of Humanistic Psychology* 9 (2):135-137; *The Highest State of Consciousness,* edited by John White (Anchor/Doubleday, 1972); *Christian Century,* January 19, 1972; *The Master Game* by Robert DeRopp (Dell, 1968); *Psychonomic Science* 27:173-175; *Science* 174:897-904 (Fischer's cartography of altered states on physiological-arousal scale); *Science* 176:1203-1210 (Tart's proposal for establishment of state-specific sciences). Further suggestions for methodology for study of altered states: *Journal of Transpersonal Psychology,* no. 3 (1971), pp. 93–124 and 125–133.

Chapter 7 MEDITATION:
"THE EYES SHALL HEAR, THE EARS SHALL SEE"

Remarks of Peter Mezan in *Esquire,* January 1972; of Maslow, in his *Religious Values and Peak Experiences* (Ohio State University Press, 1964). Meditation training of civil servants in India: Times of India News Service, April 25, 1971, and Hindustan *Times,* April 25, 1971.

Electroencephalographic studies of meditation: *Psychiatria et Neurologia Japonica* 62 (1):76-105 (English abstract); *Electroencephalography and Clinical Neurophysiology,* Supplement no. 9:51-52, no. 13:452-456; no. 7:132-149; no. 33:454; no. 18:52-53; *Behavioral Science* 6:312-323; *Proceedings of Japanese EEG Society,* 1962, pp. 77-78. Early work by Kamiyz: Lecture, UCLA, 1971, and private interview, 1971.

Phenomenon of disappearance of focal object: *On the Psychology of Meditation* by Robert Ornstein and Claudio Naranjo (Viking, 1971). Wakeful hypometabolic state in meditation: *The Physiological Effects of Transcendental Meditation,* dissertation thesis, UCLA, by Robert Keith Wallace, 1970; *American Journal of Physiology* 22 (3):795-799; *Science* 167:1751-1754; *Scientific American,* February 1972; *New England Journal of Medicine* 281:1133; *Connecticut Medicine* 34:302-303; *Federation Proceedings* 30 (2):376; *Science Digest,* February 1972.

Charles Tart's account: *Journal of Transpersonal Psychology,* no. 2 (1970), 3:462-465. Autonomic stability and meditation: *Psychosomatic Medicine,* article by David Orme-Johnson in press. Changes attributable to hatha yoga: *Journal of the American Medical Association* 220:1365.

The effect of meditation on bronchial asthma: *Clinical Research,* in press, article by Ronald Honsberger and A. F. Wilson. Blood lactate ion associated with anxiety: *New England Journal of Medicine* 277:1329-1336; *Scientific American,* February 1969. Plethysmograph changes in meditation: *Aerztliche Forschung* 21:61-65.

Additional reports on physiological changes are made available as preprints on a regular basis by MIU Mail Order Center, 1015 Gayley Avenue, Los Angeles, California 90024.

Meditation and education: *Main Currents in Modern Thought* 24:19-21; *Phi Delta Kappan,* December 1972. Meditation and criminal reform: *Kentucky Law Journal* 60 (2):411-418. Meditation and sociology: *Meaningful Leisure* by Maynard Shelly, in press; *Soldiers* 27 (2):20-22. Meditation, self-actualization, and psychotherapy: *Psychoanalytic Review* 18:129-145; *American Journal of Psychotherapy* 11:866-869; *British Journal of Psychiatry* 112:1089-1096; *Medical Journal of Australia* 51 (II), Supplement 21:844-849; *Journal of Humanistic Psychology* 5:6-16; 10:39-74; *International Journal of Parapsychology* 8:181-191; *International Journal of Psychoanalysis* 49:413-416; *Psychologia* 3:85-91; 9:2-6; 2:79-99; 12:55-58; 2:114-119; 2:236-242; *Journal of Behavior Therapy and Experimental Psychiatry* 3:97-98; *Journal of Counseling Psychology* 29 (2):139-145; *Through an Eastern Window* by Jack Huber (Houghton Mifflin, 1965); *Ways of Growth* by H. A. Otto and J. Mann (Grossman, 1968); Stanley Dean on the ultraconscious: *Behavioral Neuropsychiatry* April–May 1970. Daniel Goleman's essay on meditation as metatherapy: *Journal of Transpersonal Psychology,* no. 1 (1971), 3:1-25.

A number of bibliographies are available. "The Psychology and Physiology of Meditation and Related Phenomena" appeared in the *Journal of Transpersonal Psychology* 2 (1) 1970 (Box 4437, Stanford, California 94305). A monthly mailing of comprehensive bibliographies in German and English is produced by MIU Forschungersring für Creative Intelligence (3000 Hannover, Gretchenstrasse 36, West Germany). References are also compiled by the Biofeedback Research Society (Francine Butler, executive secretary, Psychiatry Department, No. 202, University of Colorado Medical Center, 4200 East Ninth Avenue, Denver, Colorado 80220).

Chapter 8   ALPHA—THE PARLOR GAME OF THE CENTURY

Early brainwave research: *Explorers of the Brain* by Leonard A. Stevens (Knopf, 1971). Early attempts to condition alpha rhythms: *Journal of Experimental Psychology* 28:503-508; *General Psychopathology* by K. Jaspers (University of Chicago Press, 1964). Brainwave control by biofeedback: *Psychophysiology* 6:442-452; *Experimental Medicine and Surgery* 27:13-18; *Psychology Today,* April 1968; in *Altered States of Consciousness,* edited by Charles Tart (John Wiley, 1969); lectures by

Joe Kamiya at UCLA, 1971; interview with Kamiya at Langley-Porter Neuropsychiatric Hospital, San Francisco, 1971; *Biofeedback and Self-control 1970,* annual published by Aldine-Atherton, and *Biofeedback and Self-control: An Aldine Reader,* covering research prior to 1970, both edited by Theodore X. Barber et al.

Voluntary Controls Project at Menninger Research Foundation: *Journal of Transpersonal Psychology* 2 (1), 1970; lecture by Elmer Green, De Anza State College (California), 1971; lectures by Elmer Green and Alyce Green at the International Cooperation Council Festival, Los Angeles, 1972, and at the "Science and Psi" symposia held consecutive weekends at Stanford and UCLA, 1972; *Progress of Cybernetics: Proceedings of the International Congress of Cybernetics,* edited by J. Rose (Gordon and Breech, 1970).

Smokers and alpha: *Neuropsychologia* 6:381-388; *Science* 164:969-970.

General articles on brainwave training: *Saturday Review,* April 10, 1971; *The New York Times Magazine,* September 12, 1971; *Archives of General Psychiatry* 25:429-435.

Theta training of dogs: *American Scientist* 59 (2):236-245. Brainwave training of cats: *Physiological Behavior* 3:703-707.

Comparison of biofeedback and meditative techniques in successfully altering brainwave pattern: "Zazen (Sitting Meditation) and Biofeedback Training in the Autocontrol of the Alpha Rhythm of the Brain," paper presented at symposium of the American Psychological Association, Washington, D.C., 1971, by Earl Brown, Thomas Erwin, and R. Putney of Georgia State University. See also references for Chapter 7 under the heading, "EEG studies of meditation."

Paradoxical alpha: *Journal of Transpersonal Psychology* 2 (1), 1970; *Autogenic Training,* Volume 3, edited by Wolfgang Luthe (Grune & Stratton, 1969). Flicker phenomena: *The Living Brain* by W. Grey Walter (Norton, 1953); *Flying,* January 1962; see also epilepsy references, Chapter 13.

Chapter 9   HYPNOSIS AND ASCID

General references: *Handbook of Clinical and Experimental Hypnosis,* edited by L. Cron (Macmillan, 1956); *Hypnosis,* edited by Jesse E. Gordon (Macmillan, 1967); *Hypnosis of Man and Animals* by Ferenc Andres Volgyesi (Bailliere, Tindal & Cassell, 1966); *Hypnosis Throughout the World,* edited by Frederick L. Marcuse (Thomas, 1964); *Hypnotic Susceptibility* by Ernest R. Hilgard (Harcourt, Brace, 1965); *Hypnosis: Research Development and Perspectives,* edited by E. Fromm and R. E. Shor (Aldine-Atherton, 1972); *Altered States of Consciousness,* edited by Charles Tart (John Wiley, 1969); *LSD, Marijuana, Yoga, and Hypnosis* by Theodore X. Barber (Aldine-Atherton, 1972).

Altered awareness of time: *Body Time* by Gay Gaer Luce (Pantheon, 1971); Houston and Masters' time-distortion experiments in *Intellectual*

Digest, March 1973; *Altered States of Consciousness,* see above; *Time, Experience, and Behavior* by J. E. Orme (Iliffe, 1969); *Hypnosis* by Linn Cooper and Milton Erickson (Williams and Wilkins, 1954).

Suggestology: *Psychic Discoveries Behind the Iron Curtain* by Lynn Schroeder and Sheila Ostrander (Prentice-Hall, 1970). Charles Tart's experiments with mutual hypnosis: *Altered States of Consciousness,* see above; hypnosis/clairvoyance experiments at Maimonides: Lecture by Stanley Krippner at UCLA, 1971.

Altered-states-of-consciousness-inducing devices: *Intellectual Digest,* March 1973; *Altered States of Consciousness,* see above; *The Varieties of Psychedelic Experience* by R. E. L. Masters and Jean Houston (Holt, Rinehart & Winston, 1966); *The Highest State of Consciousness,* edited by John White (Anchor/Doubleday, 1972).

Psychedelic effects of hypnosis: *Psychedelics,* edited by Bernard Aaronson and Humphry Osmond (Anchor/Doubleday, 1970); Milton Erickson's account of his session with Aldous Huxley: *American Journal of Clinical Hypnosis* 8:14-33.

Chapter 10 PSYCHEDELICS: THRILLS, TRAUMA, THERAPY

General accounts of psychedelic experience: *The Teachings of Don Juan* by Carlos Castaneda (University of California, 1968); *A Separate Reality* (Simon & Schuster, 1971) and *Journey to Ixtlan* (Simon & Schuster, 1972) by the same author; *The Beyond Within: The LSD Story* by Sidney Cohen (Atheneum, 1964); *Psychedelics,* edited by Bernard Aaronson and Humphry Osmond (Anchor/Doubleday, 1970); *The Varieties of Psychedelic Experience* by R. E. L. Masters and Jean Houston (Holt, Rinehart, 1966); *The Natural Mind* by Andrew Weil (Houghton Mifflin, 1972); *On Being Stoned* by Charles Tart (Science and Behavior Books, 1971); *The Doors of Perception* by Aldous Huxley (Harper, 1954) and *Heaven and Hell* (Chatto and Windus, 1956) by the same author.

LSD, autism, and pain: *Archives of General Psychiatry* 25:498-510. LSD and terminal illness: *Psychedelic Review* no. 11 (1971); *Altered States of Consciousness,* edited by Charles Tart (John Wiley, 1969); *Psychedelics,* see above; *LSD: The Consciousness Expanding Drug,* edited by David Solomon (Putnam's, 1964); *Journal of Drugs* 16:142-148; *Medical Times* 94:1501-1513.

LSD psychotherapy: *Journal for the Study of Consciousness,* July–December 1970; lecture by Stanislav Grof, Los Angeles, 1971; *Journal of Transpersonal Psychology* 1 (1972):45-80; *Theory and Practice of LSD Psychotherapy* by Stanislav Grof (University of Pennsylvania Press, in press).

Marijuana, general: articles by Solomon Snyder and Charles Tart, *Psychology Today,* May 1971; lecture by Richard Orkand, UCLA, 1971; *Marijuana—Deceptive Weed* by Gabriel G. Nahas (Raven, 1973);

Biochemical and Pharmacological Effects of Dependence and Reports on Marijuana Research, edited by H. M. Van Praag (De Erven F. Bohn, 1972). Marijuana disposition in long-time users: *Science* 173:72-73. THC and memory: *Science* 173:1038-1040. As substitute for alcohol: *Psychedelic Review* no. 11, 1971. THC and reaction time: *Science* 179:920-923. Accuracy in timing performance: *Science* 175:549-550. Time distortion effect of cannabis: *Science* 179:803-805.

LSD and brainstem raphe units: *Science* 161:706-708. Reports of chromosome damage: *Science* 155:1417 (original report) and *Science* 172:431-440 (refutation); *Psychedelic Review* no. 10, 1969.

Meditation as alternative to drug abuse: *Time,* October 27, 1972; *Journal of the American Medical Association* 219 (3):295-299; Mental Health Program Report (December 1971), "Physiological Effects of a Meditation Technique and a Suggestion for Curbing Drug Abuse," National Institute of Mental Health, *New England Journal of Medicine* 281:1133; *Be Here Now* by Baba Ram Dass (Richard Alpert) (Lama Foundation, 1971); *Center of the Cyclone* by John Lilly (Julian, 1972); *Today's Health,* April 1972.

Chapter 11 DRUGGING THE BRAIN: THE TROJAN HORSE

General references: *Readings in Drug Use and Abuse,* edited by Brent Q. Hafen (Brigham Young University Press, 1970); *Drugs, Development, and Cerebral Function,* edited by W. Lynn Smith (Thomas, 1972); *Narcotic Drugs: Biochemical Pharmacology,* edited by Doris H. Clouet (Plenum, 1971); *Drugs and Alcohol* by Kenneth L. Jones, Louis W. Shainberg, and Curtis O. Byer (Harper & Row, 1969); *New York State Journal of Medicine* 62 (3):332-334. Hazards of psychoactive drugs: *Science* 169:438-441; *Biochemical and Pharmacological Effects of Dependence and Reports on Marijuana Research,* edited by H. M. Van Praag (De Erven F. Bohn, 1972), for sections on opiates, amphetamines, and alcohol.

Amphetamines: *Psychology Today,* January 1972; *Science* 175:454-455; *National Observer,* March 30, 1970, and Los Angeles *Times,* February 25, 1972, amphetamine statistics.

Drugs and physiological rhythms: *Body Time* by Gay Gaer Luce (Pantheon, 1971).

Nicotine: *Smoking and Health,* Public Health Service publication; *Electroencephalography and Clinical Neurophysiology* 10:576; *Neuropsychologia* 6:381-388; *Science* 164:969-970; *Acta Neurologia* (Napoli) 12:475-493.

Heroin antagonists: *Science* 173:503-506.

Alcohol, genetic aspects: *Psychology Today,* July 1972; alcohol and gender: *Psychology Today,* June 1972; *Basic Information on Alcohol* by Roy Albion King (Narcotics Education, 1964). Alcohol and alkaloids: *Science* 167:1149-1151; 167:1005-1007. General: *Biological Aspects of Alcohol,* edited by Mary K. Roach, William M. McIsaac, and Patrick J.

Creaven (University of Texas Press, 1971); *The Biology of Alcoholism,* edited by B. Kissin and H. Begleiter (Plenum, 1972). Sleep and alcohol: *Archives of General Psychiatry* 22:406-418. Delirium tremens and dreaming: *American Journal of Psychiatry* 124:2. Effects of alcohol and caffeine on dreaming: *Science* 140:1226-1227. Ethnic differences in response to alcohol: *Science* 175:449-450.

Alcohol and brain damage: *Journal of the American Medical Association* 172:1143-1146; *Diseases of the Nervous System* 22:284-286; *Archives of Neurological Psychiatry* 52:290-295.

Side effects: *Side Effects of Drugs: A Survey of Unwanted Effects of Drugs Reported in 1968–1971,* Volume VII, edited by L. Meyler and A. Herxheimer (Excerpta Medica, 1972).

Chapter 12   SLEEP CONSCIOUSNESS AND
THE DREAMING BRAIN

General references: *Psychology of Sleep* by David Foulkes (Scribner, 1966); *Dream Psychology and the New Biology of Dreaming,* edited by Milton Kramer (Thomas, 1969); *Sleep: Physiology and Pathology,* edited by Anthony Kale (Lippincott, 1969); *The Biology of Dreaming* by Ernest Hartmann (Thomas, 1967); *Sleep* by Ian Oswald (Penguin, 1966); *The Nature of Sleep,* edited by Uros J. Jovanovic (Gustav Fischer Verlag, 1973); *Sleep and the Maturing Nervous System,* edited by C. D. Clemente, D. Purpura, and F. E. Mayer (Academic Press, 1972).

Theories about the biochemistry of sleep: *Brain and Human Behavior,* edited by A. G. Karczmar and J. C. Eccles (Springer Verlag, 1972); *Scientific American,* February 1967; *Science News,* October 3, 1970; *Pflugers Archives* 329 (3):231-243; *Current Research on Sleep and Dreaming,* publication of National Institute of Mental Health, Department of Health, Education, and Welfare; see also the general references above.

Insomnia, sleep length, naps, and sleep deprivation: *Biological Psychiatry* 2:391-399; *Brain Research* 38 (2):327-341; *Gegenbaurs Morphologishes Jahrbuch* 117 (1):107-114; *Aerospace Medicine* 43 (3):266-268; review of insomnia literature in *Psychiatric Quarterly* 45 (2):274-288; acupuncture treatment for insomnia in *Medical Tribune* 14 (3):5. Also, discussion by M. B. Sterman in *The Biology of Dreaming* (see above) and by Allan Rechtschaffen in *Sleep: Physiology and Pathology* (see above). *Biological Psychiatry* 2:391-399; *Journal of Abnormal Psychiatry* 78 (2):229-231; *Aspects of Human Efficiency: Diurnal Rhythms and Loss of Sleep,* edited by W. P. Colquhoun (English Universities Press, 1972). Time zone change (jet lag): *Archives of Neurology* 26 (1):36-48. *Journal of Consulting and Clinical Psychology* 32 (2):144-151.

Sleep patterns relating to such factors as IQ, age, mental state, psychosis: *Acta Neurologica et Psychiatrica Belgica* 68:453-459; *Brain and Early Behavior,* edited by R. J. Robinson (Academic Press, 1969).

REM sleep (rapid-eye-movement or paradoxical sleep) phenomena, periodicity, and theory; contributions by Jouvet, Rechtschaffen, and Oswald in *Sleep: Physiology and Pathology,* see above; *Archives of General Psychiatry* 15:654-659; *Brain Research* 26:49-56; *Experimental Medicine and Surgery* 27 (1–2):39-52; *Nature* 223:893-897. PGO spikes: see the general references above and *Brain Research* 48:406-411 and 412-416.

Sleep conditioning: *Science* 167:1146-1148. Electrosleep: *Newsweek,* May 17, 1971; *Nebraska Medical Journal* 58 (1):9-11.

Awareness in sleep: *Biological Psychiatry* 3:171, time estimation during sleep; *Learning and Sleep; The Theory and Practice of Hypnopaedia* by F. Rubin (John Wright, 1971); *Science News,* June 26, 1971; discussion by Ralph Berger in *Psychology Today,* June 1970.

Awareness in chemical anesthesia: *American Journal of Clinical Hypnosis* 7 (1):55-59; *Medical Proceedings* 11 (2):243-245; *Rocky Mountain Medical Journal,* January 1960; *British Journal of Anesthesia* 37 (7):544-546.

Dream theory: *Archives of General Psychiatry* 21:696-703; *Experimental Medicine and Surgery* 27 (1–2):39-52; *Memories, Dreams, Reflections* by C. G. Jung (Random House, 1961); see also general references above.

Chapter 13 HURT BRAINS: WHO IS NORMAL?

Violence and brain damage: *Violence and the Brain* by Vernon Marks and Frank Erwin (Harper & Row, 1970); "The Violent Patient in the Emergency Room," a report to the National Institute of Mental Health and the Neuro-Research Foundation; *Journal of the American Medical Association* 205 (7):503-505; 216 (6):1025-1034; *American Journal of Psychiatry* 127 (11):49-54; 128 (4):56-62; *Today's Health,* November 1970; *Science News,* March 11, 1972; "Clinical Evaluation of the Violent Patient," report to the National Commission on the Causes and Prevention of Violence.

Sociopaths and expectancy: *Science* 172:284-286; *Biological Psychiatry* 3 (1971):59-69; *Time, Experience, and Behavior* by J. E. Orme (Iliffe, 1969). Characteristic brainwave patterns: *Averaged Evoked Potentials: Methods, Results, and Evaluations,* edited by E. Donchin and D. B. Lindsley (NASA, 1969); *Les Congrès et Colloques de Université de Liege* 52:146-176 (French), colloquium reprinted as booklet, *Variations Contingentes Négatives* (Université de Liege, 1969).

Aging and the brain: *Life,* September 29, 1967 (Dilantin); *Time, Experience, and Behavior,* see above; *Time,* November 1, 1968; *Annals of Internal Medicine* 16:801; *Science* 172:959; *Nucleic Acid Therapy in Aging and Degenerative Disease* by Benjamin S. Frank (Psychological Library, 1969); *Intellectual Functioning in Adults,* edited by Lissy Jarvik, Carl Elsdorfer, June E. Blum (Springer Verlag, 1973).

Split-brain phenomena, hemisphere specialization: *American Scientist*

60 (3):311-317; Roger Sperry lecture, UCLA, 1971; *Journal of Comparative Physiological Psychology* 71:83; *Neuropsychologia* 8:110; *Psychology Today*, April 1971 and May 1973; *Science* 176:539-541.

Epilepsy: *Epilepsy Handbook* by Louis Boshes and Frederic A. Gibbs (Thomas, 1972); *Basic Mechanisms of the Epilepsies*, edited by H. H. Jasper, A. A. Ward, Jr., and Alfred Pope (Little, Brown, 1969); *Experimental Epilepsy* by Arthur Kreindler (Elsevier, 1965); *Temporal Lobe Epilepsy*, edited by Maitland Baldwin and Pearce Bailey (Thomas, 1958); *The Living Brain* by W. Grey Walter (Norton, 1953); *Living with Epileptic Seizures* by Samuel Livingston (Thomas, 1963). Conditioning of brainwave patterns in cats: *Science* 167:1146-1148; *Physiology and Behavior* 3:703-707. Children inducing seizures: Los Angeles *Times*, August 25, 1971.

Autism: *Human Intelligence*, edited by J. McVicker Hunt (TransAction Books, 1972); *Infantile Autism*, edited by D. W. Churchill, G. D. Alpern, M. K. DeMeyer (Thomas, 1971); *A Child Called Noah* by Josh Greenfeld (Holt, Rinehart & Winston, 1972). Autism and talking typewriter: Los Angeles *Times*, January 7, 1972, and interview with Smith; see also references to LSD and autism, Chapter 10.

Environmental retardation: *Human Intelligence*, see above; *Society for Research in Child Development* 31:1-68 (Monograph #105); "Adult Status of Children With Contrasting Early Life Experiences: A Follow-up Study" by Harold M. Skeels (University of Chicago Press, 1966); study conducted by Rick Heber in *Proceedings of the Second Congress of the International Association for the Scientific Study of Mental Deficiency*, Warsaw, 1970. Sleep in mongoloid children: *Journal of Neurological Science* 13:115-119. Hyperkinesis: *Human Intelligence*, see above; *A Child's Mind* by Muriel Beadle (Doubleday, 1970); *Scientific American*, April 1970. Effects of amphetamine on EEG of hyperkinetic subjects: *Science* 174:1356-1357.

Chapter 14 SCHIZOPHRENIA AND SURVIVAL

General references: *The Schizophrenias: Yours and Mine* by the Professional Committee of the Schizophrenia Foundation of New Jersey (Pyramid, 1970); *The Vital Balance* by Karl Menninger, with Martin Mayer and Paul Pruyser (Macmillan, 1967); *Biological Psychiatry* 2 (2):81-88; 2 (2):153-164; *Brain Chemistry and Mental Diseases*, edited by Beng T. Ho and William McIsaac (Plenum Press, 1971); *Schizophrenia: Current Concepts and Research*, edited by D. V. S. Sanker (PJD Publications, 1969); *The Biochemistry of Functional and Experimental Psychoses* by Hans Weil-Malherbe and Stephen I. Szara (Thomas, 1971); *Clinical Handbook of Psychopharmacology*, edited by A. Dimasci and R. I. Shader (Science House, 1970); *Biochemistry, Schizophrenias, and Affective Illnesses*, edited by H. E. Himwich (Williams & Wilkins, 1970).

Biochemical theory and research: *International Journal of Psychiatry*

3:383-403; *Journal of Nervous and Mental Diseases* 146:103-126; *Scott Medical Journal* 15:34-40; *Schizophrenia Bulletin* 4:45-66 (1971); *Canadian Psychiatric Association Journal* 15:375-388; *Behavioral Neuropsychiatry* 2 (1, 2):27-31; *Science* 171:1032-1036. Survey of Russian research: *International Review of Neurobiology* 11:199-225.

Epilepsy and schizophrenia: *Lancet* 1 (1968):398-401. Carbohydrate metabolism in schizophrenics: *International Review of Neurobiology* 11:259-290. Palmar creases: *American Journal of Diseases of Children* 120:424-431. Postcardiotomy delirium: *The Biology of Dreaming* by Ernest Hartmann (Thomas, 1967). Amines and schizophrenia: *Psychosomatics* 11:495; *Comprehensive Psychiatry* 9:155-174.

Possible neuronal malfunction in schizophrenia: *American Journal of Psychiatry* 126:149-156. Pathological immune mechanism: *Proceedings of American Psychopathology Association* 58:234-252; *Schizophrenia: Current Concepts and Research*, see above. Schizophrenia and hallucinogens: *Abstracts of World Medicine* 44:489-497. Trace-metal therapy: *Proceedings of the Twenty-sixth National Meeting of the Society of Biological Psychiatry*, Washington, D.C., 1971. (Discussion available from Brain Information Service, UCLA.)

Study of low-risk and high-risk children in Denmark: *Science News*, July 4, 1970, and *Psychology Today*, April 1971. Foster-home-reared children of schizophrenic mothers: *British Journal of Psychiatry* 112:819. · Other genetic studies: *Journal of Psychiatric Research*, 356: Supplement 1; *Biological Psychiatry* 2 (3):285-290. Value of psychotic experience: *The Vital Balance*, see above; *Psychology Today*, September 1970; *Behavioral Neuropsychiatry* 2 (314):39-42.

Mystic and symbolic elements of schizophrenic experience: *Archives of General Psychiatry* 25:481-489; *Psychedelic Review*, no. 6 (1965), pp. 7–15; *Journal for the Scientific Study of Religion* 6:246-252; *Man and His Symbols* by C. G. Jung (Aldus, 1964). Extrasensory perception and mental illness: *Parapsychological Review*, January–February 1972; Jerome Frank in *Psychology Today*, April 1973; lecture by Montague Ullman, symposium of the Society for Parapsychology, 1948; *Journal of the American Society for Psychical Research*, January 1952; lecture by Ullman to Psychiatric Forum Group, May 2, 1951; *Proceedings of the First International Conference of Parapsychological Studies*, 1955:71-74; lecture by Ullman, Sixteenth Winter Meeting of the Academy of Psychoanalysis; *Psi and Psychoanalysis* by Jule Eisenbud (Grune, 1970).

Chapter 15   BRAIN FOOD: OBESITY AND MALNUTRITION

Enzyme deficiency in the obese: *New Scientist* 55:31-33. Delayed secretion of glucagon: *Science* 178:513-516. Abnormal metabolism: *Science* 150:1051-1053; *Journal of Clinical Endocrinology* 28:106-110.

Ions and appetite: *Science* 176:1124-1125. Finicky appetites of rats with hypothalamic damage: *Brain and Behavior*, Volume 4, edited by Karl Pribram (Penguin, 1969).

Nutrition and the brain: *Biology of Brain Dysfunction,* Volume 1, edited by Gerald E. Gaul (Plenum, 1973), including discussions of glucose metabolism, malnutrition, vitamin deficiencies; *Malnutrition, Learning, and Behavior,* edited by Nevin S. Scrimshaw and John E. Gordon (Massachusetts Institute of Technology Press, 1968).

Winick-Rosso studies: *Journal of Pediatrics* 24:667-679. Starved dogs: *Czechoslovak Medicine* 14:235-245. Capetown study: *South Africa Medical Journal* 41:1027-1030. Guatemala study: *Pediatrics* 38 (2):319-372. Vitamin A deficiencies: *American Journal of Clinical Nutrition* 20:1295-1299; *European Journal of Biochemistry* 7:575-582. Deficiencies in Vitamin E: *Experientia* 24:807-808; *Acta Anatomica* 67:623-635. Trace-mineral deficiencies: *Journal of Nutrition* 97:42-52; *Proceedings of the Twenty-sixth National Meeting of the Society of Biological Psychiatry,* Washington, D.C., 1971. Vitamin C lessening brain damage in poisoned rats: *Farmakologiia i Toksikologiia* 33:622-624. Insecticides and EEG changes, unpublished report, University of Hawaii.

General effects of malnutrition on brain development: *Nutrition Review* 26:197-199; 27:251-254; 28:110-111; 28:176-177; *Nature* (London), 221:554-555; *Dimensions of Nutrition,* edited by Jacqueline Dupont (Associated University Press, 1970); *Brain Research* 6:241-251; *Annual Progress in Child Psychiatry and Child Development,* edited by S. Chess and A. Thomas (Brunner/Mazel, 1970). Prenatal effects: *Science* 160:322-323; 174:954-955.

Hypoglycemia: *Journal of Neurochemistry* 12:679-693; *Body, Mind, and Sugar* by E. M. Abrahamson and A. W. Pezet (Holt, Rinehart, 1951); *American Journal of the Medical Sciences* 261 (4):197-205; *Hypoglycemia and the Hypoglycemic Syndrome* by A. J. Kauvar and Martin G. Goldner (Thomas, 1954); *Hypoglycaemia* by Vincent Marks and F. Clifford Rose (Blackwell, 1965). Neonatal hypoglycemia: *Pediatric Research* 3:181-184.

Chapter 16   THE MOST IMPORTANT SEX ORGAN

General: *Influence of Hormones on the Nervous System,* edited by D. H. Ford (S. Karger, 1971); *Control of Human Fertility,* edited by Egon Diczfalusy and Ulf Borell (Wiley Interscience, 1971); *Critical Issues in Contemporary Sexual Behavior* (John Hopkins Press, in press).

Behavioral effects of menstrual and premenstrual hormonal changes: *Psychology Today,* February 1972; *The Pre-menstrual Syndrome* by Katherine Dalton (Thomas, 1964). Schizophrenia and the sex of fetus (physiological interaction of hormones between mother and fetus): *Journal of Psychiatric Research* 5:349-350.

Brain hemisphere and shock threshold differences in male and female infants: *The Child's Mind* by Muriel Beadle (Doubleday, 1970). Sexual differences in reaction to stimuli: *Early Childhood: The Development of Self-Regulatory Mechanisms,* edited by Dwain W. Walcher and Donald L. Peters (Academic Press, 1971). Prenatal stress, hormonal influence:

Scientific American, April 1966; *Science* 175:82-84. Hormonal differences in homosexuals: *Newsweek,* April 26, 1971; *New Scientist* 53:270-271. Periodic homosexuality: *Body Time* by Gay Gaer Luce (Pantheon, 1971). Sexual abnormalities in rats isolated in infancy: *Brain and Behavior,* Volume 1, edited by K. H. Pribram (Penguin, 1962). Hormones and MAO: *Psychology Today,* February 1972. The Pill and diminished libido: Masters and Johnson quoted in *Redbook,* January 1972. Freud's conjecture about sexual chemicals and tension, quoted in *The Mind: Biological Approaches to Its Functions,* edited by William C. Corning and Martin Balaban (John Wiley, 1968). Implanted estrogen: *Subcortical Mechanisms of Behavior* by Robert A. McCleary and Robert Y. Moore (Basic Books, 1965). Electronic stimulation of the brain and sexuality: *Physical Control of the Mind* by Jose M. R. Delgado (Harper & Row, 1969). PCPA and hypersexual behavior: *Science News,* October 3, 1970; *Rivista de Farmacologia e Terapia* 2 (1):27-34; *Science* 168:499-501; 169:1000-1001; 170:868-870; *Anatomical Record* 133:388. From the UCLA Brain Information Service, discussions by Diana Johnson of two symposia: "International Symposium on Steroids, Gonadotrophins, and Reproduction," University of Sherbrook, Quebec, 1970, and "The Influence of Hormones on the Nervous System," Downstate Medical Center, Brooklyn, 1970.

Chapter 17   FIVE SENSES . . . OR TWENTY?

Acuity of senses observed in connection with brain damage: *Mysterious Phenomena of the Human Psyche* by Leonid L. Vasiliev (University Books, 1965); *Journal of Clinical Investigation* 46 (3):429-435. Addison's disease and taste sensitivity: *Body Time* by Gay Gaer Luce (Pantheon, 1971). Potential sensitivity of the visual system: *Eye and Brain: The Psychology of Seeing* by R. L. Gregory (McGraw-Hill, 1966). Perception of pulsed microwaves: *Applied Psychology* 17 (4):689-692; *Aerospace Medicine* 32:1140-1142. Sonar system in the blind: *Science* 148:1107-1111. General perception: *The Analysis of Sensations and the Relationship of the Physical to the Psychical* (Open Court, 1914).

Structure of visual system: *Scientific American,* November 1963; *Recent Contributions in Neurophysiology,* edited by J. Cordaugh and Pierre Gloor (Elsevier, 1972), research of David Hubel and Torsten Wiesel; interview, David Hubel, Harvard Medical School, 1971; *Electroencephalography and Neurophysiology,* Supplement 31. Retinal cells as microscopic circuits: *American Journal of Medical Electronics* 1:112-121. Brain as Fourier transform: *Science* 173:74-77. Holistic transform in smell: *Discovery* 27:29-34; *Psychological Bulletin* 69:390-395. Brain as parallel coherent detector: *Science* 174:722-723. Spiral phenomenon: *Science* 165:819-821. Grating phenomenon: *Science* 168:1489-1491. Displacement phenomena: *The Psychological Review* 15 (3):139-149; 13 (4):258-275. Object moving in field of vision: *Biological*

Psychiatry 3 (3):11. Ambiguous objects: *Scientific American,* December 1971.

Eidetic imagery: *Psychology Today,* November 1970; *Journal of Psychology* 63:13-34; *Eidetic Imagery* by E. R. Jaensch (Routledge, 1930; Kegan Paul, 1950); *Scientific American,* April 1969; *The Mind of a Mnemonist* by A. R. Luria (Basic Books, 1968).

Synesthesia in mystical experience: *Watchers on the Hills* by Raynor Johnson (Harper, 1959). Attempt of Sibelius to hide his synesthesia: *Jean Sibelius* by Harold E. Johnson (Knopf, 1959). Perceptual acuity in altered states of consciousness: *An Experiment in Mindfulness* by E. H. Shattuck (Dutton, 1958). See also references on color perception and auditory phenomena for Chapters 6, 7, 9, and 10.

Visual processing at one-quarter of a second: *Scientific American,* August 1970. Distortion of words to fit context: *Scientific American,* December 1970. Auditory induction: *Science* 176:1149-1151.

Sounds associated with aurora borealis and fireballs: "Very Low Frequency Electromagnetic Fields and Behavior," dissertation by Burton Milburn, UCLA, 1970; memorandum RM 3724 APRA, The Rand Corporation, Santa Monica, California, titled "Anomalous Sounds and Electromagnetic Effects Associated With Fireball Entry"; *Electromagnetic Fields and Life* by A. S. Presman (Plenum Press, 1970).

Phenomena reported by Clarence Wieske: *Biomedical Science Instrumentation,* Volume 1 (Plenum Press, 1963). Phosphenes: *Confinia Neurologica* 23 (3):201-226; *Scientific American,* February 1970.

Dermo-optic perception (fingertip vision): *Psychological Bulletin* 63:322-337; *Biulleten Eksperimental'noi Biologii i Meditsiny* 57:16-21; *Annals of New York Academy of Sciences* 117:217-224. Human response to atmosphere ions (color phenomena, etc.): *Psychological Review* 68 (3):225-228; *Aerosol-Sorsch* 1954 (3):39-51.

Chapter 18   REVOLUTION IN THE CRADLE

General references: *The Development of Self-Regulatory Mechanisms,* edited by Dwain N. Walcher and Donald L. Peters (Academic Press, 1971); *Death at an Early Age* by Jonathan Kozol (Houghton Mifflin, 1967); *Revolution in Learning* by Maya Pines (Harper & Row, 1967); *Radical School Reform,* edited by Beatrice Gross and Ronald Gross (Simon & Schuster, 1969); *Human Intelligence,* edited by J. McVicker Hunt (TransAction Books, 1972); *Early Education,* edited by Robert Hess and Roberta Bear (Aldine, 1968); *Education and Ecstasy* by George B. Leonard (Delacorte, 1968); *The Child's Mind* by Muriel Beadle (Doubleday, 1970); *Education of the Infant and the Young Child,* edited by Victor H. Denenberg (Academic Press, 1970); *Three Babies,* edited by Joseph Church (Random House, 1966).

Rationale for early intervention: *Give Your Child a Superior Mind* by Siegfried Engelmann and Therese Engelmann (Simon & Schuster, 1966; *Modes of Biological Adaptation and Their Role in Intellectual*

Development by W. Ragan Callaway (*PCD Monographs* 1 (1), 1970, The Galton Institute, P.O. Box 35336, Preuss Station, Los Angeles, California 90035); *Cradles of Eminence* by Victor Goertzel and Mildred George Goertzel (Little, Brown, 1962); *How to Teach Your Baby to Read* by Glenn Doman (Random House, 1964); *Genetic Psychology Monographs* 66:181-283.

Effects of experience on the brain: *Journal of Comparative Physiology and Psychology* 55:801-807; *Science* 146:610-619; *Scientific American*, February 1972; *Biopsychology of Development*, edited by Ethel Tobach (Academic Press, 1971); *International Journal of Neuroscience* 2 (2):113-128; *Developmental Psychobiology* 4 (2):157-167; *Early Experience and Behavior*, edited by G. Newton and S. Levine (Thomas, 1969); *American Psychologist* 21:321-332; *Physiology and Behavior* 1:99-104; *Journal of Comparative Neurology* 123:111-119; 128:117; *Molecular Approaches to Learning and Memory*, edited by W. L. Byrne (Academic Press, 1970).

Bowers' experiments: *Scientific American*, December 1966 and October 1971. Space perception in early infancy: *Science* 172:1161-1163.

Reaction to shadow on collision course: *Science* 171:818-820. Walking response in the newborn, *Science* 176:314-315.

General references discussing innate mechanisms: *The Organization of Behavior* by D. O. Hebb (John Wiley, 1949); *Modes of Biological Adaptation and Their Role in Intellectual Development*, see above; *The Mind: Biological Approaches to Its Functions*, edited by William C. Corning and Martin Balaban (John Wiley, 1968).

Marcelle Geber's study of precocity in East African children: *Proceedings of the XIV International Congress of Applied Psychology*, 1962; *Journal of Social Psychology* 47:185-195; *Lancet* 1 (1957):1216.

South San Francisco experiment: *Pygmalion in the Classroom* by Robert Rosenthal and Lenore Jacobson (Holt, Rinehart & Winston, 1968). Remarks by Lenore Jacobson from *Early Years*, September 1971. "Sesame Street" alumni entering schools: *Newsweek*, May 22, 1972. Soviet preschools: *Lenin's Grandchildren* by Kitty D. Weaver (Simon & Schuster, 1971); Urie Bronfenbrenner in *Soviet Preschool Education*, edited by Henry Chauncey, Volume 1, "Program of Instruction" (Holt, Rinehart & Winston, 1969). See also *From Two to Five* by Kornei Chukovsky (University of California Press, 1966).

Niles Newton's discussion of breast-feeding and infant development: *Psychology Today*, July 1972. See also *Touching: The Human Significance of the Skin* by Ashley Montagu (Columbia University Press, 1971).

Jean Piaget: *The Origins of Intelligence in Children* by Jean Piaget (Norton, 1952); *Young Children's Thinking: Studies of Some Aspects of Piaget's Theory* (Teacher's College Press, Columbia University, 1966); Bruner interview in *Psychology Today*, December 1970. Prenatal stress as possible factor in later delinquency: *American Journal of Psychiatry* 118 (1962):78. Harvard Pre-school Project: *Revolution in Learning*, see above; *Woman's Day*, May 1971; *Life*, December 17, 1971; *Child-rear-*

ing practices and the development of competence: The Harvard Pre-School Project Final Report, compiled by Burton L. White, Barbara Kaban, Janice Marmor, and Bernice Shapiro for the Head Start Division of the Office of Economic Opportunity, presented in September 1972.

Chapter 19   TRANCE LEARNING AND MEMORY MOLECULES

General references: *Molecular Mechanisms in Memory and Learning,* edited by Georges Ungar (Plenum Press, 1970); *Languages of the Brain* by Karl H. Pribram (Prentice-Hall, 1971); *Chemical Transfer of Learned Information,* edited by Ejnar Fjerdingstad (North Holland, 1971); *Brain and Behavior,* edited by Karl H. Pribram, Volume 3, "Memory Mechanisms" (Penguin, 1969); *Human Brain and Psychological Processes* by A. R. Luria (Harper, 1966).

Transfer of learned behavior: *Science* 178:1219-1220; *Umschau* 16:588; *Naturwisseuschaffen,* article by Georges Ungar, in press; *Federation Proceedings* 32 (1), no. 3 (abstract), identification of specific chain of amino acids associated with learned response; *Molecular Mechanisms in Memory and Learning,* see above; personal communication from Wolfgang Parr; *Nature* 235:26; *Journal of Biological Psychology* 11 (2):20-25; *Scandinavian Journal of Psychology* 10 (1969):220-224; *Experientia* 25 (11):1215-1219; *Protein Metabolism of the Nervous System,* edited by A. Lajtha (Plenum Press, 1970). First report of learning in planarians: *American Psychologist* 14:410.

Holographic theory: *Languages of the Brain,* see above; excerpted in *Psychology Today,* September 1971; *Scientific American,* January 1969. Chimpanzee reading: *Science* 172:808-822; *Scientific American,* October 1972; lecture by David Premack, UCLA, 1971; *Psychology Today,* September 1970. Michael Gazzaniga's comment: *Think,* November-December 1970. Sign language in chimpanzee: *Science* 165:664.

Lashley's search for the engram: *Brain Mechanisms and Intelligence* by Karl Lashley (University of Chicago Press, 1929). Role of the limbic structures in learning: *Inhibition and Learning,* edited by R. A. Boakes and M. S. Halliday (Academic Press, 1972). *Limbic System Mechanisms and Autonomic Function* by C. H. Hockman (Thomas, 1972); *Proceedings of the National Academy of Sciences* 62 (3):692-696; *Autonomic-Somatic Integrations* by Ernest Gellhorn (University of Minnesota Press, 1967); *Frontiers of the Brain,* edited by John French (Columbia University Press, 1962); *Neuropsychologia* 7 (1969):235-244; *Neurosciences Research Program* 9 (2):232; *Scientific American,* April 1966; *Neurological Foundations of Psychiatry,* edited by T. Smythies (Academic Press, 1966); *Science* 173:1148-1149; *Angiology* 20:325-333; *American Scientist* 59 (2):236-245.

Suggestopedia: Lecture, Georgi Lozanov, UCLA, 1971; *Psychic Discoveries Behind the Iron Curtain* by Lynn Schroeder and Sheila Ostrander (Prentice-Hall, 1970). Biofeedback technique to enhance learning: "Some Applications of Biofeedback-Produced Twilight States," paper presented by Thomas Budzynski at American Psychological Association Convention, Washington, D.C., 1971. Neal Miller quotation from *Impact of Science on Society* 18 (3):157-167. Pygmalion-effect experiments relating to learning in adults: interview with Robert Rosenthal, Harvard University, 1971.

Holger Hydén's research: *Neurosciences Research Symposium Summaries,* Volume 1, edited by F. O. Schmitt and T. Melnechuk (M.I.T. Press, 1966); *The Anatomy of Memory,* Volume II, edited by D. P. Kimble (Science and Behavior Books, 1965); *The Human Mind,* edited by J. D. Roslansky (North Holland, 1967); *Proceedings of the American Philosophical Society* 111 (6):326-342; *Journal of Neurochemistry* 16 (5):813-821; *Naturwissenschaften* 53 (3):64-70; *Science* 159:1370-1373.

Among the relevant bibliographies available from the Brain Information Service, UCLA: *Cerebral Biochemical Changes During Memory and Learning (August 1969–August 1970); Cerebral Biochemical Changes During Memory and Learning (1966–July 1969); S-100 Protein in the Brain (August 1968–August 1971); Hippocampus and Behavior (Excluding Sleep) Stimulation, Recording, Lesions (1967–August 1970).*

Chapter 20   THE ANATOMY OF CREATIVITY

General references: *The Creative Experience,* edited by Stanley Rosner and Lawrence Abt (Grossman, 1970); *The Creative Process,* edited by Bernard Ghiselin (University of California Press, 1952); *Creativity,* edited by P. E. Vernon (Penguin, 1970); *Scientific Creativity: Its Recognition and Development* by C. W. Taylor and Frank Barron (John Wiley, 1963).

Interview with Froelich Rainey: *The Creative Experience,* see above. Frank Barron's study of writers: *Psychology Today,* July 1972.

Wallach and Kogan study and Poincaré's theory, both in *Creativity,* see above. Raynor Johnson quotation from his *The Imprisoned Splendour* (Harper, 1953). Account of Luther Woodrum from *Think,* October 26, 1971. Remarks of Erwin DiCyan: *Perspectives in Biology and Medicine* 14 (4):639-650. Importance of teaching technique and observation to young children: *Early Years,* March 1972; *Life,* December 17, 1971. Idea "fits" comparable to epileptic fits: *Brain Storms* by Wayne Barker (Grove Press, 1968). Voluntary Controls Project at Menninger Foundation: *Journal of Transpersonal Psychology* 2 (1):2-26. Description by E. H. Shattuck from his *An Experiment in Mindfulness* (Dutton, 1958). Thomas Wolfe quotation from his *The Story of a Novel* (Scribner, 1936).

Creativity in education: *Education and Ecstasy* by George Leonard (Delacorte, 1968); *Teacher* by Sylvia Ashton-Warner (Simon & Schuster, 1963); *Teaching for Creative Endeavor,* edited by William B. Michael (Indiana University Press, 1968). Versatility of the genius brain:

The Living Brain by W. Grey Walter (Norton, 1953). Leopardi passage: *Brain and Conscious Experience,* edited by John C. Eccles (Springer Verlag, 1965); original reference, Leopardi's *Zibaldone,* 30 XI, 1828. ESP and creativity: *Psychology Today,* July 1972; *Psychic,* July 1972. Tennyson excerpts from *Locksley Hall* (1842) and *The Two Voices* (1833). Henry Miller quotation: *West,* January 23, 1972. Sensory thresholds and creativity: *Prediction and Outcome* by S. K. Escalona and G. M. Heider (Basic Books, 1959).

Chapter 21   MIND AND EVOLUTION

Sperry on problem of will and consciousness: *American Scientist* 40:291-312; *Psychological Review* 76:532-536; 77:585-590; *Bulletin of Atomic Science* 22 (7):2-6; *Proceedings of the National Academy of Sciences* 63:230-231. General references on mind-brain problem: *British Journal of Psychology* 47:44-50; 58:467-476; *Brain* 88:777-786; 88:799-810; *Confinia Neurologica* 17, Supplement; 21, Supplement; 19:462-485; *Brain and Conscious Experience,* edited by John C. Eccles (Springer Verlag, 1965); *The Neurophysiological Basis of Mind* by John C. Eccles (Oxford University Press, 1953); *Review of Metaphysics* 19:24-54; *Mathematical Biosciences* 11:47-52; *Neurology India* 13:173-175; *Journal of Transpersonal Psychology* 1:4-9 (1969); *American Philosophical Quarterly* 2 (2):81-104; *Psychological Reports* 16:711-712; 16:758.

Dual (bimodal) consciousness: *American Scientist* 60 (3):311-317; *Archives of General Psychiatry* 25:481-489. Time and consciousness: *Annals of New York Academy of Science* 138:632-645.

Other quotations in this chapter are from *Man on His Nature* by Charles Sherrington (Cambridge University Press, 1951); *Eye and Brain: The Psychology of Seeing* by R. L. Gregory (McGraw-Hill, 1966); *The Imprisoned Splendour* by Raynor C. Johnson (Harper, 1953); *The Unexpected Universe* by Loren Eiseley (Harcourt, Brace, 1969); *The Invisible Pyramid* by Loren Eiseley (Scribner, 1970); *The Biology of Ultimate Concern* by Theodosius Dobzhansky (New American Library, 1967); *The Neurophysiological Basis of Mind* by John C. Eccles (Oxford University Press, 1953); *Intuition Versus Intellect* by Paul Maslow (Life Science Press, 1957); *Science and Humanism* by Erwin Schrödinger (Cambridge University Press, 1951); *Modern Man in Search of a Soul* by C. G. Jung (various editions); *How I Believe* by Pierre Teilhard de Chardin (Harper, 1969); *The Universe and Dr. Einstein* by Lincoln Barnett (William Morrow, 1948). The prayer by Kuntu Zangpo was translated from the Tibetan by Taklung Tsetul Rimpoche and appeared in *Chakra: A Journal of Tantra and Yoga,* March 1972.

Chapter 22   THE BRAIN AND PSI

Burbank prophecy: *Harvest of the Years* by Luther Burbank (Houghton Mifflin, 1927). Soviet, Czech, and Bulgarian psychic research and related western research: *Psychic Discoveries Behind the Iron Curtain* by Lynn Schroeder and Sheila Ostrander (Prentice-Hall, 1970); transcripts of 1971-1972 symposia sponsored by the Academy of Parapsychology and Medicine; further references from *Bibliography on Parapsychology (Psychoenergetics) and Related Subjects*, translated and published by the National Technical Information Service of the U.S. Department of Commerce, Springfield, Virginia; transcript of symposium sponsored by the Southern California Society for Psychical Research, Golden West College; *A. R. E. Journal*, March 1972; *Journal of Paraphysics* 4:113; *Proceedings of First Western Hemisphere Conference on High Frequency Photography, Acupuncture and the Human Aura* (Gordon and Breech, 1972); *Psychic*, May–June 1971.

Resistance to new paradigms: *The Structure of Scientific Revolutions* by Thomas S. Kuhn (University of Chicago Press, 1962, 1970). Price's acknowledgment that he accepts the existence of psychic phenomena: personal communication.

William Tiller's theories: *A. R. E. Journal*, March 1972; *Proceedings of the First Western Hemisphere Conference on High Frequency Photography, Acupuncture and the Human Aura*, see above; transcripts of symposia sponsored by Academy of Parapsychology and Medicine (De Anza College, 1971; UCLA and Stanford, 1972). Thelma Moss on healing phenomenon in Kirlian effect: the Los Angeles *Times*, July 30, 1972. Subliminal perception: *New Scientist* 53:252-255. Plethysmograph studies: *International Journal of Parapsychology* 9 (1):53-56; unpublished report by Aristide Esser and Thomas Etter on Non-Conventional Communication Project, Rockland State Hospital.

Speculation about communication system using energy radiation: *IEEE Spectrum* 1:81-95. Harold Cahn quotation from a lecture in Los Angeles, 1971. Sister Justa Smith's remarks on similarity between healing energy and magnetic fields: symposia on "Science and Psi" Stanford and UCLA, 1972. Bernard Grad's experiments with the laying on of hands: *Journal of the American Society for Psychical Research* 59 (2):95-129. Current psychokinesis research at Duke University and at the Foundation for Research on the Nature of Man: *Psychic*, July 1972. Out-of-body-experiences (OOBE) research: *ASPR Newsletter*, Spring 1972; Summer 1972; *Parapsychology*, December 1967; *Journal of the American Society for Psychical Research* 62 (1):3-27. Apparent psi in company executives: *Think*, November 1969; *Executive ESP* by Douglas Dean (Prentice-Hall, in press). Max Born remarks from his *The Restless Universe* (Dover, 1951).

Mice and jirds: *Parapsychology Review*, March–April 1972. Telepathy and precognition in dreams: paper presented to American Association for the Advancement of Science meeting in Philadelphia, December 1971, by Montague Ullman and Stanley Krippner; lecture by Krippner, UCLA, 1971; lecture by Ullman, Los Angeles, 1972; interview, Ullman, Los Angeles, 1972; *Corrective Psychiatry and Journal of Social Therapy* 12 (2):115-119; "A Nocturnal Approach to Psi," Ullman's presidential address to the Parapsychological Association, New York, 1966. Problem of precognition: *Man and Time* by J. B. Priestley (Aldus, 1964); *Time, Experience, and Behavior* by J. E. Orme (Iliffe, 1969); *ESP in Life and Lab* by Louisa E. Rhine (Macmillan, 1967); "Psi and the Problem of the Disconnections in Science," a paper presented by Jule Eisenbud at the First International Conference of Parapsychological Studies, University of Utrecht, 1953; *The Roots of Coincidence* by Arthur Koestler (Random House, 1972).

Edgar Mitchell's views: his paper, "Awareness and Science," presented at the 125th Annual Meeting of the American Psychiatric Association, Dallas, 1972; interview, Houston, 1971.

Chapter 23   TOMORROW

Predictions: *Future Shock* by Alvin Toffler (Random House, 1970); *The Biological Time Bomb* by Gordon Rattray Taylor (New American Library, 1968); *Man into Superman* by R. C. W. Ettinger (St. Martin's, 1972); *The Greening of America* by Charles A. Reich (Random House, 1970). Sigmund Koch on the future of psychology: *Psychology Today,* September 1969. Ulrich Franzen on technology: *The Creative Experience,* edited by Stanley Rosner and Lawrence Abt (Grossman, 1970).

index

Aaronson, Bernard, 113–114
Abt, Lawrence, 300–301
Abuzzahab, Faruk, 180
Academy of Parapsychology and Medicine, founding of, 45
acetylcholine (ACh), 71, 156, 210
ACTH, 71
acupuncture, 45, 333, 338; anesthesia, 52–54; Kirlian photography, 321; nerve deafness, 239
Adamenko, Victor, 319, 321
Adler, Charles, 37
adrenal gland, hormones, 251, 282; *see also* stress syndrome
adrenaline, 134, 148, 198; *see also* stress syndrome
Adrian, Edgar D., 90
aging, effects on brain, 154, 190–191
air traffic controllers, effect of stress on, 41
alcohol, 131, 136, 138–140, 175, 198; action on brain, 138–140; effect of meditation on desire, tolerance, 80; gender, 140; genetic sensitivity, 140; racial sensitivity, 140; reaction time, 138–139
alcoholism, 338; brain damage, 139–140, 170, 180; pathological intoxication, 171; therapy, 123–124
Allen, Dwight, 270
Allport, Gordon, 341
Almy, Millie, 270
Alpert, Richard, 129, 130
alpha brainwave rhythm, 78–79, 88–103, 176, 179, 241, 298, 308, 321; anesthesia, 50, 54; biofeedback training, 68, 76–77; discovery of rhythm, 89; hypnagogic state, 145; marijuana, 117; nicotine, 141; sleep deprivation, 151; timing device, 229, 280
Alpha Dynamics, 83, 99–100
alpha-2 globulin, 196
altered states of consciousness, 59–163, 179, 232, 280–281, 288, 293–294, 298, 331, 340, 344; brain structures, 59–60, 65–72; innate drive, 72; *see also* creativity, dreams, hypnosis, meditation, schizophrenia, yoga
amphetamines, 72, 132–136, 141, 172, 189, 204
amygdala, 66–67, 169, 174, 282
androgen, 217–218

sociopathic personality, 181–182, 338

sonar system in blind, 227

Soviet preschool education, 268–269

Sperry, Roger, 177, 275, 307–308

split-brain surgery, *see* hemisphere specialization

state-bound experience, 72–73

state-specific sciences, proposal for, 72

Stenevi, Ulf, 276

Sterman, Barry, 95, 147, 156

Stevens, Leonard, 90

Stewart, Kilton, 160

Stone, Irwin, 212

Stoner, Winifred Sackville, 255

Stoyva, Johann, 37

Stravinsky, Igor, 295

stress, effects of, 40–45, 84–85, 217, 250–251, 337

stress syndrome, 40–41, 84, 201

Stromeyer, Charles, 232

Structural Integration, 41–43

Strutt, John William, 316

subliminal perception, 322–323

Suggestopedia, 280–281

suicide, 27, 195, 197–198, 204, 212, 215

Swami Rama, 36, 96

Sweet, William, 167

Swoboda, Hermann, 24

synchronicity, 330

synesthesia, 60, 82, 232–234, 239

syphilitic psychosis, 204

tachyon theory, 329

Tagliamonte, Allessandro and Paolo, 222

Takata, Miki, 25

talking typewriter, *see* Edison Responsive Environment

Tantric yoga, *see* Kundalini

Taraxein, 200

Tart, Charles, 72, 80, 108–110, 163, 326

taste, 225, 331

Taylor, Gordon Rattray, 334

Teilhard de Chardin, Pierre, 312, 337, 342

telepathy, 59, 89, 110, 194, 317, 321, 324

temporal lobe, 66, 70, 168, 282, 301

temporal lobe epilepsy, 69, 168–170, 174, 176, 204, 221, 231, 338

Tennyson, Alfred, 61, 303, 335

tension headache, 37, 95

Tepperman, Jay, 208

Terman, Lewis, 153, 256, 290

testosterone, 146, 154, 172, 173, 215, 217, 219, 221

thalamus, 52, 66, 121

thalidomide, 136

THC, *see* marijuana

theta brainwave rhythm, 59, 77, 79, 81, 91, 94–96, 298

Thommen, George, 24

Thompson, J. J., 316

Thorpe, W. H., 313

Tiller, William, 316, 319–320, 329, 332

time, problems of, *see* precognition

time distortion, 110–111

Titanic, 302

Tkach, Walter, 53

tobacco, *see* nicotine

Toffler, Alvin, 333–334, 339–340

Torres, Ramon, 54

Tourette's syndrome, 180

tranquilizing drugs, 133, 136, 141, 204; effect on alpha rhythm, 94

transcendental meditation, *see* meditation

transformational linguistics, 259–260

Trehub, Arnold, 229–230

Tripp, Peter, 151

Trowill, Jay, 33

tryptamine, 198

Tunney, John, 268